Management of
the Psychiatric Emergency

Management of the Psychiatric Emergency

Stephen M. Soreff, MD
Director of Emergency and Consultation Psychiatry
Maine Medical Center
Portland, Maine

A WILEY MEDICAL PUBLICATION
JOHN WILEY & SONS
New York • Chichester • Brisbane • Toronto

Library of Congress Cataloging in Publication Data:

Soreff, Stephen M
  Management of the psychiatric emergency.

  (A Wiley medical publication)
  Includes index.
  1. Crisis intervention (Psychiatry)   2. Psychology, Pathological.   I. Title.   [DNLM:
  1. Emergencies.   2. Mental disorders.   3. Mental
  health services.   WM401 S713m]

  RC480.6.S67   616.89'025   80-22419
  ISBN 0-471-06012-7

Printed in the United States of America

10 9 8 7 6 5 4 3 2 1

To my family—
my wife, Joan,
my children, Alexandra and Benjamin—
and to Deep Structures

Foreword

In 1963, the Community Mental Health Centers Act mandated 24-hour emergency service as an essential service, and in 1973 the Emergency Medical Systems Act designed behavioral emergencies as a critical component. Yet gaps remain. All too frequently, the clinical response to a patient's request for emergency service is a tape recorded message or an answering service. Indeed, in some communities little if any clinical expertise is available. It is still a common experience for emergency medical technicians or emergency department staff to find themselves made anxious and perplexed by the emergency psychiatric patient.

The most desirable emergency response is accessible, immediate, and of the highest quality. Emergency psychiatric treatment unites the community's mental health programs with effective crisis intervention. It combines the unique opportunities of these two acts. This book brings these two together.

Dr Stephen Soreff began his work in Maine at a time during the period of the development of community mental health centers in this state. He also participated in the implementation of the state's emergency medical systems. He had an opportunity to create a highly professional program that provided services on a truly emergent basis. Because of these contributions Dr Soreff is recognized as a national leader and innovator in the delivery of emergency psychiatric services.

In this book Dr Soreff shares what he has learned from those people who are on the "front line" of emergency medical services. It is a fact that all patients experiencing a medical emergency must also be considered to have an accompanying psychiatric emergency. This book organizes and explains how to recognize and respond to these situations. The response to a psychiatric emergency should be, philosophically and in practice, part of the response to all medical emergencies.

Alan M. Elkins, MD
Chief of Psychiatry
Maine Medical Center
Portland, Maine

Preface

Emergency medical technicians (EMTs) and the emergency department (ED) staff can make decisive interventions in a psychiatric emergency and facilitate its resolution. They have the power, skill, and ability to treat successfully the patient in a psychiatric crisis. The mission of this book is to provide EMTs and ED staff with the knowledge, understanding, and techniques to deal effectively with psychiatric emergencies.

This book is predicated on the concept that the patients in psychiatric emergencies can and must be treated. These patients represent a valid use of EMTs' time and ED skills. Without prompt, proper intervention, their crises deepen. Specifically, patients who go unattended, unrecognized, and unengaged by family, EMTs, and ED staff incur increased morbidity and mortality. Their risk of suicide and homicide grows.

The book commences by defining *psychiatric emergency* and then addresses the matter of why emergency personnel are reluctant to deal with psychiatric patients. Chapter 1, What Is a Psychiatric Emergency? not only defines and describes the crisis but also explores its causes and points to methods for its resolution. Chapter 2, The Unwanted Patient, examines the characteristics of psychiatric patients in crisis and the difficulties personnel experience in treating such patients.

The book then presents a detailed, comprehensive treatment approach to each of the 12 basic types of psychiatric emergency patients. The types include the depressed patient; the anxious patient; the phobic patient; the lonely patient; the violent, paranoid patient; the disoriented patient; the suicidal patient; the patient with a thought disorder; the patient struggling to control an impulse; the patient reacting to alcohol or abused substances; the victim of a traumatic, brutal event; and, finally, the patient with no place to go.

The book takes the reader step by step through the entire psychiatric emergency for each type of crisis. First, the description of each crisis begins with the patient's moods, perceptions, and behavior. Second, it discusses the causes (intrapsychic, interpersonal, and biologic) of the psychiatric condition. Third, it covers the reactions of others to the patient. Fourth, it pinpoints the specific event which initiates the actual emergency. Fifth, it details the EMTs' response to the patient. Sixth, the book presents the emergency department evaluation: the reception, physical examination, chief complaint, psychiatric evaluation, and mental status examination. Seventh, the diagnosis, treatment plan, and immediate ED therapy

ix

are described. Eighth, each chapter concludes with the treatment course to be followed after the patient leaves the ED.

Additionally, the book addresses treatment, referral, and legal issues. Chapter 16, Crisis Mission: Treatment and Referral, outlines the various psychiatric therapies which the EMTs' and ED staff can employ to treat the patient and resolve the crisis. Further, it explores and reviews the extensive community mental health treatment network. Chapter 17, Responsibilities and Restraints: The Legal Dimensions of Intervention, examines the unique legal situations involved in psychiatric emergencies and presents an approach both to provide excellent patient treatment and to address the medicolegal concerns.

The unique feature and particular value of this volume for EMTs and ED staff is its comprehensive and specific approach to the psychiatric emergency patient. The book presents a total view of the crisis by starting with the problem from its inception in the community setting, following the patient through the ED, and concluding with a treatment program. The reader has an opportunity to discover the causes, course, and resolution of the emergency. The book furnishes specific steps for providers of emergency treatment to follow at each phase of the crisis. The book gives EMTs, ED staff members, and mental health workers the tools to treat emergency psychiatric patients.

Stephen M. Soreff, MD

Acknowledgments

A number of people have contributed generously of their ideas, efforts, and time to make this book a reality.

Patricia Olsen served as research assistant, compiling and updating much of the background information for this volume. Esther Dudley, with the assistance of Marian Fasulo, did a superb job in the manuscript preparation. E. Charles Kunkle, MD, Director of the Division of Neurology, Maine·Medical Center, made important suggestions concerning Chapter 9. Edward McGeachey, Associate Vice-President, Maine Medical Center, offered useful concepts for the preparation of Chapter 17.

Andrea Stingelin, Health Sciences Editor of John Wiley & Sons, Inc., greatly helped in the focusing and developing of this book. I also gratefully acknowledge the interest and encouragement of the Maine Emergency Medical Services Project under the medical directorship of H. Alan Hume, MD.

Finally, I thank the Department of Psychiatry and the Department of Emergency Medicine at the Maine Medical Center. Their excellent patient care has served both to initiate this book and to exemplify effective emergency psychiatric treatment.

Stephen M. Soreff, MD

Contents

1
What Is a Psychiatric Emergency?

A 26-year-old man experiences distress because "voices are arguing" in his head. He discovers his aftercare worker is away and the mental health clinic cannot see him for a week. His family has "given up" on him. He stopped his medication a month ago. He comes to the emergency department for help.

A 28-year-old, recently separated mother of two runs to her parents with fears of losing control, hurting the children, and killing herself. Her mother and father react with horror. What should they do? Whom should they call? The family physician recommends the emergency department. The parents request a rescue unit to transport their daughter.

A 30-year-old, depressed man drinks a glass of beer, goes "berserk," and wrecks the saloon. Fire officers subdue him and take him to the emergency department.

Despite the apparent diversity, these situations possess a number of important similarities and all fit the definition of psychiatric emergency. **The potential for a psychiatric emergency exists when a change in a person caused by intrapsychic, interpersonal, or biologic alterations can no longer be tolerated by that person or by significant others in the environment. The potential emergency becomes an actual emergency when either the person or the significant others seek immediate assistance.**

The definition of psychiatric emergency includes four key ideas: change, intolerance by the patient, the reaction of significant others, and immediacy of the situation. These four elements not only describe the emergency but also prescribe staff treatment approaches. The definition looks backward to the cause of the emergency and at the same time glances forward to its resolution.

1

CHANGE

The person's or significant others' awareness of a change is the first major ingredient in the emergency. This fact provides a useful way to view and understand the emergency strategically. Without such an awareness the patient, family, and emergency personnel view the psychiatric emergency as "coming out of the blue," as an act of either the devil or God, or as totally incomprehensible.

The change may originate from intrapsychic, interpersonal, or biologic influences or may result from a combination of these three. Intrapsychic change occurs within the person's mood or perceptions. The patient develops a mood disturbance.

A 25-year-old graduate student "broke down" in a physics class. He cried uncontrollably. He recalled having felt sad at this time of year for the past four years. He also remembered having had a most disquieting dream the previous night. His family history revealed that his older brother had committed suicide on this date five years ago.

Other patients experience a perceptual change.

A 65-year-old woman became preoccupied with her fear that there was electricity in the water faucet. She worried constantly about this. Her obsession grew and became a compulsion. She began to touch the faucet continually. When her touching reached the level of 500 times an hour, her husband lost patience and brought her to the emergency department (ED).

In both of these situations, the major change had taken place *within* the person's mental processes. In other incidents, interpersonal events trigger the change. Common examples include lovers' breaking up, a couple's separating, a child's leaving home, retiring, fighting within a family, and being antagonized by an employer. The relationship is the key ingredient.

When a 26-year-old man discovered that his wife was involved in an affair with his best friend, he reacted with rage, guilt, and depression. He wanted to kill the friend, then his wife, and finally himself. He cried, laughed, and blamed himself. He felt "out of control" with anger and asked a coworker to bring him to the hospital "to be safe."

The interpersonal change often reflects a loss, frequently loss of a person, a social status, or an object of perceived social significance.

A 45-year-old woman becomes overwhelmed by grief upon hearing that her husband has died of a heart attack.

A 55-year-old man contemplates suicide after being fired from his job at the post office.

A 20-year-old woman, distraught from feeling socially rejected since her hysterectomy for cervical cancer, takes an overdose of sleeping medication.

Of the three types of change, the interpersonal alteration is the easiest for both ED staff and the patient to identify as the precipitator of the psychiatric emergency.

Biologic change is the third type of alteration. Physiologic status is now recognized as one of the most significant elements in emergency psychiatry (1). The biologic changes producing alterations in patients' mental status include reactions to abused substances, reactions to alcohol, responses to prescribed medications, responses to physical illnesses, and reactions to trauma.

Abused substances that can cause the change include lysergic acid diethylamide, cocaine, and phencyclidine; these drugs produce acute psychoses. Marijuana sometimes causes panic. Amphetamines may precipitate a paranoid reaction. Discontinuation of opiates, barbiturates, and amphetamines frequently causes disturbing mental symptoms (2).

A 26-year-old law student experienced a "panic" attack after smoking some "particularly fine grass." A friend brought him to the ED. He felt anxious and scared. He paced continually, feared losing his mind, and begged constantly for reassurance. He denied using other drugs.

Alcohol can produce the change that initiates the emergency. Alcohol contributes significantly to many psychiatric emergencies and ED admissions.

A 45-year-old executive felt overwhelmed by an urge to drink. He had recently experienced his first blackout. He believed this meant he was an alcoholic. He found himself increasingly preoccupied with the "next drink." He came to the ED for control of his drinking.

Alcohol use in its three phases—initiation, continuation, and termination—can precipitate an emergency (3). In addition to being the cause of a psychiatric emergency, alcohol exacerbates a number of psychiatric conditions, including anxiety, depression, and organic mental disorders.

A growing number of prescribed medications produce side effects which constitute the change that precedes crisis. Psychotropic drugs can cause many distressing physical symptoms (4). Phenothiazines may produce akathisia (restless), Parkinson-like movements, rigidity, and some dystonia (sudden muscle movements); oculogyric crises are the most dreaded. The tricyclic antidepressants can cause acute urinary retention. Lithium carbonate produces a bothersome tremor.

A host of psychological effects accompany the use of many prescribed drugs. Antihypertensive medication, especially reserpine, can produce depression (5). Steroids have been associated with a wide spectrum of emotional reactions ranging from euphoria to depression (6).

Medical illnesses and surgical conditions sometimes result in the change that results in psychiatric emergency. Neurologic diseases ranging from epilepsy to brain tumors alter the patient's mental status. Anemias, cardiac conditions, metabolic disorders, and infections frequently result in emotional changes.

> A 50-year-old man came to the ED complaining of depression, fatigue, lethargy, and lack of interest. A psychiatrist had attributed these symptoms to the man's unhappiness about his retirement. A complete blood cell count (CBC) revealed the real cause to be a significant anemia.

Finally, trauma can cause the change that produces crisis. Head trauma with loss of consciousness is highly correlated with alterations in mental status.

> A 26-year-old student sustained a head injury while driving his motorcycle. He lost consciousness when his head, unprotected by a helmet, struck the road. Upon regaining consciousness he became violent and combative. He did not know his name, the date, or the location.

Although change represents the underlying cause of crisis, it does not fully account for the emergency. Stated another way, the change alone may not be sufficient to produce the psychiatric emergency. Often the person sustains considerable alteration in life circumstances without a crisis. For the change to evolve into an emergency, three ingredients are required: the change itself, intolerance of it, and the seeking of immediate assistance.

INTOLERANCE OF THE CHANGE

The person's intolerance of the change advances the event toward becoming an emergency. Some people tolerate the change for a long time, becoming depressed. Others become rapidly intolerant, experiencing an anxiety reaction. In the beginning of this chapter, the young man became overwhelmed by the "voices" in his head. The change consisted of the "voices," which he did not tolerate. He sought help. In the second case, the young woman felt depressed because of separation from her husband. The change produced a depression; the depression led to homicidal and suicidal ideation. She could not tolerate the depression or the thoughts. In the third incident the man went "berserk" after a glass beer. The reaction represents an extreme form of intolerance to alcohol.

The intolerance of significant others to the patient's change also advances the situation toward becoming an emergency (7). Their responses are one of the unique qualities of a psychiatric emergency. Not infrequently the patient perceives much less distress than others do. Their concern for the *patient's* treatment propels the patient into the ED.

> *A 20-year-old man recently graduated from college without any future plans. Upon returning to his home he spent more and more time in his bedroom. This situation persisted for several weeks. One afternoon he took all the contents of the freezer and placed them on the lawn. The father lost his "tolerance" for his son's behavior and brought him to the ED.*

SEEKING IMMEDIATE ASSISTANCE

The seeking of immediate assistance represents the most significant, crucial, and essential ingredient of a psychiatric emergency. The change begins the series of events. The patient's or others' intolerance of the alteration advances the crisis, but the need for immediate treatment makes it an emergency. The psychiatric literature provides diverse and occasionally divergent definitions of psychiatric emergency (8,9). However, urgency is the one element all authors agree upon.

The concept *immediacy* connotes the most important aspects of the psychiatric emergency. First, immediacy pertains to a disruptive event. Because of the urgency the patient and others cannot wait for a scheduled appointment. Second, immediacy reflects the tremendous pain of crisis for both the patient and significant others. The greater the distress, the quicker the patient or others seek relief. Third, the urgency underscores the gravity of the situation. The people involved are very concerned. They view the psychiatric emergency as a serious medical event. Fourth, immediacy emphasizes the need for rapid response.

SUMMARY

This chapter's definition of psychiatric emergency includes both description and prescription. The emergency involves a change within the person (intrapsychic), in the person's relations with others (interpersonal), or in the person's body (biologic). The emergency also includes the response of the person or significant others intolerance to that change, and the requirement for immediate assistance. This definition depicts a serious situation involving a number of people. It explains why the crisis happened at the moment it did and points toward avenues of treatment by focusing on the cause of the change.

REFERENCES

1. Fauman MA, Fauman BJ: The differential diagnosis of organic based psychiatric disturbance in emergency department. *JACEP* 6:315-323, 1977.
2. Slaby AE, Lieb J, Trancredi LR: *Handbook of Psychiatric Emergencies.* Flushing, Medical Examination Publishing Co, 1975.
3. Victor M: Treatment of alcoholic intoxication and the withdrawal syndrome. *Psychosom Med* 28:636-650, 1968.
4. Shader RI (ed): *Manual of Psychiatric Therapeutics.* Boston, Little, Brown and Co, 1978.
5. Goodwin FK, Ebert MH, Bunney WE Jr: Mental effects of resperine in man: A review, in Shader RI (ed): *Psychiatric Complications of Medical Drugs.* New York, Raven Press, 1972, pp 73-107.
6. Carpenter WT, Strauss JS, Bunney WE Jr: The psychobiology of cortisol metabolism: Clinical and theoretical implications, in Shader RI (ed): *Psychiatric Complications of Medical Drugs.* New York, Raven Press, 1972, pp 49-72.
7. Carden TS: 'Emergency'—a redefinition. *JAMA* 240:377, 1978.
8. Bartolucci G, Drayer CS: An overview of crisis intervention in the emergency rooms of general hospitals. *Am J Psychiatry* 130:953-960, 1973.
9. Frazier SH: Comprehensive management of psychiatric emergencies. *Psychosomatics* 9:7-11, 1968.

2
The Unwanted Patient

Several facts concerning psychiatric emergency patients must be confronted. First, these patients have a number of features that make them a difficult, challenging, and complicated management responsibility (1). Second, emergency medical technicians (EMTs) and the ED staff have problems dealing with psychiatric patients (2). Third, psychiatric personnel also experience difficulty working with emergency patients (3). Thus, to a degree the emergency psychiatric patient represents the *unwanted patient*.

The confrontation of the issue of unwanted patients demonstrates two of the most powerful psychiatric principles: treatment involves bringing the unconscious to consciousness, and treatment involves discussing everything that concerns the patient (4). The therapist strives to assist the patient to become aware of hidden, repressed, suppressed, denied, and avoided feelings, and of attitudes, prejudices, and the patient's history. The therapist provides a situation where patients can talk about everything that bothers them. Through the process of self-discovery, patients come to know themselves, their problems, and their capabilities, and to grow into less restricted and fuller lives.

These basic principles—that therapy includes bringing the unconscious feelings, attitudes, and history to awareness and fully exploring whatever concerns the patient—have a number of corollaries. These include (1) *anything* can be talked about, (2) discussion is emphasized instead of action, and (3) patients benefit from talking about themselves.

The first corollary is anything can be talked about. All too frequently the patient and staff view a number of subjects as taboo: sex, money, suicide, homicide, incest, and death. They avoid these issues. As a result, significant, causative material remains undiscussed and unavailable, and the emotional abscess remains unopened.

A 50-year-old woman comes to the ED terribly distraught. Her mother had died six weeks earlier after a long, painful, debilitating illness. During the last two years the patient has diligently cared for her mother 24 hours a day. The patient wrestles with anger but does not know its

7

origin. She is a religious person and believes in keeping any "negative feeling" away. During the interview she discovers her hidden resentment about having sacrificed her life for her mother. She feels relief that she can talk about her frustration.

The second corollary emphasizes that discussion is preferable to action. Psychiatric intervention aims to have the patient talk about feelings and thoughts rather than act upon them. It is preferable for the patient to come to the ED to discuss depression rather than to attempt suicide. The ED offers the patient a place to come to talk. It provides and emphasizes a verbal solution.

A 22-year-old veteran came to the ED because of despair, confusion, and loneliness. He waited a long time to be seen and did not feel the ED physician listened to him. He walked out and returned within the hour with both wrists lacerated. He said, "Now will you listen to me?"

The third corollary is therapy involves making the unconscious conscious. Patients benefit from discovering thoughts and feelings of which they have been unaware.

THE PATIENTS

The psychiatric emergency patient has a number of characteristics. These include lack of resources, intensity of symptoms, psychosis, immediate neediness, impulsiveness, violence, repetition of predicaments, inability to follow through with treatment, and helplessness. The EMTs and the ED staff must deal with these qualities and use them to develop a comprehensive treatment approach.

Psychiatric emergency patients often lack resources. They come from the lower socioeconomic groups and have few economic alternatives (5). Frequently they are unemployed. Indeed, unemployment may precipitate the crisis. Many patients have lost their social support network, family, and friends. They have few social and economic options.

Patients struggle with intense feelings and thoughts: overwhelming anxiety, crippling fear, staggering depression, alarming hallucinations, expanding delusions, and murderous impulses. The patients experience panic and perceive that life is out of control. They are on edge; all their emotions are on the surface and they sustain severe mental anguish.

Many patients exhibit mental disruptions of psychotic proportion. Their overwhelming anxiety and fears reveal underlying psychoses. Patients may have schizophrenia, manic-depressive disease, or severe organic mental disorder.

Psychiatric emergency patients seek immediate assistance. They fear impending death. In panic they ask the EMTs for transport and the ED staff for help. In desperation they demand relief.

Some patients demonstrate impulsiveness (6). They drive their vehicles wildly; they wrestle, often unsuccessfully, with strong impulses. They are oriented toward action and care little for the future. For them the difference between a thought and an action is very small.

Other patients display violence (7). In most cases it dramatically takes the form of either suicidal or homicidal behavior, or both. In other instances the patient strikes out against family, friends, people unknown to him, or property.

Some patients return several times to the ED. They repeat ineffective behavior and find themselves again in turmoil. These patients become "habitual offenders" in the ED (8,p488). They have many "rush sheets." As Talbott (9) reports, they have been in the hospital many times. They have chronic illness with periodic exacerbations.

Patients have difficulty following through on treatment recommendations. Once the crisis subsides, they return to their old patterns of behavior. They miss outpatient appointments and discontinue medications.

They demonstrate emotional neediness and helplessness. They express concern over their mental control and sanity. They ask for help to govern their minds.

EMERGENCY MEDICAL TECHNICIANS AND THE EMERGENCY DEPARTMENT STAFF

A wide variety of explanations account for the difficulties EMTs and ED staff have in the management of psychiatric emergency patients. The reasons include the characteristics of the patients, the attitudes of the personnel, and the setting.

The previously cited characteristics of psychiatric emergency patients suggest reasons why personnel reluctantly engage them. The prominent features include the patients' intensity, psychosis, violence, repeated visits, and neediness.

For the EMTs and the ED staff to deal with psychiatric emergency patients, they must confront the patients' overwhelming, painful, intense emotions. Those emotions are highly contagious. The personnel come away from the interview anxious, depressed, or confused, reflecting the patient's basic feelings. Staff members find the experience extremely disquieting, and many would prefer to avoid it.

The ED staff find themselves "over their heads" in confronting a psychosis. They cannot understand or empathize with patients who have schizophrenia. They feel the patient requires a specialist.

Not uncommonly EMTs and ED staff fear psychiatric patients. They perceive these patients as violent, hostile, combative, and dangerous. Studies indicate that some psychiatric patients do commit dangerous, violent acts (10). Personnel see psychiatric patients as a potential threat to staff members' safety (11).

Staff become reluctant to involve themselves with psychiatric patients because some patients who have been treated before come back again (12). The repeat rate means to personnel that intervention does not work and patients do not get better. The "returns" tend to discourage staff from engaging them again. When one patient came to the ED for the eighth time in two months, staff totally ignored her for several hours.

Staff often have difficulty confronting an emotionally needy person. They feel uncomfortable over the individual who has lost emotional control and asks for "mental" help. They understand a patient in pain as a result of physical trauma; they emphathize with a person in an acute grief reaction; but they have difficulty with the patient who just cries and wants help "for no reason at all."

The EMTs and ED personnel have a number of attitudes which interfere with their responses to psychiatric emergency patients. These attitudes reflect their own life experiences, their work, and their training.

The most detrimental attitude is that nothing can help the psychiatric patient. This attitude represents a therapeutic nihilism and defeatist position that totally preclude intervention. It classifies the mentally ill as unable to benefit from treatment and incapable of being rehabilitated.

Often an individual staff member's experience influences his or response. One ED physician refuses to treat alcoholic patients. His father was an alcoholic and used to beat his son when intoxicated. An ED nurse has great difficulty dealing with adolescent patients who use drugs. She has two teenagers at home and fears they will become addicts.

Lack of training is another major reason why personnel are reluctant to engage the psychiatric patient. They have had very little if any instruction in dealing with psychiatric emergencies. Most training programs emphasize the physical aspects of medicine and pay little attention to the psychological.

Staff feel they have nothing to offer the patient. They know what to do for trauma, for a myocardial infarction, or for an infection. But the results of an interview emerge as far less tangible. What good does "talking" do, or what difference does their presence make?

Staff not only feel they have nothing to offer, but they also fear doing the wrong thing with the psychiatric patient. Many personnel believe if they say the wrong thing, the patient will "go crazy." They see psychiatric patients as fragile and ready to explode. A medical student on an ED rotation voiced a fear that if she asked a patient about suicide the patient would hurt himself.

In addition, a number of factors in the emergency setting tend to influence staff interactions with psychiatric patients. These include the action orientation, the time constraints, and the legal requirements.

Emergency medicine is action medicine. It deals with visible trauma and illness.

Its treatments consist largely of tangible interventions: x-ray films, intravenous fluids, splints, blood, and electrocardiograph machines. In this kind of setting the patient requiring just talking emerges as slightly out of place. Emergency personnel rank interview skills much below the ability to start an intravenous infusion.

Time is the essence of emergency medicine. Rapid action epitomizes the emergency effort. Yet psychiatric patients require staff to spend time with them. Psychiatric intervention in the field and in the emergency department takes time. Because of the time commitment, staff are reluctant to undertake the intervention.

Finally, psychiatric intervention involves many legal considerations. Issues of whether and when to interview and transport concern the EMTs. Issues of confidentiality, restraint, and commitment concern the ED staff. The legal problems often serve to deter personnel from responding.

THE PSYCHIATRIST AND THE PSYCHIATRIC STAFF

The psychiatric staff also have difficulty with emergency patients for a variety of reasons. The reasons include certain characteristics of the patients, their own attitudes, issues of scheduling and territory, and the legal aspects of intervention.

Emergency patients have a number of attributes which cause psychiatrists to be reluctant to involve themselves in emergency psychiatry. These features include the patients' immediacy and their focus on the present, their frequent admissions, their violence, and their resourcelessness.

Emergency patients are "present oriented" and struggle with their overwhelming immediate feelings. They are not interested in a cause, a pattern, a dynamic, or an interpretation of a dream. They want immediate relief. To the psychodynamically oriented psychiatrist, the patients' problems often seem to deal too much with crushing, overwhelming reality.

Psychiatrists must cope with the high return rate. Often these physicians see the same patient in similar predicaments on many occasions. The patients are hospitalized again and again. The ED staff all too frequently remind the psychiatric consultant, "Your patient is back."

The psychiatrist and the psychiatric resident must deal with violent patients. As Madden, Lion, and Penna (13) point out, they, too, must confront the real possibility of personal assault. Patients do occasionally assault therapists (14). Psychiatrists know the physical challenge involved in emergency psychiatry (15).

The psychiatrist must deal with a number of very basic issues such as how the patient is going to obtain food, shelter, clothing, and money for medication. The therapist must develop a treatment plan appropriate to patients' requirements, respecting patients' usually limited socioeconomic options, and must match each patient's needs with the community's limited facilities. These can be very frustrating tasks.

Some psychiatrists have attitudes about treatment that lead them to avoid emergency psychiatry. They emphasize long-term, insight-oriented psychotherapy in their practices and find the emergency patient not receptive to or appropriate for that treatment (16). They tend to view these patients as poor candidates for therapy, to see them as too "present oriented," to find them uninterested in introspection, and to feel they will not follow through with treatment.

Some psychiatrists and psychiatric residents develop the attitude that there is little educational value in emergency psychiatry. They complain about the lack of diagnostic challenges. They find themselves too involved in the acute management issues, the large number of patients, and the difficulty of obtaining the proper referral. They see no academic qualities in their ED work nor any educational advantages to the time they put in.

The psychiatrist and the psychiatric resident encounter difficulty with both the schedule and the territory issue. In the former, they find themselves having to make rapid decisions, often with incomplete information, and having to see too many patients (17). ED psychiatry is the antithesis of an ordered, organized appointment schedule. In emergency psychiatry the psychiatrist must work in someone else's territory, namely the ED. The therapist functions as a consultant, often for *their* patients. As a consequence of the erratic, hectic schedule and the characteristics of the patients, some interested psychiatrists ultimately leave emergency psychiatry.

Finally, psychiatrists in the ED must confront a maze of legal issues and situations (18). Issues of confidentiality, patients' rights, restraints, and involuntary hospitalization arise continually. ED psychiatrists face potential lawsuits in many different ways. The family threatens to take legal action if the physician does not commit the patient. The patient threatens action if commitment is instituted.

REFERENCES

1. Morrice JKW: Emergency psychiatry. *Br J Psychiatry* 114:485–491, 1968.
2. Lagos JM, Perlmutter K, Saexinger H: Fear of the mentally ill: Empirical support for the common man's response. *Am J Psychiatry* 134:1134–1137, 1977.
3. Gerson S, Bassuk E: Psychiatric emergencies: An overview. *Am J Psychiatry* 137:1–11, 1980.
4. Greenson RR: *The Technique and Practice of Psychoanalysis.* New York, International Universities Press, 1968.
5. Coleman JV, Errera P: The general hospital emergency room and its psychiatric problems. *Am J Public Health* 53:1294–1301, 1963.
6. Farberow H: Crisis prevention. *Int J Psychiatry* 6:382–384, 1968.

THE UNWANTED PATIENT   13

7. Skodol AE, Karasu TB: Emergency psychiatry and the assaultive patient. *Am J Psychiatry* 135:202-205, 1978.
8. Whiteley JS, Denison DM: The psychiatric casualty. *Brit J Psychiatry* 109:488-490, 1963.
9. Talbott JA (ed): *The Chronic Mental Patient.* Washington, DC, American Psychiatric Association, 1978.
10. Grunberg F, Klinger BI, Grumet BR: Homicide and community-based psychiatry. *J Nerv Ment Dis* 166:868-874, 1978.
11. Lion JR, Bach-y-Rita G, Ervin FR: Violent patients in the emergency rooms. *Am J Psychiatry* 125:1706-1711, 1969.
12. Soreff S: Psychiatric consultation in the emergency department. *Psychiatric Annals* 8:189-194, 1978.
13. Madden DJ, Lion JR, Penna MW: Assaults on psychiatrists by patients. *Am J Psychiatry* 133:422-425, 1976.
14. Whitman RM, Armao BB, Dent OB: Assault on the therapist. *Am J Psychiatry* 133:426-429, 1976.
15. Lion JR, Pasternak SA: Countertransference reactions to violent patients. *Am J Psychiatry* 130:207-210, 1973.
16. Eisenthal S, Ferrell R, Lazare A: Attitude of psychiatric residents toward patient requests. *Am J Psychiatry* 133:1079-1081, 1976.
17. Slaby AE, Lieb J, Tancredi LR: *Handbook of Psychiatric Emergencies.* Flushing, NY, Medical Examination Publishing Co, 1975.
18. Barton WE, Sanborn CJ (eds): *Law and the Mental Health Professional: Friction at the Interface.* New York, International Universities Press, 1978.

3
Comprehensive Treatment:
An Overview

This chapter provides an overview of the comprehensive approach to psychiatric emergencies. It discusses the general principles involved in all psychiatric emergencies and details the complete psychiatric evaluation and the mental status examination. The chapter explores significant factors common to all psychiatric emergencies.

THE EMERGENCY MEDICAL TECHNICIANS' RESPONSE TO PSYCHIATRIC EMERGENCY

The response of the EMTs marks the beginning of professional intervention. The EMTs furnish much more than just transportation. Their skill and techniques can supply the basis for effective crisis management.

A number of intervention principles apply to all psychiatric emergencies: promptness, identification, time commitment, transport plan, constant attendance, involvement of significant others, and transmission of information.

Prompt EMT response diminishes the patient's and others' distress. EMTs represent help by their uniforms, patches, and jackets as well as by their vehicles. They carry with them the implication of assistance and hope.

EMTs must identify themselves to the patient and others at the scene in two ways. They must introduce themselves to the patient by their full name and their professional title. The early explanation of their role sets the stage for the intended transport, focuses the services to be provided and transmits the major message of trained, professional help. The encounter between an EMT and a patient includes formally addressing the patient and offering to shake hands. In the midst of a crisis there is still time to be polite and observe etiquette.

Psychiatric emergencies require the EMTs' time. The patient often does not fit the rapid protocol for stabilization and transportation, as would a patient with a

14

fractured extremity. It is important for the EMTs to recognize that they will have to spend time with the patient and family. By their appreciation of this time commitment, the EMTs will experience less resentment than if they had expected a quick trip.

The EMTs must state to the patient and the significant others the transport plan, then they must adhere to it. Patients need to know what is happening. Knowing they will be transported to a hospital can often relieve their apprehension. They feel treatment awaits. It is important not to lie to patients. Any deception will be amplified by the paranoid patient. EMTs must, then, follow their plan. Patients focus on the plan and use it to control their anxiety. A deviation from the schedule increases the apprehension and undermines the patient's trust in the EMTs.

From identification to completed transportation, an EMT must be with the patient at all times. The presence of an EMT reassures anxious, phobic, or depressed patients. It prevents a patient with an organic mental disorder from wandering off. It circumvents a suicide attempt.

EMTs must involve significant others in the transport. They can be of great comfort to the patient and can furnish critical information to the ED staff. They can initiate commitment papers if the patient is dangerous and declines treatment. The family, friends, and coworkers are the EMTs' allies in patient care.

The EMTs must provide the ED staff with information. The EMTs have gained a great deal of information from the patient and the significant others. They have made important observations at the scene of the intervention. They have evaluated the initial mental status of the patient. The EMTs function as the ED eyes and ears at the site of the crisis and in transport. It is imperative that the information they have acquired be passed along to the ED staff.

THE EMERGENCY DEPARTMENT EVALUATION

The decisive intervention in the psychiatric crisis occurs in the ED. The EMTs' role is completed when they have delivered the patient and pertinent information to the ED. At the ED, staff make order out of the chaos.

The evaluation of the patient involves five key steps: providing the ED reception, making a physical examination, determining the chief complaint, completing the psychiatric evaluation, and conducting the mental status examination.

The Reception

The ED reception provides the critical transition step from the community to the hospital. It continues the intervention plan initiated by the EMTs and involves certain essential approaches to the patient and those with him. An effective patient reception facilitates a thorough evaluation. If the reception is mismanaged, the patient may refuse treatment or elope (depart without permission).

The ED occupies a unique interface between the community and the hospital. Often it is located away from the main portion of the hospital, and its reception area bears more resemblance to public waiting rooms than to a medical facility. In this reception area the person goes through a process of becoming a patient. By supplying information, signing permits, and following staff directions, the person accepts the patient role. The transition to this role is critical. During the reception process, patient apprehension or staff resistance can create difficulties that carry over to the evaluation and treatment phases of the patient's care.

The principles of ED reception are as follows: promptness, identification of personnel, removal of weapons, a stated plan, constant attendance, involvement of others, and transmission of information.

Swift reception and intervention diminish anxiety. Prompt attention tells patients they are "important." The importance of promptness stems from two facts: untreated psychiatric emergencies become worse, and waiting heightens a crisis.

Staff must always greet patients. They must use proper etiquette, including offering to shake hands and addressing patients by their formal names, not just first names. They must in the process introduce themselves and identify their professional positions.

The removal of weapons is mandatory. No proper evaluation can be conducted if the patient has a weapon. Patients must surrender all weapons but can be reassured they will be returned upon completion of the evaluation. It is proper to inquire if the patient has a weapon.

The staff must next outline a plan of evaluation to the patient. Knowing what will be done and why controls the patient's apprehension. Again, this plan should be adhered to. If there are to be deviations, the patient should be notified.

Especially in the ED, the patient must not be left alone. Waiting in a busy ED can be a very stressful experience. The same fears, impulses, and apprehensions that bring patients to the ED can also precipitate their leaving prematurely. The continuous presence of a staff member serves to diminish the patient's anxiety, to provide reassurance, to monitor the patient's condition, and to forestall elopement.

One major axiom of ED reception is to keep the significant others involved. In other words, they should not leave. They provide invaluable information about the patient. They can stay with the patient and can help immensely with referral.

Staff must share information about the patient. Amazingly, within the limited confines of the ED, a great deal of pertinent patient information gets misplaced and is not transmitted (1). The secretary has received a telephone call. The triage nurse has gained some important facts. The EMTs have brought some critical observations. The family contributes vital material. Get the information; then share the information.

Several key interviewing principles must be adhered to. These techniques establish a trust and treatment relationship between physician and patient. These deal with the location of the interview, the time of the interview, the sequence of interviews, and the order of topics within the interview.

The patient desires and requires a quiet, private room for the interview. A psychiatric interview (and indeed a medical interview) is an intensely personal event. The interviewer must preserve and protect the patient's dignity. A quiet, comfortable, private setting is a prerequisite to meeting this objective.

Next, the physician must be prepared to spend time with the patient. Physicians must realize that the management of psychiatric emergencies requires time.

The physician must follow a specific sequence of interviews. This sequence will ensure gaining the maximum of information and obtaining the patient's trust. The physician must interview the patient *first, alone;* then, with the patient's permission, the interviewer should see the family, friend, or employer. Patients experience enough apprehension in coming to an ED and telling a stranger about themselves. That discomfort mounts dramatically if they believe they must not only reveal their problems but also refute information already provided by their families. The patient talks more freely when left alone with the physician. It is appropriate to begin the interview by asking the others to wait outside the room but not to leave the ED. After interviewing the patient, the interviewer should, with the patient's permission, see the others.

In proceeding through the topics of the interview, the physician gains better results by progressing from neutral to sensitive material. It is important to allow the interview to evolve before asking difficult questions. Moreover, the best interview technique permits patients to tell their story first with a minimum of interruptions. After the patient has talked, the interviewer can be more specific.

Physical Examination

The psychiatric emergency often reflects a medical illness (2). Evaluation requires an examination of the patient's physical status as well as mental status.

A complete exposition of the physical examination is beyond the scope of this book. However, the physician must pay particular attention to the neurologic and cardiovascular aspects of the examination.

Three major clinical indexes of the patient's physical state are pulse, blood pressure, and temperature. These three measurements must be obtained for all psychiatric patients.

Chief Complaint

The patient's chief complaint often crystallizes and summarizes the crisis. The chief complaint provides a great deal of information about the patient; it frequently identifies stresses, fears, and aspirations. By paying particular attention to this introductory, spontaneous remark, the interviewer makes use of a very valuable tool to understand the patient and the emergency. The chief complaint must be elicited and must be recorded verbatim.

Psychiatric Evaluation

The physician concentrates upon obtaining a complete psychiatric and medical history from the patient and from the significant others. The psychiatric history emphasizes history of present illness; social history; therapy experiences, including hospitalizations; psychotropic medications; educational, vocational, and military histories; family history; criminal justice involvements; substance and alcohol use and abuse; and activities of daily living. The medical history focuses upon illnesses, surgery, medications, and trauma.

The history of the present illness gets at the heart of the crisis. It incorporates the critical elements that initiated the emergency and the dynamics of the patient's involvement with the environment. In focusing upon the history of the present illness the interviewer must attempt to answer the question, "Why now?" As in a medical evaluation, the physician must strive for complete information, including details. "Where were you when you took the pills?" "What did your boss actually say to you?" "Is your wife involved with another person?" "How did you feel when you were diagnosed as having a peptic ulcer?"

The patient frequently resists talking about personal matters, with statements like, "That's not important," "What difference does it make, anyway?" and "Why do you care?" Yet those very details make the patient and the crisis understandable. The author's experience has shown that an interviewer's perseverance in gaining specific information will lead to better *contact* with the patient and a better appreciation of the crisis than can be achieved with only vague inquiries.

The social history emphasizes the patient's living situation and provides major clues both to the causes of the crisis and to the eventual referral. It addresses the specifics of where and with whom the patient resides, and looks at the patient's support system. Knowing a 16-year-old adolescent lives alone at the YMCA helps the examiner to understand the adolescent's predicament and the referral options.

Therapy experiences include current treatment, previous therapy, and psychiatric hospitalizations. This part of the psychiatric history highlights one major finding in the psychiatric emergency population — these patients often are not new to treatment. Thus, it becomes even more important to inquire about therapy. Many patients are already in therapy at the time of their ED admission. Kass, Karasu, and Walsh (3) reported 36 out of 100 psychiatric patients in one ED were currently in treatment. In these cases it is important to determine the nature of the treatment and to be in contact with the therapist. A history of therapeutic experiences and their successes will suggest which kind of referral will be best for the patient. Finally, as one of the by-products of deinstitutionalization—the discharge of patients from the state hospitals into the community—many ED patients will have had at least one psychiatric hospitalization (4). Clearly, the psychiatric emergency patient often is not new to the system or to therapy. Much useful information is available from the history.

A history of psychotropic medication use is important for several reasons. First, a significant number of ED patients—LePoidevin and Reid (5) report 46 percent and Atkins (6) reports 54 percent—are already taking these medications. These drugs can actually precipitate the crisis or can help to control it. The physician must ascertain the patient's response to these preparations. Second, many patients have experienced similar psychiatric episodes and have been successfully treated with medications. By inquiring about the patient's medication history, the physician obtains valuable clues as to which preparation should now be prescribed. Third, some patients have developed very disquieting side effects from certain medications. A physician's knowledge of these reactions can prevent a recurrence.

An educational, vocational, and military history reveals a great deal about patients, their development, and their current situations. The physician must ask adolescents about their school background. It is appropriate to explore with high school and college students how they are doing in school. The patient's job or lack of it provides vital information. Unemployment, position termination, and retirement all correlate with psychiatric crises. Job stresses cause and contribute to emotional problems. Conversely, emotional crises are reflected in the patient's work. Finally, the patient's military history provides information. In some instances military experience may have caused the crisis. The type of military discharge often determines whether a Veterans Administration hospital will accept the patient by referral.

A family history provides further information. Schizophrenia has familial correlations (7). Manic-depressive illness has been demonstrated to be a genetically determined disease. The family history offers a longitudinal view of the patient and supplies key developmental information.

The patient can be involved with the criminal justice system in several ways. Bizarre, inappropriate behavior may have precipitated police intervention. In such cases the patient is rarely under arrest but rather in protective custody. Psychiatric illnesses may lead to criminal activity. Incarceration results in significant psychiatric disturbances for many people. In all three situations the interviewer must inquire concerning the nature of the charges pending. In certain situations the actual charge will determine the type of referral available.

A substance and alcohol history must be obtained in all psychiatric emergencies. Use of alcohol and other drugs correlates highly with ED admissions and ED psychiatric populations (8).

A history of the patient's patterns of sleep, appetite, and sexual activity yields useful material. Sleep increases in certain depressions. In other depressions early morning waking is found. Anxiety and paranoia lead to diminished sleep. Various emotional problems affect the appetite. Significant weight loss occurs in severe depressions. Sexual activity is disturbed in many psychiatric problems. Increased libido often accompanies mania; decreased libido occurs in depressions.

A medical history involves inquiry into illnesses, medications, trauma, and surgery. Not only do certain illnesses present as psychiatric problems, but patients also react emotionally to their medical diagnoses. Recent illnesses are particularly significant. The list of medications affecting mental status grows daily. The physician must know all the drugs the patient is taking. Trauma, especially to the head, causes psychiatric manifestations; subdural hematoma are frequently overlooked. Surgery also correlates with crises.

Mental Status Examination

The last step in the psychiatric evaluation involves a formal mental status examination. This provides a comprehensive mental picture at the time of the patient's ED admission. The mental status examination has been termed the psychiatric equivalent of the physical examination.

Although the actual mental inventory should be done toward the end of the patient interview, much of the information will have been derived during the interactions with the patient. The following discussion details the nine parts of the mental status examination: appearance, affect, thought content, suicidal intent, homicidal thoughts, intelligence, judgment, insight, and sensorium.

Appearance.   This term refers to the patient's physical appearance, eye contact, kinesics, and apparel. Appearance is one of the most under-used pieces of patient information. The power of observation enables the examiner to derive a number of clues about the patient's dynamics and diagnosis.

Physical appearance includes evidences of the patient's self-care habits, presence of tattoos, use of makeup, and body type. The patient's hygiene reflects his or her problem. The interviewer should pay particular attention to condition of fingernails and hair and should also notice whether the patient has shaved recently. Tattoos often reveal characteristics of the patient—hates and loves or hopes and failures. Makeup and the appropriateness of its application supply further clues. Finally, body types offer information. A very tall, thin man triggers a consideration of Klinefelter's syndrome; a very thin, young woman, anorexia nervosa.

The patient's eye contact, or lack of it, communicates additional information. Some paranoid persons make no eye contact with the interviewer; others wear sun glasses to prevent people from seeing their eyes.

The patient's body movements during the interview reveal a great deal. It is important to notice whether the patient sits, stands, or paces. Some patients become extremely animated during the interview; others remain immobile.

Clothing does help make the diagnosis. Is the attire appropriate, buttoned, coordinated, neat, and clean? Shabby, dirty, ill-fitting garments suggest that the patient is depressed or has an organic mental syndrome.

Affect. The patient's feelings are significant indicators of the mental status. Patients both describe and demonstrate their emotional reactions. These range from depression to jubilation, from rage to apathy, and from excitement to a "flat" response.

The interviewer must assess the appropriateness of the affect to the context of the speech. A person who laughs while depicting a funeral scene arouses a certain degree of concern.

The interviewer must also monitor his or her own emotional responses to the patient. Emotional states are contagious, and by recognizing the feelings the patient engenders in himself, the interviewer can begin to comprehend the emotions the patient is struggling with. If the interviewer feels sad when talking with a patient, then most likely that patient is depressed.

Thought Content. Patients reveal a great deal about themselves by the expression of their thoughts. Thought content refers to the rate of verbal productions; the organization of thoughts; and the presence or absence of delusions, obsessions, hallucinations, and illusions.

The rate of speech is important and must be noted. A manic patient often talks with "pressured" speech: one thought immediately follows another. At the other extreme, the depressed patient seemingly takes all day to express a simple idea.

The organization of the communication pattern is consistent with the patient's diagnosis. In normal discourse one can usually follow the logic and the flow of a person's statements. The first idea is related, relevant, and linked to the next. However, in many patients' conversation, the order of ideas is illogical and disorganized. Such patients exhibit "flight of ideas," "loose associations," or "derailment"; they move randomly from one topic to another. An acutely schizophrenic patient speaks in a series of rhythms, in a sing-song fashion. A patient with an organic mental disorder speaks totally incoherently.

Some patients demonstrate "circumstantiality." They answer a question by following an extremely long and convoluted route. But they ultimately answer the original question (it is important in these situations for the interviewer to remember the question). In contrast, the "tangential" patients supply volumes of information in response to an inquiry but never actually address themselves to the original question.

Delusions are false ideas maintained in contradiction to fact or reason. By definition, any challenge to them (pointing out reality, for example,) meets with failure. Delusions offer a number of diagnostic possibilities. Paranoid patients believe people are after them. Depressed patients feel people should punish them for relatively minor indiscretions. Manic patients see themselves as the world's saviors.

Obsessions are ideas the patient focuses on almost to the exclusion of all other ideas. Obsessive patients become preoccupied with a concept, a thought, or a fear and spend all their time dwelling on it. Obsessions appear commonly in a number of diagnoses, especially the thought disorders, the depressions, and the anxiety reactions.

Hallucinations are false perceptions. Patients sense something in the environment that is not there. To the patient the experience appears genuine. The common hallucinations are auditory (usually hearing voices), visual, olfactory (smelling something not present), and tactile (feeling a sensation). The interviewer must ask when, where, and under what circumstances the hallucinations occur. It is also important to ask about the quality of the hallucinations and the patient's reaction to them.

Illusions are misinterpretations of some object, sound, or smell actually present in the environment. For example, a patient may mistake a stick for a snake. When the examiner points out what the object really is, the patient corrects the misinterpretations.

Suicidal Intent. The physician must ask all ED psychiatric patients about suicide. Suicide concerns account for 11 percent (6) to 53 percent (9) of all ED psychiatric admissions.

This inquiry must include thoughts of suicide, plans to kill oneself, history of attempts, and family history of suicide. The questions must be specific and the details pursued. Staff express reluctance to introduce this subject, considering it rude or erroneously thinking that it will give the patient the idea. Actually, most patients appreciate the question and view it as evidence of the interviewer's concern.

Homicidal Thoughts. As with suicide, the interviewer must explore the possibility of homicide. Many patients do turn to the ED to control their impulse to kill (10). The interviewer must ask about thoughts of homicide, specific plans, history of assault or homicide, and family history of violence. Crises produce extreme behavior. Since some stressed patients do kill, no mental status evaluation can be complete without an inquiry about homicide (11).

Intelligence. This part of the mental status evaluation requires the interviewer to estimate—"guess"—the patient's basic intelligence. The level of the patient's mental ability determines to some extent the treatment approach.

Judgment. How has the patient handled life? How has he or she dealt with the current stresses? The answers to these questions offer information about the patient's judgment. They provide more useful material than questions such as "What would you do if you found an addressed, stamped envelope on the street?"

Insight. This category looks at the amount of insight the patient possesses about the current situation. Many patients in crisis have some strong potential to understand the predicament. Their level of insight gives a useful guideline as to what type of therapy would be of greatest benefit to them.

Sensorium. This portion of the interview checks out the state of the computer—the brain—and its level of function. The evaluation of sensorium furnishes the major evidence to establish the diagnosis of organic mental disorder. The assessment consists of four parts: orientation, recall, calculations, and abstractions.

Orientation encompasses three spheres: person, place, and time. The first is the patient's name. The second is where he is. The third means the day, the time of day, the date, the month, and the year. Time orientation is lost first and person orientation is the last to become lost as an organic mental disorder develops.

Memory also must be checked in three areas: immediate, recent, and distant. To test immediate memory, the interviewer gives the patient three unrelated objects to memorize (table, red, 63 Broadway). Then in one minute the interviewer asks the patient to repeat them. In the area of recent recall, the physician inquires about events within the last 24 hours. The history of the present illness also supplies information about recent recall. To assess distant memory the interviewer focuses the questioning on past events. In organic mental disorder the patient loses recent recall first, then distant recollection.

Calculations provide a useful test of brain function. Here the interviewer asks the patient to subtract in serial fashion 7 from 100 (100-93-86-79-72-65-58-51-44-37-30-23-16-9-2). This calculation should be done within one minute and without the use of paper and pencil.

Finally, the interviewer must give the patient a couple of proverbs or abstractions to interpret. This exercise furnishes information about the patient's ability to understand abstract ideas. Useful proverbs include the following: "A stitch in time saves nine"; "People in glass houses should not throw stones"; "The tongue is the enemy of the neck"; "He who hesitates is lost"; and "The golden sword beat down the iron door."

Patients often are either overly abstract in their explanation of a proverb or too concrete in their interpretation of it. In the overly abstract situation, the patient waxes eloquent, evolves a lofty response, and displays circumstantiality. One encounters this behavior in schizophrenic patients, manic people, and patients with severe obsessive-compulsive personality. As an example of a concrete answer, a patient might reply to the proverb "People in glass houses should not throw stones," with "They will break the window." One finds concrete thinking in schizophrenic patients and patients with an organic mental disorder.

The interviewer not only must perform the mental status examination but also must *record* it.

DIAGNOSIS, TREATMENT PLAN, AND IMMEDIATE EMERGENCY DEPARTMENT THERAPY

This section presents the three elements—diagnosis, treatment plan, and immediate therapy—which serve as a turning point in the course of the psychiatric emergency. All the previously obtained information contributes to the diagnosis. The treatment plan looks to the future. The immediate therapy furnishes a bridge from the emergency department crisis to a community referral.

Diagnosis

In order to ensure proper treatment for the psychiatric emergency patient, the physician must determine a diagnosis. A diagnosis provides the pivotal point in the crisis. To reach the diagnosis the physician must employ all the information gained from the patient's physical examination, psychiatric evaluation, and mental status evaluation; the EMTs' reports; and the significant others' observations. From this diagnosis the physician formulates a treatment plan. Specific treatment must be based on a specific diagnosis.

This book employs the diagnoses used in the *Diagnostic and Statistical Manual of Mental Disorders, ed 3* (DSM III) (12). The DSM III presents the most recent and far-reaching diagnostic classification in American psychiatry.

One further comment should be made concerning the accuracy of the ED diagnosis of psychiatric patients. Diagnoses can be extremely accurate and can be substantiated through follow-up studies. Indeed, Robins, Gentry, Munoz, and Marten (13) report a correct diagnosis in 89 percent of cases. This accuracy reflects the amount and availability of information in a crisis. Material that may rarely surface under normal circumstances is often dramatically exposed during an emergency.

Treatment Plan

The treatment plan is the working blueprint for the patient's future course of therapy. The treatment plan is based on the patient's diagnosis, the patient's support system, and the community resources.

Immediate Emergency Department Therapy

ED intervention provides immediate therapy, as well as evaluation and referral. The therapy includes the following: the interview, control of impulses, medications, conjunction sessions, and family sessions.

First and foremost, the initial interview by the physician benefits a great many psychiatric patients. They feel they are being listened to and understood. Their withdrawal and isolation have been breached. The function of "just listening" and asking questions must not be underestimated. The patient feels, "Well, someone finally cares!"

The second major form of immediate therapy is control. The ED and its staff can help the patient gain physical control of impulses. The staff asserts control in the following manner and sequence: promptness, geographic isolation, interpersonal distance, security personnel, and physical restraints.

Promptness cuts anxiety and heightens the opportunity to control the patient. Delay increases apprehension and accelerates the patient's losing control.

A quiet, neat, attractive office away from the main part of the ED offers a geographic isolation which helps control patients. Control is also facilitated by being enclosed within the transport vehicle. Physical space limitations assist patients in finding their emotional boundaries.

Each person is surrounded by a body buffer zone ("personal space"), which is greatest in back, least in front, and intermediate on the sides (14). By taking care not to intrude into that zone, the physician can avoid provoking the patient into uncontrolled behavior. The important thing is that the interviewer's physical presence at a distance controls many patients.

The converse is also true with other patients, for whom closeness and hand holding provide a measure of control. This is especially true of anxious and depressed patients.

Security personnel play an important part in the modern ED. By their uniforms and presence they demonstrate control. Force must be displayed before it is employed: the display alone has controlled many a situation. The security personnel are part of the medical and psychiatric management of the patient. They act under a physician's direction.

Physical restraints at the extremities and waist can be employed to control violent patients. Before instituting restraints, the physician must have enough personnel. Only one person must be in charge of putting the patient in restraints and only that individual must initiate the team activities to apply them.

Medications benefit the patient while in the ED. One technique involves the physician's giving the patient medication in the ED, having the patient wait an hour, and then evaluating the effect. The dystonic reaction some people experience after receiving phenothiazines requires drug intervention. Acutely anxious and agitated patients require intramuscular (IM) medication so that relief may begin quickly. The author has found haloperidol (Haldol) 2 to 5 mg IM every half hour extremely effective.

ED conjunction therapy can resolve significant differences between partners of a love relationship—husband and wife, lovers of the same sex, and couples living together. In those instances the physician deals directly with both partners together.

Finally, family crises can be resolved by the physician's working with the entire family together. This requires the family to sit down and talk over the dispute in the ED.

CARE AFTER THE EMERGENCY

This section discusses the patient's progress and course of treatment after the ED evaluation. It completes one of the main themes of this book, namely that a psychiatric emergency involves a continuum of intervention from the community to the ED and then back to the community. The remainder of the chapter reinforces the concept that the ED is a key facility but only a part of the community's treatment network.

The emergency department physician can make appointments for patients with community agencies. One occasionally hears the notion that psychiatric patients must call for their own appointments. The author believes that in many instances it is appropriate and desirable that the ED physician arrange a referral appointment. Often the patient is too disorganized or too depressed to do it. The physician's referral ensures a definite follow-up for the patient. It also gives the patient the message that further help will be available and hope should be maintained.

The treatment involves a well orchestrated application of the community resources network over time. In the acute phase of the crisis patients may require hospitalization, home visits, partial hospital programs, frequent psychotherapy sessions, and regular medication reviews. As patients stabilize they may attend weekly individual or group therapy sessions. Still later they may require only occasional appointments, reduction or discontinuation of medications, and few home visits.

A significant number of ED psychiatric patients in crisis require hospitalization. Atkins (6), Satloff and Worby (15), and Coleman and Errera (16) report high hospital admission rates for psychiatric patients from the emergency department. This fact highlights the point that a psychiatric crisis is a major disruption of the patient's life and, as Spitz (17) notes, a serious event.

The following seven Ds depict the general indications for psychiatric hospitalization: *destructiveness, disorganization, dysphoria, disorientation, deviancy, detoxification,* and *doctors.*

Destructiveness means suicide and homicide. Dangerousness to self or others marks one of the few absolute criteria for hospitalization. Indeed, in these cases the state governments have demanded that physicians act as the patient's agent and restrain (if necessary) and commit the patient to a hospital even without the patient's consent.

Disorganization describes a state of total loss of mental control. The patient demonstrates no ego boundaries, talks in loose associations, shows derailment, and exhibits flight of ideas. The patient with a thought disorder (schizophrenia), the patient who is acutely intoxicated, and the anxious patient typify this situation.

Dysphoria describes severe depression. In deep depression the patient has ceased to function and just barely exists. The severely depressed patient meets this criterion.

Disorientation describes the patient with a severe organic mental disorder. Hospitalization would permit physical control of the patient and allow a comprehensive physical investigation into the cause of the condition.

Deviancy pertains to those situations in which a superficial crime and arrest are indicative of an underlying severe psychiatric crisis. The depressed patient who steals an obviously insignificant item in order to get caught and gain help typifies this phenomenon. For many patients in crisis, hospitalization and treatment are far more appropriate than incarceration in a jail.

Detoxification is the sixth indication for admission. The hospitalization provides medical management of the withdrawal and prevents reintroduction of the intoxicating substance.

In the last category, *Doctor,* the patient's therapist recommends or requests admission. This therapist, who has been working with the patient, may recognize certain danger signs indicating that admission is advisable; these indications may or may not be apparent to the ED physician. This admission category emphasizes the importance of the ED physician's contacting the patient's community therapist.

The eventual crisis resolution through treatment rests upon several psychiatric principles. First, the majority of patients not only voluntarily seek ED assistance but also actively pursue inpatient and outpatient treatment (18). Patients are motivated to obtain help. Second, individual psychotherapy involves an intensely powerful relationship between a patient and a therapist covering a significant time period (19). The therapist's contributions to the therapeutic relationship are expertise, skills, active listening, interpretations, and respect for the patient. The patient contributes experiences and feelings. They work together. Third, patients with specific diagnoses require specific medications in significant dosages and with appropriate medical monitoring (20).

REFERENCES

1. Soreff S: Psychiatric consultation in the emergency department. *Psychiatric Annals* 8:189–194, 1978.
2. Hall RCW, Popkin MK, Devaul RA, et al: Physical illness presenting as psychiatric disease. *Arch Gen Psychiatry* 35:1315–1320, 1978.
3. Kass F, Karasu TB, Walsh T: Emergency room patients in concurrent therapy: A neglected clinical phenomenon. *Am J Psychiatry* 136:91–92, 1979.

4. Talbott JA: Care of the chronically mentally ill—still a national disgrace. *Am J Psychiatry* 136:688–689, 1979.

5. LePoidevin D, Reid AH: Emergency psychiatric referrals to the casualty department of a general hospital. *Scot Med J* 13:306–311, 1968.

6. Atkins RW: Psychiatric emergency service. *Arch Gen Psychiatry* 17:176–182, 1967.

7. Kolb LC: *Modern Clinical Psychiatry,* ed 8. Philadelphia, WB Saunders Co, 1973.

8. Galanter M, Karasu TB, Wilder JF: Alcohol and drug abuse consultation in the general hospital: A systems approach. *Am J Psychiatry* 133:930–934, 1976.

9. Watson JP: Psychiatric problems in accident department. *Lancet* 1:877–879, 1969.

10. Lion JR, Bach-Y-Rita G, Ervin FR: Violent patients in the emergency room. *Am J Psychiatry* 125:1706–1711, 1969.

11. Gronberg FK, Klinger BI, Grumet BR: Homicide and community-based psychiatry. *J Nerv Men Dis* 66:868–874, 1978.

12. *Diagnostic and Statistical Manual of Mental Disorders,* ed 3. Washington, DC, American Psychiatric Association, 1980.

13. Robins E, Gentry KH, Munoz RA, et al: A contrast of the three more common illnesses with the ten less common in a study and 18-month follow-up of 314 psychiatric emergency room patients. *Arch Gen Psychiatry* 34:285–291, 1977.

14. Hall ET: *The Hidden Dimension.* Garden City NY, Doubleday & Co, 1966.

15. Satloff A, Worby CM: The psychiatric emergency service: Mirror of change. *Am J Psychiatry* 126:1628–1632, 1970.

16. Coleman SV, Errera P: The general hospital emergency room and its psychiatric problems. *Am J Public Health* 53:1294–1301, 1963.

17. Spitz L: The evolution of a psychiatric emergency crisis intervention service in a medical emergency room setting. *Compr Psychiatry* 17:99–113, 1976.

18. Whiteley JS, Denison DM: The psychiatric casualty. *Br J Psychiatry* 109:488–490, 1963.

19. Fromm-Reichmann F: *Principles of Intensive Psychotherapy.* Chicago, Phoenix, 1964.

20. Shader RI (ed): *Manual of Psychiatric Therapeutics.* Boston, Little Brown & Co, 1978.

4
The Depressed Patient

THE PATIENT

Feelings of worthlessness, shame, and dread permeate the lives of depressed people. Sadness, lack of color, and chronic fatigue dominate their existence. They view their world as hopeless and their plight as helpless.

> *Paul Jones has noticed something wrong with himself ever since he and his wife separated. He experiences difficulty at work because of loss of interest and an inability to concentrate. He cannot fall asleep, and when he does he awakes early without a sense of being refreshed. He worries a great deal, drinks too much, does not eat, has lost twenty pounds, lacks interest in sex, and feels unhappy. He finds his days intolerable, interminable, and oppressive. He views his future with despair and wonders about suicide. He feels guilty for a variety of past and present indiscretions and obsessively reflects upon his separation from his wife and two children. He alternately blames himself and his wife. He misses his children. His mood is sad; his world, empty; and his future, bleak. Paul Jones is depressed.*

Depression is the most commonly encountered type of psychiatric emergency (1). This fact reflects the prevalence of depression in the United States (2). Depression affects the patient's mood, it colors perceptions, and it governs behavior.

The Patient's Mood

First and foremost, depression is a disturbance of mood. The person feels sad and experiences profound unhappiness. The sadness either remains constant throughout the day or fluctuates during the day. In fluctuating depression, the patient may awake with optimism and enthusiasm, but as the day unfolds the depression returns. Other patients report morning "blues" which subside during the day. Patients describe their moods in a variety of terms: "the blues," "the uglies," "the

29

miseries," "wicked," "the black cloud," "confusion," "mud in the head," or "the thing." Depressed people sustain tremendous emotional pain. They feel the anguish, despair, apprehension, and distress that accompany depression. The sadness hurts. They experience helplessness and hopelessness (3). Paul Jones suffers.

The Patient's Perceptions

The depression colors the patient's perceptions. Perceptual changes include a sense of alienation, pessimism, guilt, loss of the future, and distorted perception of time.

Depressed patients develop a sense of alienation from those about them. They see others as distant, disinterested, or hostile. They see themselves as apart and isolated.

Depressed people become pessimistic. Everything seems like failure: work is poorly done, interpersonal relations are unsatisfactory, and the future looks black. This pessimism extends to views of the past. People who are depressed recall life events with a sense of failure and displeasure. They focus on their past indiscretions and dwell on their mistakes. Paul Jones remembers all the things he did wrong in his marriage. He feels guilty. He sees himself as the cause of the predicament and the villain. He also believes he is a needless burden on his family and society.

The perceived loss of the future looms as one of the most important features of depression. Depressed people expect their present emotional agony to persist indefinitely, and they lack any vision of "a light at the end of the tunnel."

Time passes slowly, with hours seeming like days and days feeling like an eternity. For Paul Jones time has become a burden.

The Patient's Behavior

The depressed patient exhibits a variety of behavior disturbances. These involve the patient's sleep, appetite, sexual activity, alcohol and drug use, dreams, energy level, and ability to concentrate. The depression not infrequently leads to suicidal behavior; occasionally it results in a homicidal act.

Sleep disturbances plague the depressed patient (4). Some patients sleep virtually all the time, preferring bed to any activity. Despite a prodigious amount of rest, they still complain of being tired. Others find great difficulty in getting to sleep. They cannot fall asleep, and when they do, they rise too early. Early morning waking is one of the cardinal symptoms of depression.

Sleep deprivation potentiates depression by producing lethargy, difficulty in concentration, and chronic fatigue. Paul Jones, exhausted, works inefficiently and ineffectively. Sleeplessness has compounded his situation.

Depression affects appetite. Although some patients gain weight, the majority complain of weight loss. Not infrequently the patient reports having lost up to 40 pounds within several months. The sad person does not want to eat. Food becomes insipid; mealtime is meaningless and meal preparation is avoided.

Sexual activity undergoes the same kind of change as appetite. Occasionally a person responds to depression with an increase in sexual activity, attempting to fill the emptiness and drive away the sadness with sensual adventures. However, most depressed patients simply lose interest in sex and avoid it.

Alcohol consumption becomes involved in the depression in a variety of ways (5). First, alcohol in and of itself acts as a depressant. Second, people with alcohol problems frequently also have histories of depression. Alcohol use and depression contribute to each other. Third, depressed people commonly increase their alcohol use. Fourth, the patient's sense of shame over heightened drinking further contributes to the feeling of worthlessness.

Insomnia, fatigue, and emptiness cause the patient to turn to both prescription and street drugs. Patients experiment with a variety of sleeping preparations, including barbiturates or minor tranquilizers. Some patients attempt to counteract the depression with stimulants. Occasionally a depressed person discovers that "diet" pills, especially amphetamines, relieve the depression and supply "energy." Some people use bronchial dilators to feel better; the ephedrine improves mental status.

Dreams reflect the depression. An elderly gentleman with manic-depressive illness dreamed about being frustrated in a classroom situation. This dream always signaled the onset of a depressive episode. One depressed woman reported "blue" dreams with images of being trapped and isolated.

Depressed patients complain of lack of energy, enthusiasm, drive, and interest in work and home. They do not want to get up, go to work, or return home at night. At work they "go through the motions" without involvement. They live at home without any sense of commitment. They avoid recreational activities.

Depressed people are unable to concentrate. They cannot read a book or even an article. They do not undertake any projects.

The sadness, hopelessness, helplessness, lack of future, absence of energy, loss of interest, sleeplessness, isolation, and pain combine to make suicidal behavior another cardinal feature of depressed patients (6). They think about suicide, they attempt to kill themselves, or they actually commit suicide. Paul Jones wonders about suicide.

Often, depressed patients pursue a passive death. They stop eating. They do not take required medications such as digitalis or insulin. They cross streets without looking. They smoke in bed. They drink to excess and then drive. They take extra sleeping pills. "But not to kill myself; I just wish I would never wake up," one patient explained in the emergency department after ingesting too many pills.

There is one other very nasty element of depression—homicide. One extremely depressed woman saw the world as so bleak that she planned to kill her two children and then herself. She felt the world was so terrible that she could not allow her children to live in it. She believed they would "all be better off dead."

THE CAUSES OF DEPRESSION

The three basic causes of depression are: intrapsychic, interpersonal, and biologic. These factors work separately or in combination to produce the depression.

Loss is the basis for both the intrapsychic and interpersonal causes. Identification of the loss not only supplies the staff with an explanation for the depression but also suggests what treatment will resolve the problem.

Intrapsychic Causes of Depression

The intrapsychic cause consists of the loss of an ideal or of an imagined relationship.

Sometimes people set impossible personal goals or adhere to unattainably lofty standards. Such people often become depressed when they do not achieve their goal or conform to their standard. Interestingly, in many instances these people who feel they have failed are perceived by others as quite successful.

> A 38-year-old woman complained bitterly about her life. She was married to a young executive, had two attractive, healthy children, and dwelled in a modern home. She expected to "control" everything and expected herself to be "perfect." Indeed, before marriage and again when the first child was very young, she had felt in complete control. However, as the children developed, they challenged her authority. She perceived herself as no longer in control or perfect. The loss of her ideal made her depressed.

The loss of imagined relationships is another intrapsychic cause of depression. Not uncommonly a person develops an intense mental relationship with another person, who is unaware of the first person's feelings. In the extreme, the individual feels uniquely involved with a public figure. A number of people committed suicide after President Kennedy's assassination, believing they could no longer live without the relationship. People who fabricate these relationships build an entire fantasy system to verify the relationships. They misinterpret gestures as directed toward themselves.

> A 20-year-old college student became infatuated with an attractive young woman at his school. He believed her to be secretly in love with him. Although he pursued her throughout the campus, he was always

too shy to talk to her. He wrote her anonymous love letters. He sat gazing at her in the library and felt her casual smiles were meant for him. When he discovered that she was "pinned," he became distraught. He cried, tore up his room, and wanted to commit suicide. His roommate brought him to the infirmary. The young woman never even knew who he was.

Interpersonal Causes of Depression

The interpersonal causes of depression take a number of forms (7). Broken relationships (death, divorce, and separation) may cause depression. Other depressions arise from protracted conflicts. Still others occur as a reaction to loss of economic security or of physical integrity.

Death represents the ultimate loss of relationship (8). It leaves an indelible mark on the survivors. The bereaved respond both physically and emotionally. As Lindemann (9) notes, people who are mourning feel "sick," hurt in the pits of their stomachs, lose their appetites, and experience profound sadness. They painfully review all aspects of the relationship. They feel guilt. Did they do enough for the loved one before the end? Did they in some way cause the death? The grief reaction usually lasts from six months to a year. Prolonged reactions go on for years.

Divorces and marital separations produce depression. Paul Jones recoils from his separation. Approximately 50 percent of marriages in many areas of the United States now terminate in divorce (10). Divorce causes significant morbidity for both partners and for their children. Marriage represents the most important interpersonal decision a person makes. The rupture of this relationship produces profound personal distress. A similar dynamic occurs when homosexual relationships terminate.

Many other types of separations precipitate depressions. A 22-year-old woman became bitter and sad when her husband began a military tour of duty which left her alone for a year. She had one two-year-old son and was pregnant again. When a child leaves home for school or marriage, a parent often feels sad. Young adults often become intensely depressed upon leaving home for college, military service, employment, or marriage.

Protracted conflicts at home lead to depression. Disputes between parents and children are common. These assume even broader dimensions if more than two generations reside within the same household. Stresses among grandparents, parents, and children can produce unbearable tensions. Marital conflicts are one of the most common distresses.

A 13-year-old boy was brought to the ED by his parents. They complained that he seemed withdrawn and that his school grades had dropped. The ED physician discovered him to be significantly depressed. The boy felt caught in his parents' battles. His father abused alcohol and occasionally threatened to hurt his mother and himself. His mother continually threatened to leave. The boy felt it was his responsibility to keep the family together. As his parents' conflict intensified, his depression deepened.

Employment problems cause depression in a number of ways. Loss and lack of work correlate with depression. Our society prizes achievement and work. Employment is a major source of status as well as income. Not uncommonly, job loss produces an acute depression. Employment stresses result in depression. Common job-related stresses include conflict with colleagues or superiors, the need to relocate, the perception of being underemployed, and feeling trapped in a certain job.

People react to illnesses and surgery with depression. It is usual to view oneself and one's body as perfect and to respond with anger and sadness if a physician says something is wrong with it. Some people see their illnesses as socially detrimental and consider themselves no longer socially acceptable.

One 50-year-old, married man with four children, a construction manager, became profoundly depressed when his physician told him he had diabetes. He believed his wife would not want him and his children would not respect him.

Patients react with depression to serious medical conditions. These commonly include chronic obstructive pulmonary disease, cancer, end stage renal disease requiring dialysis, myocardial infarction, and rheumatoid arthritis. Similarly, patients respond to a number of surgical procedures with depression: colostomies, amputations, gastrectomies, and hysterectomies. Finally, trauma, with its resultant disfiguration and impairment, precipitates depression. Depression frequently occurs after an accident resulting in paraplegia, after severe trauma, and after an extensive burn.

A 42-year-old, successful salesman, married and the father of three, began dialysis. This treatment required his hospitalization for five hours, three times a week. Although he had known for several years that he had kidney disease, he experienced shock and despair when he started dialysis. He felt his position in the family and in the community was contracted and denigrated.

Biologic Causes of Depression

Medical disorders, organic mental disorders, medications, and manic-depressive illnesses are the major biologic causes of depression.

Hypothyroidism, anemias, and pancreatic tumors serve as examples of medical disorders which may first appear as depression. Patients with these disorders often complain of weight alterations, loss of interest and energy, difficulty with work, and fatigue. In myxedema (hypothyroidism) the patient has edema, slow healing of wounds, an enlarged thyroid gland, decreased cardiac output, constipation, and dry, brittle hair (11). Many anemias first clinically reveal themselves as depression. Cancer of the pancreas is associated with depression (12).

A 50-year-old man came at the request of his family doctor to the ED for treatment of his depression. He recently had retired from working as a baker and found it difficult to adjust to his new life. Several months before admission to the ED, he had had cardiac surgery for the insertion of a prosthetic valve. The prosthesis had damaged his red blood cells and had produced anemia.

Head trauma, electrolyte imbalances, tumors of the central nervous system, intracranial infections, and substance abuse can cause organic mental disorder, which may first appear as a depression. Associated characteristics are disorientation, lability of affect, impaired judgment, and fatigue.

A number of medications cause depression. The most cited has been the antihypertensive medication, reserpine (13). Both the initiation and discontinuation of birth control pills have also been implicated in depression (14).

Manic-depressive illness is a genetically transmitted, biochemical disorder characterized by dramatic mood swings (15). Manic-depressive patients report that depression "comes out of the blue" and persists for months. During the low period these patients experience profound loss of interest, energy, and appetite; they become suicidal; they often cease to function; and they require hospitalization. As the depression lifts, patients may go into a "high." They have excessive energy; sexual interest increases; they engage in many activities; they overspend; they place many long-distance telephone calls; and they sleep, if at all, only a few hours each night. Research indicates that manic-depressive illness occurs in families, and color blindness has been associated with this disease. Often other family members may have histories of alcohol abuse. The biochemical mechanism involves norepinephrine and serotonin: a decrease triggers the depression and an increase initiates a manic episode.

A husband brought his 32-year-old wife, a nurse and mother of three, to the ED because she was "not functioning." She spent the day in bed, did not cook, felt empty and worthless, and contemplated suicide. She had been hospitalized one year ago for a similar episode. In the intervening summer she had been "high," according to her husband's report; she felt that she had been all right then. Her sister and grandmother had spent years in and out of state hospitals. She had manic-depressive illness and was in the depressed phase.

THE REACTIONS OF OTHERS

Depression is a remarkably contagious mood. The patient's melancholic feeling infects other people, and they begin to mirror the patient's feelings of worthlessness and hopelessness. They react in several ways: anger, avoidance, or appropriate concern.

People become angry with depressed patients. The family is annoyed by the person's absence at meals, sullenness, constant fatigue, and protracted negative attitude. Friends become angry at the patient's "always" being down and constantly complaining. Coworkers become frustrated when the patient does not contribute as expected on the job.

People express their anger in a variety of ways. Families fight with the patient. They argue and make impossible demands. They even wish the patient would die. Friends find themselves confronting the patient with admonitions to "shape up." Employers may dismiss the depressed worker.

A 55-year-old custodian became depressed when his last child left home to be married. Providing for the family had been the focus of his life. Now he felt unnecessary. He accelerated his alcohol use. His wife quarreled with him. His work performance deteriorated. He denied having any problems. After several months, his boss terminated his employment.

At the other extreme family, friends, and coworkers may avoid the depressed person. People simply feel the patient's pain and prefer to avoid it. Not uncommonly, the patient is ignored by the family and eventually lives virtually alone within the house. Such a person dines alone and retires early, also alone.

A 40-year-old woman with a family history of manic-depressive illness gradually became depressed. As she abandoned her usual household tasks, the family filled her role. The older children did the shopping, cooking, and cleaning. The husband cared for the younger children. She ultimately took to her bed.

Friends no longer seek the patient's company. Similarly, at work colleagues prefer to do the patient's share and avoid him or her rather than to have to deal with the depression. The avoidance by others supports the patient's basic postulate of self-worthlessness.

Fortunately, appropriate concern and action offer a constructive third alternative. In this instance the others respond by getting the patient to seek help. The family applies pressure to go for assistance. Family members involve the family physician or clergyman in the quest. These professionals, without anger or avoidance, suggest intervention. They make an appointment with a psychotherapist and they accompany the patient to that interview. They express their love and their desire that the person get better, and they make it clear that the patient is needed. Those are things the patient needs to hear. Friends and coworkers make similar pleas. A good friend can offer some common sense, practical advice about where to go for help, perhaps telling the patient of others with similar problems who have benefitted from treatment. Employers may make treatment a condition of continued employment. Or, by adjusting work schedules, they can make therapy possible. The concern of the family, friends, and coworkers can be decisive in the patient's seeking and obtaining treatment.

THE INITIATION OF THE EMERGENCY

Certain events convert a depression into an emergency. A depression can be a prolonged situation with the patient and those in the patient's social milieu struggling for several years with the sadness. Yet depression does create situations which require immediate intervention. These involve termination of employment, severe impairment of function, suicidal behavior, eruption of conflict, insomnia, and overwhelming psychic pain.

Inability to go to work generates an instant psychiatric emergency. Regardless of the depression's cause, not going to the job is a highly significant development. The depression has reached such severity that the patient cannot function. Profound sadness, feelings of worthlessness, hopelessness, and fatigue have made the person give up. Paul Jones seeks immediate help when he cannot go to his job.

Severely impaired functioning leads the patient, and especially others, to seek assistance. At work decreased activity means diminished income. At home reduced performance creates a chaotic household. Often the patient recognizes this diminished productivity and looks for help. More often family and employers demand that the person seek therapy.

Thoughts and threats, as well as acts of suicide, dramatically precipitate a psychiatric emergency. Often, depressed patients become startled by their own thoughts of suicide. One patient stated, "I knew things were bad when the idea of suicide occurred to me. I never thought I would ever reach that level." It was because of the suicidal thoughts that she went to the ED. Threats of suicide trigger responses from family, friends, and coworkers. In fact, if they do not respond to statements about self-destruction, the patient may indeed be driven to acts of suicide. Suicidal talk is always "a cry for help" (16).

Depression sometimes produces open conflict that sets off the crisis. Depressed patients may gain insight from the hostile responses they have provoked and may then seek treatment. Or, the patient may realize from others' anger that something must be done about the depression. The open conflict demands resolution. The depression might be tolerated, but the conflict cannot be.

Insomnia sometimes precipitates the psychiatric emergency. The patient does not tolerate lack of sleep. Insomnia develops rapidly into around-the-clock distress and impairment. The chief complaint given in the ED reflects this problem: "I cannot sleep"; "Sleeplessness"; or "Give me something to make me sleep."

When the pain of the depression becomes overwhelming to patients, they seek help. The experience of emptiness, hopelessness, worthlessness, and loneliness dominate the patient's existence. The pain of being so depressed hurts too much. People in such pain must seek some relief and escape. Alcohol, drugs, sex, and sleep have not provided refuge. The patient turns to the ED.

THE EMTs' RESPONSE TO THE EMERGENCY

The EMTs must respond to the depressed patient in a firm, organized manner. They must challenge the patient's hopelessness and helplessness with a well defined treatment approach. Their intervention must include a prompt response, identification of themselves, a stated plan, removal of any potential suicide weapons, provision for participation of the family and friends, and constant accompaniment of the patient.

The prompt response underscores the importance of the patient and the crisis. It provides a clear message of help and hope to the patient and the family. It underlines the EMTs' commitment to providing treatment.

The intervention commences with EMTs' identifying themselves to the patient and significant others. They do this by stating their formal names and their title. They emphasize the patient's worthiness with a handshake. Their introduction signifies that professional help has arrived. Their greeting challenges the isolation, and their identification of themselves introduces hope.

The EMTs must state a treatment plan. Doing this informs the patient about the sequence of events to follow. Often the patient not only is reluctant to accept help but also feels undeserving of it. The formulation of a treatment plan asserts the EMTs' confidence in the patient's ability to reverse the depression.

EMTs must remove potential suicide implements from the patient. These include guns, knives, razors, and pills. Not uncommonly, patients hurt themselves during the intervention.

EMTs must elicit the family's and friends' participation in the intervention. These people offer accompaniment to the patient, provide information to the ED staff, and help in the referral process. They are allies in the treatment process.

EMTs must be aware of their own reactions to the depressed person. They must not share the patient's belief that there is no way out, and they must not feel helpless in the face of the person's despair. They must not become impatient about the slow answers and helpless behavior. They must maintain a professional, treatment-oriented approach.

EMTs must accompany the patient throughout the intervention and transport. Their presence precludes elopement and self-destructive behavior, confronts the loneliness and depression, and fosters the patient's belief that help has arrived.

THE EMERGENCY DEPARTMENT EVALUATION

At the ED the decisive intervention occurs. There, the staff encounters the patient; deals with the family, friends, and coworkers; and challenges the depression. The evaluation includes the reception, conducting the physical examination, noting the patient's chief complaint, conducting the psychiatric evaluation, and making a mental status examination.

The Reception

The initial ED contact with the depressed patient must advance the positive interaction established by the EMTs and set the stage for an effective therapeutic interaction. The staff must meet and greet the patient. This procedure includes introducing themselves and explaining what will happen next.

Delays in the emergency department are detrimental for depressed patients. If they are kept waiting too long, the delay tends to confirm the patient's self-appraisal of worthlessness. The longer the delay in evaluation, the more difficulty staff have in reaching the patient and convincing the patient they have something to offer.

Staff or family must be with the patient throughout the ED intervention. The depressed patient finds the ED confusing, overwhelming, and frightening. Unattended patients may elope, believing that others need help more than they themselves. The ED may create anxiety because it confronts the depression the patient has sought to avoid by alcohol, work, or sleep. Not uncommonly, depressed patients fear commitment. Or they feel trapped by the ED. Having someone with the patient diminishes all these possibilities.

Staff must enlist the appropriate participation of family members and friends. These people care about the patient, have valuable information, and help in the implementation of the treatment plan.

Time is an important element in the evaluation of the depressed patient. Because they speak and move slowly, depressed patients often require more time than other patients. They answer questions only after long silences; their thoughts come slowly; they volunteer little information; and they lack spontaneity. The prolonged interview provides a clue to the patient's diagnosis.

Physical Examination

The physician must perform a physical examination. Temperature, pulse, and blood pressure must be measured. Although it is beyond the scope of this volume to describe the examination, the physician must pay particular attention to the neurologic examination.

> A concerned son brought his recently widowed, 65-year-old father to the ED because he was "depressed and just sat there." The examining physician noted ophthalmoscopic evidence of papilledema of the left eye. Subsequent investigation discovered the presence of a left frontal mass.

The physician must also order appropriate laboratory studies.

Chief Complaint

The patient's chief complaint highlights and encapsulates the various aspects of the depressed patient's dynamics and crisis. The patient frequently makes direct statements: "I'm depressed, I want help"; "I cannot cope anymore"; "I want to die"; or "I feel crazy." In other cases, the patient emphasizes the symptoms: "I can't sleep," or "I can't go on anymore." In still others, the chief complaint reflects a different kind of reason for the admission: "My wife said I must come."

Psychiatric Evaluation

A number of specific areas of the psychiatric history require exploration in the assessment of depressed patients. These are history of present illness (HPI), history of previous episodes of depression as well as periods of euphoria, a family history of depression, medical history, history of past and present use of medications, use of alcohol, abuse of other substances, sleep pattern, weight changes, and history of suicidal behavior.

The HPI is the principle means of discovering and understanding the crisis which produced the psychiatric emergency. The HPI may show a recent loss: separation, divorce, death, or termination of an intense relationship. Or the HPI may reveal a significant conflict within the family, with the spouse, or at work. A thorough HPI indicates the cause of the depression in the majority of patients.

The depressed patient frequently has a history of depression. Both *unipolar* and *bipolar* illnesses are characterized by recurrent depression. In the former, patients experience periodic depression. In the latter, patients have not only periodic depressions but also episodes of mania. A history of depression also indicates the manner in which the person handles stresses and reveals the form the previous depressions assumed, their length, and their treatments. A history of mania provides another major diagnostic clue: bipolar manic-depressive illness features a history of alternating "highs" and "lows."

Depressive illness can be inherited (17). Unipolar and bipolar depressive illnesses are now understood to be genetic diseases. The family history of mental illness, especially depression and mania, becomes highly significant. Color blindness has been linked to manic-depressive inheritance patterns (18).

The physician must focus upon recent illnesses, surgery, allergies, thyroid problems, and trauma. Diseases and surgery are correlated with depression in two ways. First, many medical conditions such as anemia, heart disease, cancer, and diabetes produce a depression-like syndrome characterized by fatigue, lack of motivation, and withdrawal. Second, patients feel depressed upon discovering they are ill. The physician must inquire about allergies before prescribing medication.

The patient's medication history is particularly important. Certain drugs, for example, reserpine antihypertensives, precipitate depression. Studies indicate at least half the patients seen in psychiatric crisis have already been taking a psychotropic medication (19). The physician must find out what drugs the patient has taken and for what period of time, and must evaluate the dosage and effectiveness of each medication. By discovering which antidepressants have helped before, the physician can most effectively prescribe the proper antidepressant now.

Patterns of alcohol use and substance abuse must be explored. Patients experience "a crash" when they stop using amphetamines. Acute sadness and anxiety occur when the effects of opiates wear off.

The physician must inquire into the patient's sleep pattern. Sleep disturbances both mirror and potentiate depression.

The physician must assess the patient's dietary practices. Weight changes also provide a barometer to the diagnosis and the depth of a depression. As a general rule of thumb, the greater the weight loss, the greater the depression.

The physician must investigate suicidal behavior. Suicide, suicide attempts, and suicidal gestures all result from depression.

Mental Status Examination

The mental status examination provides important clues in the evaluation of depressed patients. The physician must pay particular attention to the patient's appearance, affect, thought content and production, suicidal ideation, homicidal wishes, insight, judgment, and sensorium.

The patient's appearance in many instances points to the diagnosis of depression. Clothes are often disheveled, dirty, ill-matched, and in poor repair. Patients wear dark, bland, drab apparel. Personal hygiene reflects the depression: depressed people often do not bathe, use makeup, wash their hair, or trim their fingernails. Their eyes show signs of crying, worry, and sleeplessness. Depressed patients have difficulty looking at the examiner, preferring instead to gaze at the floor. They move slowly.

Affect is the hallmark of depression. The patient emanates a feeling of despair, doom, and gloom. This mood becomes infectious, influencing family, coworkers, and the interviewer.

Depression influences the thought processes in a number of ways. Thought production appears to be slowed down. The patient answers questions reluctantly, hesitantly, and with few words. The mind seems to put forth few ideas. The patient's discourse lacks spontaneity. The thoughts the patient does advance reflect a neglective world view. The negative attitude produces thoughts of self-worthlessness that occasionally become delusions of total valuelessness. Finally, a sense of guilt permeates the patient's thoughts. In extreme depression the sense of worthlessness and guilt reaches psychotic proportions.

Depressed patients' belief that others would be better off without them leads to the risk of suicide. If the patient has considered suicide, the physician must seek details. If the patient has actually made suicidal plans, the interviewer must pursue the particulars of implementation. The physician must elicit a history of suicidal behavior—attempts, results, and reactions.

Homicide is within the potential of depressed patients. The physician must elicit, as for suicide, information concerning thoughts and plans of homicide.

The physician must explore the patient's insight about the crisis. This assessment helps not only in the evaluation of mental status but also in the selection of the most appropriate referral. The patient's level of insight varies. Some patients do not even recognize their depression until the crisis has fully developed. Others, like Paul Jones, appreciate the problem and actively seek help.

The patient's judgment is a critical component of the mental status examination. How does the patient view the depression? Has self-esteem been dangerously eroded? In essence, how has the patient handled the depression; can this person be trusted?

Finally, the interviewer must be concerned with the patient's sensorium. The physician assesses whether patients are oriented to person, place, and time; whether they can subtract from 100 by serial 7s; whether they recall immediate, recent, and distant events; and how well they can handle abstractions. The sensorium is important in two ways. First, depression produces a pseudodementia; namely, the patient appears to have organic deficiencies which in reality are manifestations of the depression (20). Second, organic mental disorder produces depression.

DIAGNOSIS, TREATMENT PLAN, AND IMMEDIATE EMERGENCY DEPARTMENT THERAPY

Diagnosis

The diagnosis serves as the pivotal point in the treatment of the depressed patient in crisis. It is the product of information gained from the patient's physical examination, chief complaint, psychiatric evaluation, mental status examination, and data derived from the EMTs and significant others. From the diagnosis the physician determines a treatment plan.

Three major diagnoses dominate the picture for the depressed patient. Adjustment reaction with depression is the first category; episodic depression, the second; and organic mental disorders, the third (21).

Adjustment reaction with depression occurs in association with a social crisis, as has previously been discussed. In this situation the examiner can isolate and define the interpersonal event which triggered the depression. The physician diagnoses Paul Jones as experiencing an adjustment reaction of adult life with depression.

Depressive episode is a diagnostic subcategory of episodic affective disorders and either occurs as a depressive disorder (single or recurrent) or as part of bipolar affective disorder, alternating with episodes of mania. The diagnostic criteria involve a number of considerations. First, these patients exhibit a predominant, pervasive, depressive mood. Second, they have four of the following eight symptoms: appetite alteration, sleep disturbance, loss of energy, agitation or psychomotor retardation, loss of interest in activities, or diminished sexual drive, excessive guilt, inability to concentrate, and recurrent thoughts of death or suicide. Third, this condition must have persisted for more than a week. Fourth, the patient does not display the delusions or hallucinations typical of schizophrenia. Fifth, the patient does not have an organic mental disorder. Finally, the patient has neither residual subtype of schizophrenia nor a grief reaction.

In organic mental disorders with depression, identifying the cause provides the key to treatment (22). If the patient has hypothyroidism, thyroid replacement is required. If alcohol depresses the patient, then alcohol must be eliminated.

From the diagnosis, the physician must formulate and then implement a treatment plan.

Treatment Plan

This plan must encompass three aspects of the patient's crisis: the immediate treatment to be rendered in the ED, the specific cause of the situation, and the referral.

Immediate Emergency Department Therapy

Much of the immediate treatment for depression is accomplished during the evaluation interview, for in that interaction the patient begins to realize people care and listen. Patients recognize that they suffer from a medical problem called depression. Further, they become aware that this illness has an identifiable cause and, most important, that depression can be treated.

The immediate treatment, in addition to an exploratory, empathic evaluation interview, must include: (1) interjection of hope, (2) prescription of the correct medication, and (3) establishment of a definite referral.

Hope is the major ingredient which makes everything else happen. Without hope, suicide looms as a real choice.

Medications provide one of the most effective modes of treating depression. Their use raises several critical questions. First, when is their use indicated? Second, when must the physician start them? Third, which preparation is most appropriate? Fourth, how much must be prescribed?

The physician employs medications when the depression has become severe enough to interfere with eating, sleeping, and living. Indications include weight loss, protracted sleep disturbance, and persistence of painful sadness. Uncontrollable crying is another reason for drug intervention.

If the patient requires medication, it must be initiated at that visit to the ED.

Tricyclic antidepressants remain the best first choice drug treatment for depression. Minor tranquilizers have little value. In fact, some have been noted to produce dysphoric effects of their own. The monoamine oxidase inhibitors are excellent antidepressants but rarely are the first choice because of the dietary restrictions that must be followed when these drugs are used. Electroconvulsive therapy is used after antidepressant therapy proves ineffective. Lithium carbonate has relieved some depressions although its principle use is as a mood leveler.

The decision about which tricyclic antidepressant to prescribe depends on the level of the patient's anxiety. The patient experiencing a significant amount of agitation benefits from amitriptyline (Elavil). This drug has antianxiety as well as antidepressant qualities and also promotes sleep. When the patient feels little or no anxiety, imipramine (Tofranil) is most effective. This drug has proved useful for control of the episodic depressions. Doxepin (Sinequan) has similar sedation qualities but fewer of the cardiovascular side effects than the other preparations.

The patient's medication history and the family's history provide other valuable clues in prescribing the correct antidepressant. Often the patient or a family member has experienced other episodes of depression. Finding out which antidepressants were effective provides valuable information. Very often several members of a family respond in the same way to the same medications.

If an antidepressant is prescribed, it must be begun at a low dosage and supplied to the patient in a limited quantity. Since depressed patients often take overdoses, it behooves the physician not to prescribe a lethal amount of medication.

Finally, the physician must establish a definite referral. The medication's effect must be monitored, and the depression requires treatment beyond the ED evaluation.

CARE AFTER THE EMERGENCY

Paul Jones accepts the ED physician's recommendation and enters the psychiatric unit of a general hospital. Deepening depression, increasing incapacitation, growing isolation, emerging suicide potential, and accelerating alcohol consumption make psychiatric hospitalization the treatment of choice for Paul Jones.

His admitting psychiatrist performs a thorough physical examination; orders thyroid studies, an EEG, a CBC, electrolytes, BUN, and an ECG; and commences regular individual sessions with Mr Jones. Paul Jones also participates in group therapy sessions and occupational therapy activities on the unit. Because he begins to respond positively to the hospital treatment, his psychiatrist elects not to use any medications. Paul Jones discovers he is not alone, people do care, and others listen to him. He sleeps and eats well again; he sees a future. The hospital provides him with help and hope and reverses the depression.

Upon discharge he resumes his work and continues to see his psychiatrist in regularly scheduled sessions. There he not only discusses his feelings about the separation but also explores the roots of his difficulty with his wife. He discovers a number of the "distancing" techniques he has used in his interactions with her. She later joins Mr Jones and his therapist. Ultimately the couple reconciles and resumes living together.

There are a number of appropriate therapies for depressed patients. The treatment chosen for any particular patient depends on the level of the depression and the extent of the patient's support system. Treatment modalities include psychiatric hospitalization, day treatment programs, outpatient psychotherapy, and home psychiatric intervention.

Hospitalization

In addition to the general reasons for psychiatric hospitalization outlined earlier in the book, the depressed patient has several specific requirements for an inpatient experience (23). These include self-destructive potential, inability to function, severe sadness, and protracted insomnia.

When the risk of suicide becomes great, the patient must be hospitalized. Each year, over 25,000 Americans commit suicide (24). The majority of these patients experienced a desperate depression before killing themselves. Self-destructive patients require the safety and protection of an inpatient unit.

Often depressed patients view themselves as hopeless and helpless. They feel all efforts to help them are preordained to fail. Hence, these patients not only make plans to kill themselves but also consider worthless any attempt to treat them. In such situations the physician must initiate involuntary hospitalization (25).

As in the case of Paul Jones, the inability to function is another indication for an inpatient experience (26). Paul Jones cannot go to work. His depression has incapacitated him.

The affect of sadness hurts. It pains the patient greatly and oppresses the family, friends, and coworkers. Inpatient treatment provides intensive help and relief. In the hospital unit, others help shoulder the burden. Overwhelming sadness is the third indicator for admission.

Finally, insomnia, especially when protracted, is a great potentiator of depression. By allowing patients to escape from their usual environment and by providing medications in higher doses than can be used at home, the inpatient unit becomes one place to address the problem of sleeplessness.

Day Treatment

For patients whose depression is moderately severe and incapacitating, if they have no plans of suicide or homicide and also have a very supportive, caring, interested, and involved social support system, day treatment offers a number of treatment advantages (27). It provides the day-long intensive therapy experience of an inpatient unit — individual and group therapy and occupational therapy activities — and permits the patient to remain at home at night. Day treatment stresses support but furnishes more patient autonomy than does hospitalization.

Outpatient Psychotherapy

Most patients benefit from outpatient psychotherapy, either through individual or group sessions (28,29). Paul Jones continues in outpatient treatment after hospitalization. For insightful patients who are not too severely depressed, who have a low suicide risk, and who are still able to function, outpatient therapy is the treatment of choice.

Outpatient therapy must be multifaceted. First, the ED referral must be definite — an appointment with a therapist, not just a telephone number to call. Second, the sessions must be regularly scheduled. The patient benefits from knowing when the next appointment is. Third, the therapist must skillfully combine support with insight and interpretations. Fourth, a physician must monitor the patient's response to medications.

Home Psychiatric Intervention

For some patients, mental health workers who visit the patient at home can serve as an important adjunct to the other treatments. A home visitor can help overwhelmed patients to organize their lives. A depressed patient who has difficulty in even getting out of the house can be helped to arrange and keep therapy session appointments. Mental health workers who see the patient at home can provide valuable information concerning the home conditions.

REFERENCES

1. Frazier SH: Comprehensive management of psychiatric emergencies. *Psychosomatics* 9:7-11, 1968.
2. Lehman HE: Epidemiology of depressive disorders, in Fieve RR (ed): *Depression in the 1970s: Modern Theory and Research.* The Hague, Exerpta Medica, 1971, pp 21-30.
3. Seligman MEP: *Helplessness.* San Francisco, WH Freeman & Co, 1975.
4. Hawkins DR: Depression and sleep research: Basic science and clinical perspectives, in Usdin G (ed): *Depression: Clinical, Biological, and Psychological Perspectives.* New York, Brunner/Mazel, 1977, pp 198-234.
5. Pottenger M, McKernon J, Patrie LE, et al: The frequency and persistence of depressive symptoms in the alcohol abuser. *J Nerv Ment Dis* 166:562-570, 1978.
6. Miles CP: Conditions predisposing to suicide: A review. *J Nerv Ment Dis* 164:231-246, 1977.
7. Bartolucci G, Drayer CS: An overview of crisis intervention in the emergency rooms of general hospitals. *Am J Psychiatry* 130:953-960, 1973.
8. Becker E: *The Denial of Death.* New York, The Free Press, 1973.
9. Lindemann E: Symptomatology and management of acute grief. *Am J Psychiatry* 101:141-148, 1944.
10. *Statistical Abstract of the United States: 1978* ed 99. Washington DC, United States Bureau of the Census, 1978.
11. Brodie HKH: Central control in endocrine systems, in Usdin G (ed): *Psychiatric Medicine.* New York, Brunner/Mazel, 1977, pp 73-94.
12. Snodgrass PJ: Diseases of the pancreas, in Wintrobe MM, Thorn GW, Adams RD, et al (eds): *Harrison's Principles of Internal Medicine,* ed 6. New York, McGraw-Hill Book Co, 1970, pp 1576-1587.
13. Goodwin FK, Ebert MH, Bunney WE Jr: Mental effects of reserpine in man: A review, in Shader RI (ed): *Psychiatric Complications of Medical Drugs.* New York, Raven Press, 1972, pp 73-107.
14. Glick ID, Bennett SE: Psychiatric effects of progesterone and oral contraceptives, in Shader RI (ed): *Psychiatric Complications of Medical Drugs.* New York, Raven Press, 1972.

15. Cadoret RT, Tanna VL: Genetics of affective disorders, in Usdin G (ed): *Depression: Clinical, Biological, and Psychological Perspectives.* New York, Brunner/Mazel, 1977.

16. Farberow NC, Shneidman ES (eds): *The Cry for Help.* New York, McGraw-Hill Book Co, 1965.

17. Kolb LC: *Modern Clinical Psychiatry,* ed 8. Philadelphia, WB Saunders Co, 1973.

18. Mendlewicz J, Linkowski P, Guroff JJ, et al: Color blindness linkage to bipolar manic-depressive illness. *Arch Gen Psychiatry* 36:1442-1447, 1979.

19. Atkins RW: Psychiatric emergency service. *Arch Gen Psychiatry* 17:176-182, 1967.

20. Wells CE: Pseudodementia. *Am J Psychiatry* 136:895-900, 1979.

21. *Diagnostic and Statistical Manual of Mental Disorders,* ed 3. Washington DC, American Psychiatric Association, 1980.

22. Fauman MA, Fauman BJ: The differential diagnosis of organic based psychiatric disturbance in the emergency department. *JACEP* 6:315-323, 1977.

23. Rabiner CJ, Lurie A: The case for psychiatric hospitalization. *Am J Psychiatry* 131:761-764, 1974.

24. Murphy GE: Suicide and attempted suicide. *Hosp Pract* 12:73-81, 1977.

25. Monahan J: Prediction research and the emergency commitment of dangerous mentally ill persons: A reconsideration. *Am J Psychiatry* 135:198-201, 1978.

26. Cumming J, Cumming E: *Ego & Milieu.* New York, Atherton Press, 1970.

27. Fink EB, Longabaugh R, Stout R: The paradoxical underutilization of partial hospitalization. *Am J Psychiatry* 136:149-155, 1978.

28. Karasu TB: Psychotherapies: An overview. *Am J Psychiatry* 134:851-863, 1977.

29. Marmor J: Short-term dynamic psychotherapy. *Am J Psychiatry* 136:149-155, 1979.

5

The Anxious Patient

THE PATIENT

Anxiety emerges as the key feature and pivotal quality in all of emergency psychiatry. This most disturbing emotion both propels the patient to seek help and leads people in the patient's social milieu to call for assistance. Anxiety generates the immediacy in the emergency.

> Mario Amato brings his wife, Mary, to the ED, reporting he "can not take her anymore." This ED admission culminates a stressful month during which Mrs Amato has become progressively more anxious. Although she describes herself as a "tense" person and takes pride in being an immaculate housekeeper, both qualities have dramatically escalated since her last child, Paula, left home for marriage. Since then she has had trouble sleeping, has demanded that her husband spend all his time with her, compulsively and thoroughly cleans the house, and worries a great deal. She has been to several physicians for vague complaints and concerns. None has found anything wrong, although one started her on a minor tranquilizer. She restricts her life to the home and "cannot sit still."
>
> Mr Amato becomes increasingly concerned. His wife makes him, their friends, and the children uneasy by her pacing, cleaning, and worrying. Activity brings her no relief. Finally, she decides that electricity is in the water faucet and commences to touch the faucet continually. At this development her husband brings her to the ED.
>
> Mrs Amato experiences increasingly overwhelming anxiety. It permeates her entire life and affects those about her. Anxiety precipitates the emergency.

Anxious patients struggle with an intensely powerful, painful feeling. They find the emotion colors all their activities and dramatically alters their lives. It rapidly becomes the focus of their lives, dwarfing family relations and work responsibilities. Anxiety immediately affects mood, perceptions, and behavior.

The Patient's Mood

Everyone has experienced moments of anxiety. Before an important test, a sports event, or a social occasion, people feel anxious. However, this normal anxiety differs significantly in both quality and quantity from the anxiety that dominates the anxious patient. A number of features describes this more severe anxiety: a sensation of panic; feelings of deep discomfort, desperation, apprehension, and perplexity; and the urge to do something. The anxiety that propels Mr and Mrs Amato to the ED is a very intense emotion.

Have you ever experienced a wild, headlong plunge through a woods when you thought you were lost, felt an overwhelming sensation when you smelled the faint odor of smoke in a theater, or been on a sailboat seemingly heeling too much and about to take on water? Each instance creates moments of panic. Most, fortunately, are of short duration. Yet the feeling of panic looms as a very powerful, well remembered experience. The anxious patient experiences a sustained sense of panic. Through an appreciation of the feeling of being panicked, one can momentarily enter the world of the anxious patient.

Anxious patients experience deep discomfort. Patients report feelings of being profoundly ill at ease. The sensation of anxiety pierces right to the person's core.

Anxious patients rapidly come to appreciate the dyad of anxiety: apprehension and desperation. Life, for them, becomes eclipsed by anxiety. They perceive no future, no relief, and no meaning to life. One anxious patient reported "life is hell" and "without any hope." His confidence had been shaken to its core; his defenses had been breached and he had begun to doubt himself.

Anxious patients are also perplexed. By definition, anxiety is "the anticipation of danger, the source of which is largely unknown or unrecognized" (1). Patients feel panicked, uncomfortable, apprehensive, and desperate, but the reason for their anxiety is not clear to them. People can endure a host of painful emotions if they at least know the source. But the patient suffers without knowing why. Mrs Amato does not know why she is so distressed.

Panic, discomfort, desperation, and perplexity all contribute to a pervasive characteristic of anxious patients, their urgent demand for relief. In contrast to depressed patients, who often delay seeking treatment, and paranoid patients who avoid intervention, anxious patients demand help. They want assistance and they want it now. They are impatient. Mrs Amato demanded her husband be with her at all times.

The Patient's Perceptions

Anxiety rapidly moves from being just a feeling to affecting the patients' entire world view. It colors all their perceptions, alters their assumptions, and distorts their logic. The anxiety finds expression in these patients' appreciation of time, in their belief that being alone will exacerbate their plight, in their preoccupation with physical complaints, in their level of consciousness, in their attention span, and in their apprehension concerning their sanity.

Anxiety significantly alters one's perception of time in two ways. First, many patients report that time passes too slowly.

A 30-year-old housewife, mother of two, experienced a major anxiety attack. She could not sleep for one week, went continuously to neighbors for help, and became preoccupied with time. She said each minute seemed like a hour. She complained that the days were too long and that she could not "fill them."

Second, doom and dread dominate the anxious patient's view of time. The housewife just cited contemplated suicide as her anxiety mounted. She saw no future except pain. The perception of "impending disaster" made her seek a way out (2,p111).

Anxious patients fear being alone, believing their condition will further deteriorate. They hope the presence of family or friends will remove or reduce the sense of dread and doom. Other people can at least share the burden of anxiety.

Anxious patients channel their anxiety into concern about their physical health. They consult a series of physicians in search of a medical explanation for their distress. Typically, the patients report a number of vague complaints. The physicians find nothing wrong, yet the patients remain "symptomatic" and dissatisfied. Mrs. Amato follows this pattern. Some patients focus all their apprehension on one concern such as a fear of cancer, of choking, or of a heart attack. A woman experiencing a severe anxiety attack believed she was dying; she lay on the stretcher expecting the end.

Anxiety produces a number of altered states of consciousness. Patients, responding to intense anxiety, experience one of several dissociative states. In the *fugue* condition patients disappear from their usual haunts to escape an anxiety-provoking conflict (3,p101). Amnesia for the flight usually accompanies this state.

The author vividly recalls treating in the ED a 28-year-old woman who had abruptly left her husband and two children and traveled 2,000 miles by bus. Ultimately people from Travelers Aid brought her to the ED. She expressed wonderment at being there and had no recollection of the trip or the reason for it. A telephone call to the worried family quickly ascertained that the flight had been preceded by a major domestic altercation.

Other patients experience *depersonalization* and perceive everything around them as strange and unreal. One patient struggling with severe anxiety reported everything about him appeared to be made of cardboard. Another response to overwhelming anxiety is Ganser's syndrome. In this condition a patient who is trapped, for example, imprisoned, portrays a mental status featuring nonsense or approximate answers to simple questions. In answer to the query, "Who is the current President of the United States?" such a patient would say, "Woodrow Wilson." The person with Ganser's syndrome might report that the sum of two and two is five. Still other patients handle intolerable stress, conflict, and anxiety by developing amnesia. They remove the stress and the symptoms by forgetting them—blocking them from consciousness. Finally, conversion reactions are a neurotic response to overwhelming anxiety (4).

Anxious patients notice that their level of thinking and attention is altered. They find their thoughts racing and cannot control them. They experience difficulty in concentration on reading, conversation, or work. They continually scan the environment and remain vigilant.

All these perceptions culminate in the patients' questioning their sanity. This uncertainty finds expression in statements like "I'm losing my mind," "Am I cracking up?" or "I'm breaking up." The anxiety challenges the patients' view of themselves and their mental well-being.

The Patient's Behavior

The patient's behavior dramatically reflects the intense feeling of anxiety and the alterations of perception. The panic, discomfort, desperation, apprehension, and urgency, coupled with the distorted view of time, fear of illness, and concern for sanity, are rapidly translated into actions. The patient reacts physiologically and responds with activity, clinging, and demanding.

Anxiety affects physiology. Anxious patients' respirations increase. Some people develop a hyperventilation syndrome marked by decreased blood carbon dioxide level and felt by the patient as faintness, tingling in the extremities, palpitations, and breathing difficulty. The pulse quickens and the blood pressure elevates. The patient sweats. The muscles become tense.

Patients respond with activity. Depressed patients stop functioning, phobic patients retreat from society, but anxious patients *do something*. They pace. They clean their homes and order their belongings. Mrs Amato is very active. She cannot sit still, nor can she sleep.

The fear of being alone and the dread of the future compel the patient to cling to other people. Mrs Amato wants her husband with her at all times. She seeks out people to be with her. She needs people. She firmly refuses to be alone.

Finally, the urgency, desperation, dread, and panic all lead the patient to demand help. Anxious patients are not passive, obscure people. They impatiently assert their right to relief. They want help and they want it now.

THE CAUSES OF ANXIETY

Intrapsychic, interpersonal, and biologic causes produce anxiety.

Intrapsychic Causes of Anxiety

Anxiety is the signal that a deep mental process has become more nearly available to the conscious mind. All people carry in their unconscious minds many thoughts and assumptions about themselves, their experiences, their family backgrounds, and their environments. Some of these thoughts and assumptions are quite pleasant, such as "I am a good person." Others are disquieting, like "I hate my brother," or "I hate myself." These produce discomfort and anxiety when they emerge into consciousness.

Each person uses a variety of mechanisms to keep some unconscious thoughts from consciousness. People use repression to keep from remembering painful experiences. People also employ reaction formation by doing or saying the opposite of what they feel. Isolation is used to separate emotions from events. Denial permits one to avoid an entire situation, feeling, or thought by negating it. But when a thought or feeling that has been kept in the unconscious does break through to conscious awareness, it produces anxiety and perplexity because the patient had struggled to remain unaware of its very existence.

A number of situations are responsible for bringing unconscious mental constructs to preconsciousness and consciousness and producing anxiety. These include alterations of the patient's environment, media events, thought disorders, and dreams.

Throughout life people experience a wide variety of social, vocational, recreational, and political events, any one of which can trigger a series of recollections and feelings. For example, people attending a wedding naturally reflect upon their own marriages. However, in psychiatric emergencies a significant amount of anxiety accompanies the remembrance.

A 35-year-old business executive, married with three children, received a promotion. His very pleased employer had made him a branch manager and substantially enhanced his salary. But the advance made the patient "mildly uneasy." His apprehension increased as his coworkers and subordinates praised him and foretold even greater future steps. The second morning on the new job he had an anxiety attack. Other employees assumed he was having a heart attack and summoned the rescue unit.

After medical clearance in the ED, a psychiatric evaluation revealed an intense fear of success. All his life his parents had made him feel he was a failure. They always focused upon his few mistakes and never commented upon his successes. In fact, they acknowledged his good deeds with, "Well, do better next time." As a result, his promotion troubled him deeply. He felt it was not deserved and believed he could not possibly do the assignment. The anxiety became the signal for a host of remembrances of failures.

Another source responsible for triggering intrapsychic anxiety attacks is the media. Movies, especially, but also books, newspapers, and television programs can set off an episode. A recent movie dealing with exorcism led a number of people to seek help in the ED. The author vividly recalls a young man who experienced an anxiety episode of a severity to warrant hospitalization after viewing a television program dealing with the execution of a United States Army soldier in World War II. Still other patients experience extreme discomfort after watching or reading certain horror stories and mysteries.

Anxiety may be the predominant feature of a schizophrenic episode. Here the patient clearly responds to internal forces, such as hallucinations or delusions, with apprehension and fear.

Finally, a dream can be the source of an anxiety attack (5).

Bill Peters, 48 years old, awoke from a dream in a cold sweat, his heart pounding and his thoughts racing. The dream so disturbed him that he did not go to work that day. Ordinarily he functioned well as a highly competent marketing executive, husband, and father of two. Recently he had received from his older brother a letter inviting him and his family to his niece's wedding. As he reflected upon the dream, which involved "bloody images" of his brother and his brother's family, his anxiety mounted. At the insistence of his wife and family physician he went to an emergency department.

A psychiatrist who consulted Mr Peters in the ED found a number of significant pieces of information. Mr Peters was the second of three children; he had an older brother and a younger sister. Mr Peters strongly asserted he loved his older brother, never resented being "pushed around by him," and was not jealous of the forthcoming marriage, although neither of his own daughters was married. It became clear to the physician that an unconscious feeling of rivalry, jealousy, and hostility had surfaced in the dream. The patient denied that the dream had any connection with reality. He did, however, express relief after the interview and felt "talking" did help. The dream had brought to consciousness things the patient preferred to repress. This awareness had caused anxiety.

Interpersonal Causes of Anxiety

Anxiety may arise as a distress signal that a social situation is becoming overwhelming for the patient. In contrast to the intrapsychic cause, the precipitating stressor is a recent event and is linked to an interpersonal situation. Six interpersonal events commonly cause anxiety responses: separation, loss, death, conflict, confinement, and closeness.

A separation threatens to disrupt the social matrix and the relationship. With that threat, anxiety emerges. Separation occurs under a variety of circumstances: lovers temporarily live apart, a child goes to school, a son joins the service, a husband takes an overseas assignment without the family, or a family member enters a hospital for surgery (6). In many of these situations the anxiety is mutual, but one of the parties more demonstratively expresses the distress.

A 21-year-old pregnant woman came to the ED with massive anxiety because her husband was to be stationed on a ship at sea for the next four months. She believed she could not survive without him, and she was panicked. Compassionate reassignment of the husband dramatically relieved her symptoms.

Loss accounts for Mrs Amato's anxiety. The marriage of her last child, a daughter, makes her very uncomfortable. She has centered her career as a housewife upon taking care of her children. Suddenly the focus of her life is gone. Also, she is particularly fond of Paula, has enjoyed doing many things with her, and often confides in her. Symbolically she demands that her husband remain with her to make up for the loss of her daughter.

Death is the ultimate separation and loss. It is small wonder that the grief reaction includes anxiety. The survivors feel apprehension and dread, see no future, and cannot concentrate. For many people struggling with a death, anxiety emerges as the basic reaction. Since deaths also occur in the ED, it is particularly important for the staff to appreciate the survivor's anxiety (7). Furthermore, most people contemplate their own death with apprehension. One's personal death is also the ultimate termination of all relationships.

Conflict generates anxiety. Struggles within the family, school, religious institution, and work place produce anxiety. As the conflict increases, the anxiety mounts.

A husband and wife brought their 13-year-old son to the ED. He had recently threatened to run away and to hurt himself. During the interview he demonstrated massive anxiety. His parents' constant fights and mutual threats of divorce made him very uncomfortable, and he sought flight to avoid his discomfort.

Confinement produces anxiety. Dramatic panic attacks occasionally occur when a person is placed in jail. The Ganser's syndrome cited earlier is a vivid illustration of anxiety precipitated by penal confinement. Other physically limited spaces such as elevators and airplanes produce anxiety. Expanding the notion of confinement from its purely physical connotations, one encounters people "trapped" in a variety of social predicaments. These include bad marriages and dead-end jobs. Often people become aware of the anxiety first and only later recognize the trap that has caused it.

Finally, physical closeness to other people generates anxiety. People require space (8). When they are impinged upon, they feel anxious. A 65-year-old wife sensed increased anxiety within herself in direct response to her husband's retirement. Since he had stopped work and spent all his time at home, she felt "no room" for herself there. Again, prison triggers this reaction. Hospitalization, with its multiple intrusions and roommates, can produce anxiety. The classic "homosexual panic" in actuality may be caused by impingement upon one's life space rather than by sexual fear.

Biologic Causes of Anxiety

A number of biologic conditions cause significant anxiety. The resultant anxiety resembles that derived from intrapsychic and interpersonal causes. This fact underscores the need for staff to explore carefully and fully the medical as well as the psychological and social bases for a patient's anxiety. The biologic causes fall into five categories: natural precipitants, medical illnesses, medication effects, abused substances, and reactions to psychotropic drugs.

Caffeine has been widely implicated in the medical and psychiatric literature as a cause and certainly as a potentiator of anxiety (9). Doses of 50 to 200 mg are sufficient to make a person experience the pharmacologic effects of caffeine. The average cup of brewed coffee contains 100 to 150 mg of caffeine; a glass of cola, 40 to 60 mg; and many aspirin preparations, 32 mg. Caffeinism is characterized by tremulousness, tachypnea, insomnia, irritability, and anxiety.

> *A 55-year-old man came to the ED with severe anxiety. There were two dynamic factors involved: his only child, a son, lived 6,000 miles away; and his business had failed. He also consumed 10 cups of coffee each morning and several cola drinks each afternoon. He commented that without his morning coffee he was "a wreck." Subsequent therapy, with discussion of the losses, did little to relieve his symptoms; however, a reduction of his caffeine use dramatically decreased his anxiety.*

Anxiety is an early symptom of many medical illnesses. Excessive thyroid hormone in hyperthyroidism and thyrotoxicosis causes nervousness, irritability, and insomnia (10). A pheochromocytoma can initially manifest itself as an anxiety attack (11). Anxiety is common in respiratory difficulty, especially in asthmatic attacks and acute respiratory distress. Mitral valve prolapse syndromes produce panic attacks (12). Anxiety often accompanies paroxysmal atrial tachycardia (13).

A host of medications produce anxiety, either as direct effects or as side effects. The substance L-dopa (L-dihydroxyphenylalanine), a major drug for the treatment of parkinsonism, has been associated with overactivity, restlessness, and agitation (14). Adrenocortical steroids cause and sustain anxiety states (15). Patients report restlessness, inability to concentrate, and insomnia when receiving corticosteroids. The author evaluated a patient who had successfully undergone a renal transplant and who complained of "an inability to sit still," insomnia, and "racing thoughts." These symptoms were a direct manifestation of the prednisone dosage required to control the rejection phenomenon. The higher this patient's prednisone dosage, the more he felt anxious. An excessive dose of thyroid preparation is reflected in the patient's anxiety level. Many of the bronchodilators cause anxiety (16).

A number of street drugs and alcohol are responsible for unleashing dramatic acute episodes of anxiety. The patient develops massive apprehension and the classic picture of the panic state. The patient and friends find the symptoms completely intolerable. Atlhough the variety of abused substances appears ever increasing, several drugs stand out as precipitants of anxiety attacks: marijuana, lysergic acid diethylamide (LSD), amphetamines, and phencyclidine (PCP). Additionally, alcohol use precipitates anxiety attacks.

Marijuana can cause panic attacks in some people. Although marijuana is widely used and often assumed safe, it has been involved in a number of psychiatric emergencies (17). Some patients' reaction to the drug induced temporal disintegration, loss of control, and regression to a relaxed state with panic (18).

A law student panicked after smoking some grass. His very concerned friend rushed him to an ED. The student expressed the fear of "losing my mind." He recalled it was "unusually fine" grass. Impending law school examinations had recently made him nervous. This was also the first time in his life he had lived away from home. In the ED he begged for reassurance of his sanity. Later, he experienced a recurring fear of another panic attack and subsequently avoided marijuana.

LSD, amphetamines, and PCP are associated with anxiety reactions. LSD causes the infamous "bad trip" or "freak-out" (19). This panic lasts about 24 hours. The patient finds the experience terrifying. Amphetamines produce anxiety in two ways: first, when patients take the drug, either orally or intravenously; and second, when they are unable to obtain the drug (20). Their lives have been so centered upon the substance that they are frantic until they reestablish a supply. PCP ("Angel Dust"), in addition to a wide variety of neurologic symptoms and delusions, produces significant anxiety in some patients (21).

Withdrawal from alcohol often begins with tremors and resembles an anxiety attack. One of the common symptoms of alcohol abuse is tremulousness. The patient also experiences a sense of urgency, doom, and panic which leads to the next drink.

Psychotropic drugs trigger anxiety responses under two circumstances: phenothiazines induce akathisia and antidepressants precipitate mania and schizophrenia. In the first instance, the phenothiazines (e.g., Thorazine and Stelazine), the thioxanthenes (e.g., Navane), and the butyrophenones (e.g., Haldol), among others, produce akathisia. This extrapyramidal symptom consists of inability to sit still, restlessness, and a vague sense of uneasiness. The patient complains of "restless feet" and a desire to "jump out of my skin." In the second instance, tricyclic antidepressants can precipitate a manic episode in a manic-depressive patient overtreated in the depressed phase; tricyclic antidepressants can also cause a schizophrenic reaction in a patient with an underlying thought disorder.

THE REACTIONS OF OTHERS

Anxiety is contagious. Anxious patients infect those about them at home and at work with their panic, apprehension, and immediacy. Mr Amato feels his wife's anxiety. He becomes involved in her experience. As she worries, he worries. Rarely does anxiety remain isolated. The social milieu shares the feeling. Those about the patient become uneasy and uncomfortable.

People resent the demands of the anxious patient. Mr Amato dislikes his wife's requests not to leave her alone. He has become a prisoner of her fear and apprehension. Clinging behavior elicits frustration. People feel they can never do enough to satisfy the patient. No matter what they do the patient wants more.

Those about the patient become caught up in the person's great urgency. Anxious patients perceive their world collapsing and feel panicked, and so do their significant others. The others sense something must be done immediately. Mr Amato wants immediate help.

The social environment does not tolerate an anxious person. Other people may try to avoid the person. But, as noted, the patient pursues them. Ultimately, the involved people actively seek help. They want relief from their own patient-induced pain, discomfort, apprehension, dread, insomnia, worries, and frustrations. In essence, they want help with their shared anxiety.

THE INITIATION OF THE EMERGENCY

Panic, a fear of a fatal illness, hyperventilation, an incapacity to function, an impulse toward self-destruction, and an inability to be alone—all these situations convert the anxious person into an emergency patient. The patient is intolerant of the anxiety and seeks immediate assistance.

Panic is intensified anxiety; it combines intensity, dread, and immediacy. Abused substance reactions epitomize the panic situation. The sudden anxiety engulfs and overwhelms the patient. The person comes to the ED.

Anxiety in the form of a fear of dying drives some patients to the ED. The patients believe they are having a heart attack or choking to death. Mrs Amato worries a great deal about her health. She has sought medical attention. Not infrequently, a patient comes to the ED complaining of chest pain and is admitted to the cardiac intensive care unit. After appropriate observation, laboratory studies, and consultation, the diagnosis of anxiety attack is made.

Patients experiencing dizziness, dyspnea, and tingling sensations in their extremities seek immediate help. The hyperventilation syndrome, usually perceived by the patient as a dreadful disease, engenders a tremendous sense of urgency.

Anxiety becomes incapacitating if it persists for any time. It rules Mrs Amato's life. With her health concerns, her compulsions, and her insomnia, she ceases to function at home. This kind of functional incapacity ultimately makes patients seek help. They frequently report, "I can't cope," and wonder what has happened to their lives.

The 30-year-old, very anxious housewife considers suicide. The pain of her anxiety makes her contemplate death as an escape. The very thought of suicide mobilizes her to seek immediate help. She notes, "I know I am in deep trouble when I actually consider suicide."

Finally, being left alone heightens patients' anxiety. Mrs Amato controls her symptoms as long as her husband remains with her. Without him, her apprehension mounts. The patients perceive their utter survival depends on someone else—anyone. The absence of a significant person not only causes the anxiety initially but also precipitates the emergency.

People around the anxious patient call for immediate intervention for the following reasons: (1) their own discomfort, (2) the obviously inappropriate behavior of the patient, (3) concerns about the patient's ability to function, and (4) fears for their own sanity. *Their* inability to tolerate the patient's anxiety and *their* anxiety derived from the patient initiate the actual emergency.

When those about the patient become significantly disturbed, they do something. Mr Amato brings his wife to the ED. Her behavior is intolerable to him. Like the patient, the significant others demand intervention. But they also want to gain some distance from the patient. Their pain is less if someone else deals with the patient.

Significant others also seek intervention because of their concern about the patient's obviously bizarre, inappropriate behavior. Ganser's syndrome offers an example of this situation.

A 45-year-old woman in the ED gives obviously inappropriate answers to questions. She calls the city by a wrong name and says white is black. The history reveals that friends brought her to the ED after "rescuing" her from her house. There she had acted very strangely, demonstrating inappropriate answers and severe anxiety. She felt trapped at home where her alcoholic husband had threatened to kill her if she left, and had beaten her when she stayed. Her home had become her prison. The friends became distressed and intervened.

In the third situation, spouses, friends, and employers react to the anxiety's crippling effect upon the patient. The anxious person in these environments ceases to be productive and becomes a disquieting influence. Not infrequently an employer sends a patient to the ED "to see someone and do something" before the patient can return to work. Whereas the depressed person simply does not accomplish anything, the anxious patient not only achieves little but also disrupts a great deal.

Finally, in extreme anxiety the significant others start doubting themselves. They feel so much of the patient's apprehension, discomfort, panic, and dread that they begin to wonder about their sanity. They demand help not only for the patient's sake but also for their own. Often both the patient and the significant other are tense, nervous, "up-tight" people. One gets anxious; the other becomes anxious. The first person's anxiety escalates in response to the other's apprehension. A vicious cycle of anxiety develops. Ultimately, one person's self-doubt leads to seeking help for both.

A 65-year-old woman began to feel a "rumbling in her stomach" (her code expression for anxiety). Insomnia and apprehension followed. Her husband worried about her and in turn became concerned about his heart. She then feared he would have another heart attack. Each person's anxiety fueled the other's. Finally, the husband brought his wife to the ED.

THE EMTs' RESPONSE TO THE EMERGENCY

The EMTs' approach to the anxiety crisis requires an appreciation of and a consideration for the unique features of the patient and the significant others. The patient's panic, apprehension, concern about time, demands, and restlessness dictate a particular kind of EMT intervention. Similarly, the reflected anxiety of the significant others calls for a specific involvement. The EMT response must incorporate the following principles: (1) an immediate and firm presence, (2) self-understanding, (3) a structure and a structured reaction, (4) provision of treatment, (5) control, (6) a future orientation, and (7) participation of the family.

The immediate physical presence of the EMTs commences the intervention. This response must be prompt. Rapidity of response acknowledges the importance of the crisis and the significance of its control. The EMTs must introduce themselves by their formal names and their professional role. Their uniform, their badges, and their vehicle all signify a trained, professional approach. The EMTs must continue the intervention by remaining with the patient throughout the transport process.

Second, EMTs must recognize the emotions an anxious patient generates in themselves. They quickly discover themselves caught up in the crisis. They too become anxious. However, before their anxiety disrupts their intervention, they must appreciate it as just another piece of evidence about what is occurring within the patient. EMT discomfort with the anxiety crisis underscores the importance of having a planned, structured protocol.

A structure and a structured approach diminish anxiety. Structure here refers to a physical containment, which serves to check the patients' feelings of losing their minds. The rescue vehicle serves both to provide boundaries to the patient and to offer the hope of medical attention. A structured approach is a planned procedure for providing help. The EMTs must tell the patient of the intervention plan in order to convey to the patient that something can be done but that it requires time. The use of a structured plan controls both the patient's and the EMTs' apprehensions.

Fourth, EMTs provide treatment to the anxious patient. Their immediate presence and their structured plan begin the treatment process. By their continual interaction with the patient they provide the human contact so desperately required.

Fifth, control is the most important ingredient in the EMTs' response. They must act as if they are in full control of the situation. In Mrs Amato's situation, as Mr Amato demonstrates less and less control at home with his wife, her anxiety grows. The patient wants and needs someone else to assume responsibility throughout the entire crisis. An authoritative approach diminishes anxiety.

Sixth, EMTs must demonstrate to the patient and family a *future orientation*. Treatment will relieve the symptoms. Dread will not win. Intervention leads to improvement.

Finally, the EMTs must ensure the family's involvement and participation in the intervention. The family can stay with the patient and provide valuable information.

THE EMERGENCY DEPARTMENT EVALUATION

ED evaluation and treatment of the anxious patient require a prompt, firm reception; a physical examination; an appreciation of the chief complaint; a thorough psychiatric evaluation; and a mental status examination. While these things are being done, the attention decreases the anxiety and begins the treatment.

The Reception

ED intervention follows and enlarges upon the principles advanced for the EMTs' management. These include a prompt response; direct, firm, immediate staff involvement; and control.

A prompt staff response diminishes patients' apprehension and circumvents their demands. Since the patients believe their very lives are threatened, any delay heightens their fears. Their demands escalate if they feel they are being ignored. Rapid intervention serves also to minimize the patient's disruption of the rest of the ED.

Staff must greet the patient personally and firmly, involve themselves with the person, and see that the patient is not left alone. They must ensure the family's participation in the evaluation.

First, staff must introduce themselves with a handshake and identify themselves. Their uniform presents tangible evidence to the patient and family that professional help is being rendered. The staff must intervene with firmness. They must arrange for someone to be with the patient throughout the evaluation process. Family and friends often function in this capacity.

The most important facet of initial ED intervention is that staff assert and establish their control over the patient and the situation. Their firm, immediate presence commences the control process. Although staff will undoubtedly feel themselves becoming uneasy and uncomfortable with the anxious patient, they must move with deliberate speed to emphasize their command of the crisis. They must outline to the patient and family the evaluation approach to be undertaken, and then periodically they must remind the patient of the plan and provide reassurance. Staff project the message that the patient can be controlled. Anxiety must be met with composure, command, and confidence.

Control must be gained structurally as well as by staff. The architecture of the ED setting must provide boundaries. The anxious patient requires spatial limits. The structure asserts the control. An office with some pacing space, out of the major area of the ED and with limited sensory input, helps the anxious patient.

Physical Examination

The physical examination for anxious patients must include measurement of temperature, pulse, blood pressure; observation of skin appearance and hair condition; and auscultation of the chest. Elevated temperature is one of the important signs of a serious alcohol withdrawal syndrome. A rapid pulse rate not only provides an immediate measure of the anxiety level but also demonstrates any change during ED intervention. Abnormal heart rates are associated with a number of medical conditions, including paroxysmal atrial tachycardia and hyperthyroidism. A significantly heightened blood pressure of 200/100 mm Hg occurs with pheochromocytomas. Warm, moist skin and fine hair suggest hyperthyroidism. Mitral regurgitation causes the mitral valve prolapse syndromes; auscultation reveals a midsystolic click and a pansystolic murmur (22).

Chief Complaint

The chief complaint provides an important clue to the nature of the crisis and the urgency of the situation. Patients often begin with "I can't take it any more." They complain of being nervous all the time. Others signify the magnitude of the emergency with "I'm losing my mind," or "I'm panicked." Some simply say, "I'm afraid—help me."

Psychiatric Evaluation

Thorough psychiatric and medical history point toward the cause of the anxiety attack. The physician must obtain a history of present illness (HPI), a social history, a family history, a psychiatric history, a history of alcohol and substance use, a work history, and a medical history, including medications used.

The HPI provides an explanation of why the crisis occurred at this time. The physician must examine recent events, conflicts, and changes and must investigate current influences and stresses. Mrs Amato has two problems, her daughter's leaving home and her husband's growing intolerance and increasing remoteness.

The social history supplies a picture of the patient's current living situation. It answers the questions of where the person lives and with whom. It not only furnishes valuable information concerning the roots of the crisis but also points to the availability of family and friends to aid in the emergency's resolution.

The family history provides further developmental data and genetic information. The family history furnishes a longitudinal view of the patient and focuses upon family origins of the crisis. An early loss of a parent often seems to promote the later emergence of insecurity and anxiety. A family history of mental illness supplies further diagnostic clues, since manic-depressive illness has a marked genetic component.

The physician must elicit a psychiatric history. This includes a history involving current therapy and previous treatment, including psychiatric hospitalizations. It is important to inquire about the use of psychotropic medications. A doctor had started Mrs Amato on a minor tranquilizer.

It is necessary to inquire about the patient's use of alcohol and abused substances. These substances produce anxiety during all three phases of their use: intoxication, chronic usage, and withdrawal. Many patients experience severe anxiety when they terminate alcohol consumption.

A work history provides further information. It offers a picture of how the patient functions and supplies data concerning current vocational stresses.

The physician must take a careful medical history, emphasizing diet, illnesses, and medications. The extensive consumption of coffee, tea, and cola points toward a diagnosis of caffeinism. A history of cardiac disease suggests a need to rule out paroxysmal atrial tachycardia and mitral valve prolapse syndromes. A patient who reports having had thyroid disease may be suffering from endogenous thyroid hormone excess as well as overmedication with one of the various thyroid preparations. A number of medications are implicated in producing anxiety attacks: L-dopa, adrenocortical steroids, and bronchodilators.

Mental Status Examination

Certain sections of the mental state examination are particularly significant in the assessment of anxious patients. Although a complete mental examination must be obtained for each patient, appearance, affect, thought process, suicide potential, judgment, insight, and sensorium are emphasized.

The physician can gain much insight through simple observation of the patient's appearance. Kinesis provides dramatic clues. Anxious patients pace, cling to others, move rapidly from one activity to another, smoke excessively, and talk endlessly. They look frightened.

The affect of anxiety is the hallmark of anxious patients. They describe feelings of panic, dread, apprehension, and loss of control. More important, physicians must appreciate their own emotional reactions to the patient. The physician's reacting with a disquieting, intense, anxious feeling as a result of interacting with a patient should be recognized as a major clue to the patient's underlying emotion.

The thought processes reflect the anxiety in several ways. First, the thoughts come "too fast." The patient either jumps from one topic to another or pursues one subject in infinite detail. The overly detailed speaker seems afraid to omit one piece of information, as if mastery of the details can control the anxiety. Second, anxious patients become preoccupied with their health, their physical complaints, and death. Third, the patients' thoughts are centered on themselves. Their horizons are circumscribed and their interests are inner-directed.

Clearly, the physician must inquire about suicide potential. Suicide becomes a possibility in the face of overwhelming anxiety. Protracted anxiety especially raises the patient's suicide risk.

Judgment and insight are major casualties of anxiety. Urgency and panic distort patients' assessment of themselves, the future, and reality. The fear of imminent death makes people behave in unlikely ways. Anxiety often precludes insight; the patient's perplexity vividly highlights this effect.

Finally, the physician must assess the patient's sensorium. Is the patient oriented to person, place and time? Is the patient's recall—immediate, recent, and distant—intact? The sensorium indicates whether the anxiety represents delirium. Delirium occurs in drug use and alcohol withdrawal.

DIAGNOSIS, TREATMENT PLAN, AND IMMEDIATE EMERGENCY DEPARTMENT THERAPY

After the initial ED intervention and the medical and psychiatric examinations, the physician must reach a diagnosis, formulate a treatment plan, and render immediate therapy. All the information derived during the evaluation is used in determining the diagnosis. The physician must take into account data from the family and observations reported by the EMTs as well as information from the patient interview.

Diagnosis

An impressive list of health disorders are first noticeable as anxiety. These disorders range from medical illnesses to situational disturbances. The most prominently encountered diagnoses for anxious patients in emergencies are adjustment disorders, dissociative disorders, episodic affective disorders, depression, schizophrenic disorders, drug induced disorders, and medical problems (23).

Adjustment disorders are frequently diagnosed in anxiety attacks. This diagnostic category is formally called adjustment disorder with anxious mood. Staff often can identify a particular intrapsychic phenomenon or interpersonal stress that has precipitated the crisis.

Dissociative disorders include amnesia, fugue, and depersonalization states. The history discloses a conflict and a trap. The anxiety becomes channeled into loss of memory, flight, or detachment, and away from the stress. The symptom, the stress, and the mental status suggest this diagnosis.

Anxiety disorders include panic disorder and generalized anxiety disorder. In the former the patient has experienced at least three panic attacks within three weeks. In the latter, the anxiety persists for at least six months and often commences in adolescence or young adulthood. Generalized anxiety disorder is distinguishable from the adjustment disorders in that the former relates more to chronic conflicts and long-term stresses.

Anxiety can be the predominant feature of a manic episode. Mania is classified under the diagnostic heading episodic affective disorder, which contains the subcategories manic disorder and bipolar affective disorder. In manic disorder the patient's history reveals only manic experiences, either one or several. In bipolar affective disorder the history includes episodes of both mania and depression.

Expansiveness, hyperactivity, elation, insomnia, and grandiosity characterize the manic patient. Psychiatric history and family history of mental illness are very important in the diagnostic evaluation of manic patients. Although in susceptible persons interpersonal stress can set off a manic episode, the principle cause is biochemical alterations in the central nervous system (24).

Anxiety can be the major manifestation of a depression. The underlying depression then must be diagnosed. Mrs Amato's major problem is depression. Her losses cause her anxiety.

Schizophrenic disorders often manifest themselves as intense anxiety reactions. Although anxiety may dominate the clinical picture, the patient also demonstrates elements of thought disorder. This diagnosis will be extensively discussed in Chapter 11.

The diagnosis of drug induced organic mental disorder depends upon the drug involved. History, physical examination, and mental status are important here. LSD, amphetamine, and PCP intoxications cause anxiety, as do alcohol withdrawal and caffeinism. Numerous medications — L-dopa, adrenocortical steroids, thyroid, antipsychotic drugs, and antidepressants — cause anxiety.

Finally, in situations where the anxiety is a manifestation of a medical illness, that illness must be diagnosed. Examples include thyroid disorders, mitral valve prolapse syndromes, and pheochromocytomas.

Treatment Plan

The treatment plan involves a two-step process. First, staff must confront, control, evaluate, and diminish the anxiety. Second, they must formulate a referral program to continue the treatment beyond the ED. The referral must take into account the patient's symptoms, diagnosis, and dynamics, the support system, and the patient's resources. The referral must be definite.

Immediate Emergency Department Therapy

The immediate task of the ED physician and staff is to confront, control, and then relieve the patient's anxiety. The control of the anxiety results from staff interaction and architectural boundaries. The physical examination and the psychiatric evaluation focus the patient's attention on treatment, not on apprehension. By being enclosed in an office the patient can begin to perceive bounds to the fear of losing control.

Relief comes from a variety of specific techniques and medications. Hyperventilation must be circumvented. The physician's talking with the patient about the diagnosis and interpretations helps diminish anxiety. Medications reduce symptoms. Proper referral promises ongoing treatment.

Hyperventilation syndrome can be interrupted by identifying it, employing a breathing bag, talking, and helping patients become aware of their respiratory rate and depth (25). When staff and patient recognize the hyperventilation syndrome, the patient feels relief that there is a cause for the distressing symptoms. Having the patient breathe into a brown bag has been noted to be effective. The interview can refocus the patient's attention and alter the breathing pattern. In another method the physician involves the patient in controlling the rate and depth of breathing (26); here the patient gains control of the process.

Either a diagnosis or an interpretation of symptoms dramatically diminishes anxiety. In the first instance, when the physician diagnoses an anxiety state, the patient realizes the distressing symptoms are attributable to a known disease. There is an explanation for the dread, doom, terror, and apprehension. The diagnosis also starts the patient trying to identify a cause. In the second case, when the physician makes an interpretation — a connection between the anxiety and an event — the patient begins to see that the panic did not come out of the blue and gains insight into the crisis. In a case similar to but less severe than Mrs Amato's, a 45-year-old housewife experienced immediate relief when an ED physician linked the onset of her anxiety to her daughter's going away to college.

A number of medications are useful to control anxiety. The drug of choice varies with the severity of the anxiety and its cause. For mild to moderate anxiety and in drug-induced anxiety attacks, diazepam (Valium) is quite effective in doses of 5 to 10 mg PO, with repetitions as indicated (27,p27–38). This medication is particularly useful in the immediate treatment of intoxication from a street drug, since one can never be sure of the exact substance ingested. In severe anxiety states reaching the psychotic level, chlorpromazine hydrochloride (Thorazine) 25 to 50 mg PO initially or thioridazine (Mellaril) 50 to 100 mg PO are very effective. For intramuscular administration, haloperidol (Haldol) 2 to 5 mg is extremely effective.

Akathisia requires the use of antiparkinsonian preparations: trihexyphenidyl (Artane) 2 to 5 mg PO tid and benztropine mesylate (Cogentin) 2 to 5 mg PO tid or diphenhydramine hydrochloride (Benadryl) 50 mg PO tid. Alcohol withdrawal is treated with chlordiazepoxide hydrochloride (Librium) 25 mg tid.

Finally, by arranging an appropriate referral, such as hospitalization, the physician points the way toward continued relief and treatment.

CARE AFTER THE EMERGENCY

Mrs Amato enters the hospital with fear and trepidation. Her husband expresses ambivalent relief about the admission. Once she is in the hospital several things work to diminish her anxiety. Her doctor conducts a thorough physical examination. This reassures her of her physical well-being. Then he starts giving her Elavil 25 mg tid and 50 mg qhs. The drug diminishes her anxiety during the day, helps her sleep at night, and begins pharmacologically to reverse her depression. She appreciates seeing other patients with similar problems and benefits from the staff interaction. Finally, her daughter visits her. In her dread, she has come to believe her family has rejected her. The hospital schedule structures her life.

After several weeks of hospital treatment, Mrs Amato's anxiety comes under control. She begins to feel confident again. She then starts in the day treatment program and remains in it for two months. This program continues the structure and therapy initiated in the hospital. Finally, she is discharged from day care and referred to a psychiatrist to monitor her Elavil effect and to complete her course of psychotherapy.

The anxiety crisis generally requires therapy beyond the ED. The ED intervention is the pivotal point in the evaluation and treatment of the anxious patient. However, quite often the ED admission does not resolve the symptoms or the crisis. Effective ED management includes making the appropriate referral.

Three major options emerge as treatments of choice for anxious patients: hospitalization, day treatment, and outpatient psychotherapy. The severity of symptoms, the patient's insight, and the environmental support determine the approach for each patient.

Hospitalization

A number of considerations determine whether a patient needs hospitalization. These include the severity of the anxiety, the patient's response to ED therapy, the patient's sense of control, the risk of suicide, and the adequacy of the support system.

Severe anxiety such as Mrs Amato's mandates hospitalization. Extreme anxiety totally disrupts the patient's life. This inability to function at home or at work is an indication for hospitalization (28). A manic episode, with its severe agitation, necessitates hospitalization.

If the anxiety does not respond to ED treatment, the physician must consider hospitalization. This is especially true of patients experiencing drug intoxication. Some patients' anxiety increases in the ED. Such a crescendo further indicates hospitalization.

Patients ask for hospitalization for control. They experience "nervous breakdown" and complain of losing their minds. Panic overwhelms them. They look to the hospital to provide the external control the anxiety has obliterated.

As anxiety increases, and especially as it continues, the risk of suicide grows.

The 30-year-old housewife seriously considered suicide as an escape from the extreme discomfort of a prolonged panic. The chief complaint of "I can't take it anymore" becomes a message for others to take control by hospitalization.

On occasion a patient is hospitalized in order to provide necessary relief for the patient's family. Anxious patients disrupt their environment and exhaust the people around them. Mrs Amato enters the hospital not only because of her extreme anxiety but also as a relief to her family. Hospitalization also permits the patient to gain a respite from the family. If the family has intense stress and conflict, the patient benefits by getting away even for a brief time. The hospital offers the patient a way out of the trap.

Hospitalization provides the anxious patient with control, medications, and intensive therapy. The physical constraints of the unit and the immediate availability of the staff combine powerfully to control the anxiety. The hospital extends the program of architectural and personnel intervention begun in transport and continued in the ED. Hospitalized patients receive medication in higher amounts than they would at home, and with more consistency because of professional monitoring.

Lithium carbonate therapy for manic patients is best begun in the hospital. There, staff can conduct a complete physical examination, acquire appropriate laboratory studies, and monitor the patient's response. The hospital staff provides intensive psychotherapy, including individual, group, and community therapy. The staff also offers an occupational program to refocus the patient's attention and assist the patient to experience success. Hospitalization affords the most powerful therapeutic tool to control anxiety.

Day Treatment

Day Treatment offers an excellent intermediate program for anxious patients. To qualify for day treatment, patients must have a supportive social environment and some control of their lives. Day treatment provides the structure of hospitalization and gives the patient some autonomy. It also supplies daily, intensive psychotherapy.

Outpatient Psychotherapy

Many patients with moderate but controlled anxiety benefit from psychotherapy. Medications can be of value in the outpatient setting, but proper exploration of the roots of the anxiety can be even more effective. The first step is to link the patient's anxiety to events, feelings, or thoughts. The second step is to examine those events, feelings, and thoughts for their meaning to the patient. This process also helps the patient to understand that the symptoms did not come out of the blue and that seemingly irrational things actually do make sense.

Where depression underlies the anxiety, antidepressant medications provide a valuable adjunct to therapy. Amitriptyline hydrochloride (Elavil) and doxepin hydrochloride (Sinequan) offer control of anxiety and also have antidepressant actions. The medications can be used in dosages of 25 to 50 mg tid or qid very effectively.

Anxiety is a powerful, distressing, and incapacitating symptom. It compels the patient and significant others to seek and demand help. It must be confronted with a firm, structured, and confident approach. It must be treated.

REFERENCES

1. Frazier SH (ed): *A Psychiatric Glossary,* ed 4. Washington DC, American Psychiatric Association, 1975.

2. Kolb LC: *Modern Clinical Psychiatry,* ed 8. Philadelphia, WB Saunders Co, 1973.

3. Drever J: *A Dictionary of Psychology.* Baltimore, Penguin Books, 1960.

4. Freedman AM, Kaplan HI, Sadock BJ: *Modern Synopsis of Comprehensive Textbook of Psychiatry.* Baltimore, Williams & Wilkins Co, 1972.

5. Cavenar JO, Sullivan JL: A recurrent dream as a precipitant. *Am J Psychiatry* 135:378-379, 1978.

6. Soreff S: The last child to school. *Primary Care* 4:335-365, 1977.

7. Soreff S: Sudden death in the emergency department. *Crit Care Med* 7:321-323, 1979.

8. Hall ET: *The Hidden Dimension.* Garden City NY, Doubleday & Co, 1966.

9. Creden JF: Anxiety or caffeinism: A diagnostic dilemma. *Am J Psychiatry* 131:1089-1092, 1974.

10. Ingbar SH, Woeber KA: The thyroid gland, in Williams RH (ed): *Textbook of Endocrinology* ed 4. Philadelphia, WB Saunders Co, 1968, pp 105-286.

11. Goldberg LI: Pheochromocytoma, in Hurst JW, Loque RB (eds): *The Heart.* New York, McGraw-Hill Book Co, 1966, pp 777-784.

12. Pariser SF: Panic attacks: Diagnostic evaluations of 17 patients. *Am J Psychiatry* 136:105-106, 1979.

13. Dorney ER: Paroxysmal atrial and nodal tachycardia in adults, in Hurst JW, Loque RB (eds): *The Heart.* New York, McGraw-Hill Book Co, 1966, pp 295-299.

14. Goodwin FK: Behavioral effects of L-DOPA in man, in Shader RI (ed): *Psychiatric Complications of Medical Drugs.* New York, Raven Press, 1972, pp 149-174.

15. Carpenter WT Jr, Strauss JS, Bonney WE: The psychobiology of cortisol metabolism: Clinical and theoretical implications, in Shader RI (ed): *Psychiatric Complications of Medical Drugs.* New York, Raven Press, 1972, pp 49-72.

16. Innes IR, Nickerson M: Drugs acting on postganglionic adrenergic nerve endings and structures innervated by them (sympathomimetic drugs), in Goodman LS, Gilman A (eds): *The Pharmacological Basis of Therapeutics,* ed 3. New York, Macmillan Co, 1965, pp 477-520.

17. Slaby AE, Lieb J, Tancredi LR: *Handbook of Psychiatric Emergencies.* Flushing NY, Medical Examination Publishing Co, 1975.

THE ANXIOUS PATIENT 71

18. Melges FT, Tinklenberg JR, Hollister LE, et al: Temporal disintegration and depersonalization during marihuana intoxication. *Arch Gen Psychiatry* 23:204–210, 1970.

19. Balis GU: The use of psychotomimetic and related conscious-altering drugs, in Arieti S, Brody EB (eds): *American Handbook of Psychiatry,* ed 2, vol 3. New York, Basic Books, 1974, pp 404–446.

20. Angrist BM: Toxic manifestations of amphetamine. *Psychiatric Annals* 8:443–446, 1978.

21. Allen RM, Young SJ: Phencyclidine–induced psychosis. *Am J Psychiatry* 135:1081–1084, 1978.

22. Cobbs BW: Clinical recognition and medical management of rheumatic fever and valvular heart disease, in Hurst JW, Loque RB (eds): *The Heart.* New York, McGraw-Hill Book Co, 1966, pp 519–610.

23. *Diagnostic and Statistical Manual of Mental Disorders,* ed 3. Washington DC, American Psychiatric Association, 1980.

24. Manzep GA: Four cases of mania associated with bereavement. *J Nerv Ment Dis* 165:255–262, 1977.

25. Waites TF: Hyperventilation—chronic and acute. *Arch Intern Med* 138:1700–1701, 1978.

26. Missri JC, Alexander S: Hyperventilation syndrome. *JAMA* 240:2093–2096, 1978.

27. Shader RI, Greenblatt DJ: The psychopharmacologic treatment of anxiety states, in Shader RI (ed): *Manual of Psychiatric Therapeutics.* Boston, Little, Brown & Co, 1978, pp 27–38.

28. Cumming J, Cumming E: *Ego and Milieu.* New York, Atherton Press, 1970.

6
The Phobic Patient

The phobic patient focuses fear upon an object or situation. While the thing that is feared remains insignificant or avoidable, the patient functions. When the object becomes too important or the situation must be confronted, the patient's anxiety escalates and a crisis develops.

THE PATIENT

Mrs Mary Burnheart has developed an overwhelming fear of leaving her house. When she even thinks of a trip to the store, she feels anxious; when she finds herself outside, she panics. As a result, she now refuses to go out and has become a prisoner in her own home. Her family has grown very concerned about her behavior and urges her to get help. This is the crisis: she and her family want her to go out, but she cannot.

Mrs Burnheart's fears began three years ago when this 35-year old housewife and mother of three experienced an episode of dizziness and nearly fainted while driving alone to a new market. At that moment she had thought she was going to die. Despite her family physician's pronouncement of excellent health and his prescription of Valium, she dreads another attack and vows never to drive alone. Her family and friends understand and provide her with traveling companions.

About the time of the dizziness episode, she and her 44-year-old, civil engineer husband had quarreled about their relationship, and their last child had entered first grade. Mrs Burnheart had participated extensively in the activities of her church. Her widowed mother, who lives in a neighboring community, disapproved of Mrs Burnheart's plans to complete college. Mrs Burnheart had experienced a number of phobias as a child. Her mother also has a history of phobias.

Mrs Burnheart's fears have grown. She became uncomfortable in stores and looked for exit signs. She worried about being in the super-market check-out line, and she sat by the door in restaurants. She stopped visiting her friends. Then she ceased driving.

Her husband, with the support of the family physician and the min-ister, calls the local rescue unit for help. Her agoraphobia has become intolerable. The phobia affects the patient's mood, perceptions, and behavior.

The Patient's Mood

Phobic patients develop significant emotional reactions. These responses include anxiety, depression, and panic.

Phobic patients display a wide range of affects depending upon the proximity of the feared object. When successful in avoiding the dreaded subject, the patients feel fine and function well. As they anticipate the object, they become anxious, frightened, and depressed. When actually confronting the object, they experience overwhelming terror and panic. Mrs Burnheart functions without symptoms at home. However, if she even envisions a trip to the store, she becomes anxious. If she does venture out, she panics.

Anxiety is the central emotional experience for the phobic patient. The anxiety is intense: the person is filled with apprehension and dread. In contrast to the affective experience of the anxious patient, who feels uncomfortable but does not know why, the phobic patient experiences anxiety and knows why. Mrs Burnheart clearly understands what her problem is: going out.

The phobic patient feels depressed. In contrast to the depressed patient, who responds with melancholia to past losses, the phobic patient feels sad because of future events. Mrs Burnheart experiences loss of her future.

Phobic patients fear emotional disintegration. As they approach the feared object, they panic. They believe the encounter will result in their annihilation, insanity, loss of control, or death. This belief accounts for the tenacity with which Mrs Burnheart clings to her home.

The Patient's Perceptions

Obsession is the major perceptional focus of phobic patients. It dominates their mental activity. They obsessively anticipate encountering the object. The feared object takes on a referential quality. Obsession eventually precludes all other types of thinking. It extends to preoccupations about health.

Phobic patients dwell on the phobia. Even if they avoid the feared object or situation, mentally, they deal with it continually. The acrophobic patient thinks about high places; the ailurophobic individual worries about cats; the claustrophobic person dreams about closed places; and the mysophobic individual reflects about germs. Mrs Burnheart worries all the time about going out.

The feared object invades and dominates the patients' future orientation. Whatever they want to do, they anticipate that the feared object will interfere. They elevate the power of the object and permit it to control their future.

Phobic patients develop ideas of reference about the feared object and believe it has special importance to them. This phenomenon parallels the psychoanalytic theory which describes the phobia as having symbolic significance (1). Occasionally the patient ascribes human attributes to the object. One 29-year-old housewife had an intense fear of bees. She would not go outside during bee season. She believed the bees were out to get her and stared at her before their attack.

As the phobic obsession grows, it excludes other mental activity. Patients cannot concentrate on their work or have a job. The preoccupation becomes the occupation. Mrs Burnheart ultimately does not function at home.

Finally, the obsessional thinking extends from the feared object to preoccupation with one's health. The patient wonders if there might be something physically wrong. Every symptom is suspected of indicating some medical disease. Mrs Burnheart remains secretly convinced her doctor has missed something. She knows her dizziness is the real problem.

The Patient's Behavior

The behavior disturbances stand as the sine qua non of the phobic disorders. The feared object alters and dominates behavior. The patient develops major avoidance patterns, employs a companion system, and exhibits the physical sequelae of anxiety.

The phobic patient centers all activities on avoidance of the feared object. A 24-year-old claustrophobic man had a fear of being trapped on a long bridge. He would drive thirty-five miles out of his way to avoid crossing a particular bridge on the turnpike. In other situations, the patient finds ways around taking an elevator or airplane. Mrs Burnheart controls her anxiety by not leaving the house.

But the avoidance method fails under two circumstances: first, if the patient simply cannot avoid the object (for example, if flying becomes mandatory for business reasons), and second, if the dreaded object becomes so ubiquitous that the patient can no longer avoid it. Mrs Burnheart's original symptoms had occurred only when she drove alone. Then they had happened in stores and, finally, whenever she left the house. The extension of the feared situations precludes successful avoidance.

The phobic patient develops and relies upon a companion (2). The patient demands that the partner accompany him or her everywhere. This person sympathizes with the patient's basic fears. Originally, Mrs Burnheart's family supports her and believes in the danger of another dizzy spell. The companion also prevents the patient from experiencing the conflicting thoughts or feelings which belie the phobia. If Mrs Burnheart had sought to run away from home, her traveling partner would have precluded that possibility.

Behavior reflects the anxiety. Phobic patients pace, sweat, develop tachycardia, and have elevated blood pressure. They display hyperventilation syndrome, with rapid respiration, tingling sensations in the extremities, and dizziness (3). Mrs Burnheart's dizziness three years before this crisis had been a hyperventilation episode.

THE CAUSES OF PHOBIA

Intrapsychic factors and interpersonal stresses are major causes of phobia. Their influences frequently overlap and merge. Under certain conditions they do cause phobic behavior.

Intrapsychic Causes of Phobia

Intrapsychic influences lead to the development of phobia in several ways. First, they furnish a psychodynamic formulation for its evolution. Second, childhood experiences help to explain the manifestations of the phobia. Third, intrapsychic factors account for the patient's being fearful even in the absence of any external precipitants.

The following psychodynamic mechanism describes the development of a phobia. The person experiences (beyond awareness) an unacceptable feeling or thought. Normally, repression simply prevents the offending idea from reaching conscious recognition. However, in the person who will become phobic, repression proves inadequate. The patient attaches the unacceptable feeling or thought to an object. Now all that is necessary is avoid that object. The mental dilemma has been displaced onto an external subject and avoided. The phobic person's object choice frequently has a symbolic quality and solves more than one mental conflict.

Patients struggle with a limitless variety of unacceptable feelings and thoughts. They have sexual reactions to people they know they should not feel that way about. They develop angry and resentful feelings when they should not. They want to be taken care of but feel they should not be. They desire to flee but know they should stay. Mrs Burnheart struggles with unacceptable feelings of resentment toward her mother and has thoughts of running away from home. The church teaches her "honor thy father and mother" and society says she must stay home. But all she is consciously aware of is fear of another dizzy spell.

Earlier phobias contribute to the current symptomatology (4). Children frequently have phobias. Such experiences can lead to reliance upon phobic solutions to later problems. Mrs Burnheart has a history of childhood phobias and had retreated to her bedroom at times of stress. For people who had childhood phobias, a current problem may reactivate a dormant fear. One 30-year-old woman had nearly drowned in the ocean at the age of 3½ years. Her husband surprised her with the announcement that he had purchased their "dream house" overlooking the ocean. Her old fear flooded her; she dreamt of drowning and she developed a dread of going in the car. If she could not get there, she did not have to live there.

Further evidence for the intrapsychic contribution to phobias comes from the observation that often people have long-standing fears for objects remote from their lives. They fear snakes although they rarely if ever deal with snakes. Or they express phobic reactions toward heights, but in daily living they are rarely exposed to any high places. The intrapsychic mechanism provides the basis for this phobic reaction.

Interpersonal Causes of Phobia

Interpersonal factors are a more obvious and immediate cause of phobic behavior. These involve issues of dependency and hostility. They include the interpersonal transmission of anxiety as well as the person's reaction to loss.

In the first instance, a person has difficulty expressing and experiencing dependency. Slater (5) observes that our society prizes personal independence above all else. The patient learns to hide any dependent yearnings. Yet, through phobic behavior and alliance with the companion the patient does achieve the same end. Mrs Burnheart knows she should not be too involved with her husband and his career. He tells her not to be. She secretly resents this exclusion. Her fear of driving results in his accompanying her everywhere.

A phobic reaction provides a way to express interpersonal hostility. Anger and resentment are unacceptable emotions that the patient does not display directly. Mrs Burnheart does not like her mother. Yet to her as a regular church attender, this resentment is indicative of hypocrisy. By not being able to drive she avoids visiting her mother.

Interpersonal transmission of anxiety produces both school (6) and work phobias. In school phobia a child, usually in the first grade, expresses fears of going to school, complains of stomach aches, and stays home. Careful investigation reveals that the mother's anxiety over the child's leaving *her* alone is the cause. The child's "phobia" reflects the mother's separation fears. According to Eisenberg (7), the parent's anxiety is transmitted to the child. Work phobia represents a similar dynamic situation in which the spouse's anxiety precipitates the other's fear of going to the job (8).

Not uncommonly, a person handles a loss through a phobic reaction. The grief resulting from a severed relationship leads to avoidance of subsequent ones. The phobic symptom prevents the person from becoming involved again. A college student felt tremendous pain when her steady "dumped" her. For a year she avoided anyplace where she might meet anyone.

Mrs Burnheart's agoraphobia represents the confluence of intrapsychic causes and interpersonal stresses. She has a history of phobias and characteristically avoids unacceptable feelings and thoughts. In the last three years a number of stresses have confronted her: hostility toward her mother, dissatisfaction with her husband, a perceived diminishment of her maternal role, and an educational aspiration. Her phobia "solved" these conflicts.

Biologic Causes of Phobia

In a number of situations biologic factors cause phobic behavior. These factors include certain medications, abused substances, and medical-surgical illnesses.

Certain drugs produce photosensitivity as a major side effect. Chlorpromazine (Thorazine) causes this reaction. As a result, some patients taking this preparation do develop phobic-like behavior to avoid the sun.

Amphetamine withdrawal and excessive use of marijuana have sometimes been accompanied by phobic-like behavior. The patient avoids others during the withdrawal stage.

Some people, in reaction to a medical illness or surgical procedure, withdraw and display phobic behavior. This phenomenon has been seen in patients with tuberculosis and cancer. It has also been noticed in patients who have an amputation or a colostomy.

THE REACTIONS OF OTHERS

Patients with significant phobic symptoms impact upon their social environment. The symptomology and mood are of such intensity and quality that they directly affect other people about the patient. The milieu cannot avoid the patient's problem.

Family and friends react to the phobic patient and the symptoms in several ways; their responses follow a particular sequence. First, they accommodate to the symptoms. Second, they grudgingly acquiesce to the patient's requirements. Finally, they either accept the symptomology indefinitely or confront the patient.

In the first phase, the family and friends agree with, believe they understand, and accommodate to the patient. They go along with the patient's fear because at least initially it has a rational basis. Indeed, if Mrs Burnheart experiences dizziness and almost faints while driving, she should not be allowed to be alone in the car. The phobic patient's partner finds himself in emotional symphony with the patient and actively participates in the companion role. The family and friends willingly develop a support system for the patient. Neighbors offer assistance with transportation and the children work out a schedule for being available.

Then, they begin only grudgingly to participate in the problem. They question the basis of the behavior. After all, the physician says there is nothing wrong with mother. They become annoyed with the patient's intrusion into their lives. They discover that supporting the symptoms is inconvenient. Yet the patient still displays significant distress upon venturing into any of the forbidden areas. The family and friends find themselves in a dilemma.

Ultimately, they resolve this dilemma by either accepting the patient's condition or having a confrontation about it. In the former eventuality the family and friends develop an extended support system. One family only travels by car or train for vacations since the wife refuses to go on an airplane. In the other option the family finally demands that the patient get help. They refuse to alter their lives any longer. Mrs Burnheart's family now confronts and challenges her housebound behavior.

THE INITIATION OF THE EMERGENCY

Several events convert a person living with significant phobic symptoms into a patient experiencing a psychiatric emergency. These events arise when (1) the patient cannot avoid dealing with the feared object, (2) the patient can no longer tolerate the symptoms, (3) the phobia expands to intrude upon the family and patient, and (4) the social support system confronts the patient.

Avoidance is the cornerstone of the phobic condition. However, if avoidance fails and the person must confront the feared object or situation, anxiety dramatically increases and panic ensues. Often this confrontation occurs without the patient's expecting it.

> A 35-year-old housewife feared confined spaces. When she was a child her parents had punished her by locking her in the closet. She refused to go into elevators, but since she lived in the country this fear of elevators caused no problems. She and her husband planned a combination business and vacation trip. She overlooked the plane trip involved. She went to the airport and boarded the aircraft. As she sat in the cabin her anxiety mounted. Suddenly she felt dizzy and faint and thought she was going to die. In a panic she ran from the plane with her bewildered husband in pursuit.

In the second situation the patients become intolerant of their own behavior. They find life too restricted by their fears. They discover that career and social options are precluded by the symptoms. Mrs Burnheart does not like the end result of her agoraphobia—being trapped at home. She feels like a prisoner. She resolves to do something.

In the third situation the phobic symptoms expand to eclipse the patient's entire life. The fearfulness places intolerable demands on both the patient and the people in the environment. Clearly this occurred with Mrs Burnheart.

Finally, family and friends become angry and cease to tolerate the patient's behavior. They no longer support it. They confront the patient, saying the behavior is exasperating and the fear is "all in your head," and they insist that the patient get help. Mrs Burnheart's family insists she go to the hospital. Her husband takes a firm hand.

THE EMTs' RESPONSE TO THE EMERGENCY

Mr Burnheart calls the rescue unit after all family efforts to coax Mrs Burnheart to leave the house and go for help have failed. The rescue unit faces a difficult task. She does not want to go with them. One of the EMTs expresses disbelief when she describes her fears of dying if she leaves the house.

They make another attempt. This time they proceed more slowly, advise the patient before each step in the transport process, include the youngest child in the intervention, and continually reassure the patient. Mrs Burnheart, with anxiety, accompanies them.

The EMT response must be based on the unique features of the phobic patient. EMTs must provide reassurance during each phase of the transport process. To intervene effectively the EMTs must base their approach on three considerations: the specific application of the protocol, the recognition of their own reactions, and the utilization of appropriate family members and friends.

Intervention Protocol

The EMTs follow the general protocol but with emphasis upon reassuring the patient continually, telling the patient what the intervention sequence will be, rehearsing and reviewing that plan with the patient, and keeping someone with the patient at all times. The successful management of the phobic patient requires the EMTs' skills and involves their time.

The EMTs' intervention begins with their identification of themselves. They must introduce themselves by name and by professional role. The name emphasizes the personal nature of the contact: personalizing the relationship helps to diffuse the anxiety and to establish trust. Telling the patient one's role underscores the professional nature of the intervention. The EMT badge and jacket signify assistance by trained workers.

The EMTs' major role is to reassure the patient. This can be achieved by several methods. First, they give the promise of relief and deliver the message that the patient can be helped. Second, they assure the patient that he or she will not die or go insane. Third, they maintain a firm, controlled, confident posture during the crisis. This enables the patient to have perseverance. Fourth, they make the patient aware of rapid breathing to avoid the emergency of hyperventilation syndrome. Fifth, reassurance comes from a stated intervention plan.

The EMTs must tell the patient what they hope to accomplish and how they plan to achieve it. This stated plan becomes the focus of the intervention and serves a number of purposes. It informs the patient and the family as to the exact nature of the proceedings. Although the patient may experience initial anxiety upon hearing the plan, ultimately it is helpful to know what *is* happening. The plan provides structure for the intervention. It gives the patient something to focus on. It permits the patient, the family, and the EMTs to recognize certain milestones in the transport process: leaving the house, getting into the rescue vehicle, traveling in the vehicle, and going into the ED.

The intervention plan functions also as a source of discussion and rehearsal. Before setting out, the EMTs and the patient review the steps involved. Together they anticipate and rehearse each phase. The patient talks about the fears to be expected. This leads to the patient's actually taking the steps and discovering they were not so bad as anticipated.

The patient must be accompanied during the entire intervention. The companion or the EMT shares and checks the increased anxiety. The presence of this person prevents a panic attack and keeps the patient from fleeing from assistance. Mrs Burnheart desperately wants to return to the house as she walks to the ambulance and during the trip to the ED.

The EMTs' Reactions to the Phobic Patient

The EMTs experience a number of personal reactions to the phobic patient which interfere with their trained approach. These include disbelief, underestimation of psychopathology, impatience, and frustration.

Many EMTs do not believe the fear is real or that it can be as significant as the patient and family say. To be afraid of going outside, of closed spaces, and of animals sounds ridiculous to them.

The EMTs' intervention with the phobic patient takes time. It requires a commitment to a process. This process moves slowly, requires discussion, and involves rehearsal. It necessitates their dealing closely with a very anxious person over a prolonged time period.

The severity of the symptoms, the reluctance of the patient, the time involved—all produce feelings of frustration.

Utilization of Others

The participation of family members and friends in the intervention process is essential. The presence of the phobic person's companion often is the key element that allows the patient to confront the anxiety. EMTs must encourage these people's involvement. Mrs Burnheart's youngest child remains by her side during the trip and in the ED.

THE EMERGENCY DEPARTMENT EVALUATION

The ED evaluation involves the reception, the physical examination, the chief complaint, the psychiatric evaluation, and the mental status examination.

The Reception

The ED staff approach to the phobic patient requires a number of specific considerations. The reception must be prompt. They must reassure the patient, accompany the patient at all times, and involve the family. They must monitor their own reactions to the patient.

The ED admission and an effective evaluation hinge upon a prompt reception. The patient remains reluctant and anxious and desires home and flight. Any delay in the ED not only increases apprehension but also provides the excuse to leave. The process by which a phobic patient actually wants and accepts help has been difficult and long. The patient's presence in the ED is both tentative and fragile.

The ED staff must continue to amplify the reassurance begun by the EMTs. Their professional roles, their uniforms, and the medical setting combine to offer the message of help. They reassure the patient and the family by a firm, confident approach. A formal and professional identification by staff, coupled with a handshake, lays the foundation for the patient to feel secure.

Anxiety is checked and elopement forestalled by having someone with the patient at all times. The entire ED situation is very stressful to the patient, and the temptation is strong to use the traditional method of dealing with anxiety— avoidance. The uninterrupted presence of a staff member helps to control apprehension and flight.

The family and friends serve as the key individuals in the ED evaluation. In the case of phobic patients it may be preferable to interview the patient with a family member or friend. The phobic patient may not be able to tolerate separation from the companion. The family or friend supplies important information about the patient and the development of the condition. These significant others facilitate referral planning and help to implement it.

Staff experience similar reactions to phobic patients as did the EMTs. They often fail to appreciate the seriousness and the depth of the symptoms. They, too, feel impatient and frustrated about the time involved.

The evaluation process itself is therapeutic. It allows phobic patients actually to articulate their fears. In doing so they discover that they can talk about their fears without being destroyed. They find a new method to handle phobia—talk, not avoidance.

Physical Examination

Initial screening for the phobic patient generally includes pulse, blood pressure, and temperature. Additionally, the physician must perform a complete physical examination in order to assure the patient about his or her physical health.

Chief Complaint

The chief complaint reflects many of the dynamics of the phobic patient and the crisis. Patients state the problem directly: "I'm afraid to go out"; or "I'm terrified by the airplane." or they focus on their reaction: "I'm panicked"; or "I am out of control." They display insight: "I am trapped by my own fears."

Psychiatric Evaluation

The physician pays particular attention to certain aspects of the psychiatric evaluation. The history of present illness (HPI), social history, and family history are especially pertinent. It is important to note developmental events, vocational history, and previous psychiatric treatment. The physician also explores the use of medication, substances, and alcohol, and secures a medical history.

The HPI provides very useful information in the evaluation process. It describes the evolution of the crisis. The physician focuses upon the emergence of each fear and the patient's reaction to it. The HPI traces the events occurring at the commencement of each symptom. The physician studies the impact of these fears upon the patient's life and pursues the reason why the crisis developed when it did rather than at some other time.

The physician then examines the patient's social situation. This information offers a view of where and with whom the patient resides. More significantly, it supplies a glimpse of how the social milieu had responded to the patient and the symptoms.

The family history provides further historical dimensions. Phobias occur in families. Commonly a mother and then a daughter develop similar fears. Mrs Burn-heart's mother has a history of phobias.

The developmental history furnishes a longitudinal perspective. The phobic patient frequently has had childhood phobias.

From the vocational history the physician gains several pieces of information. First, the vocational history reveals the impact of the phobias on the patient's level of functioning. Mrs Burnheart's symptoms grossly interfere with her performance of many roles. Second, the influence of the phobia on the total work history can be discovered. An executive changed jobs frequently in order to avoid flying. Third, the physician discovers job pressures which have motivated the patient to seek therapy; fears may too often have restricted options and advancements.

The history of psychiatric treatment is important. Frequently, the patient has experienced and been treated for similar episodes. One patient developed major phobic symptoms whenever she became severely stressed. The history of previous therapy often points out effective treatments.

The physician must inquire about the use of psychotropic medications. Many patients are already taking at least one drug at the time of the ED evaluation (9). The family physician has prescribed Valium for Mrs Burnheart.

Additionally, it is necessary to investigate the patient's use of abused substances and alcohol. Phobic patients frequently try a variety of drugs to control their fears. They also use alcohol to excess in an endeavor to master their dilemma.

Finally, an investigation of medical problems explores for other causes for the behavior. Not infrequently the patient has developed the phobia in response to medications or because of an illness.

Mental Status Examination

The physician emphasizes several parts of the mental status examination in assessing the phobic patient. These include affect, thought content, suicide, judgment, and insight.

Phobic patients experience a major disturbance of affect. They develop extreme anxiety and depression. Panic in the emergency situation characterizes phobic patients. They feel terrified. Depression often accompanies their apprehension. The physician feels these emotions of anxiety and depression during the interview and comes away disquieted by the encounter and sensitive to the patient's anguish.

Phobic thinking dominates these patients' thought content. They obsessively review and preview their lives, always in terms of the fear. Phobic patients do not have hallucinations or delusions. The fears seem almost delusional because of the tenacity with which patients hold to them, but patients always know they are only fears.

The physician must ask about the patient's potential for suicide. Although rare as a cause of suicide, phobias certainly account for depression. Suicide is one way out of the phobic trap.

The HPI offers clues about the patient's judgment. Have the fears been allowed to control the person's life? How has the patient dealt with the fears?

Insight is a critical determinant of the treatment. Before seeking assistance, the patient has often come to understand much of the phobic behavior intellectually. Patients understand the irrationality of their fears but feel helpless to control themselves.

DIAGNOSIS, TREATMENT PLAN, AND IMMEDIATE EMERGENCY DEPARTMENT THERAPY

All the information gained from the interview with the patient, the family's observations, and the EMTs' experiences contribute to the physician's reaching a diagnosis and determining a treatment plan. Therapy is begun in the ED.

Diagnosis

The ED physician diagnoses Mrs Burnheart as having agoraphobia with panic attacks.

The American Psychiatric Association's *Diagnostic and Statistical Manual of Mental Disorders,* ed 3 (DSM III) lists four major criteria for the diagnosis of agoraphobia (10). First, the patient avoids situations where he or she will be alone. Second, the person avoids at least one of the following five situations: (a) open or closed spaces, (b) traveling alone, (c) being more than five miles from home, (d) walking alone, or (e) being alone. Third, the patient anticipates anxiety in the preceding situations. Fourth, the phobia symptoms do not represent a major depressive disorder, an obsessive compulsive disorder, or schizophrenia. The DSM III further subdivides agoraphobia as occurring with and without panic attack.

The DSM III includes two other diagnoses under the heading phobic disorder. A person who fears public scrutiny and anticipates this type of exposure with anxiety is said to have *social phobia*. This patient eats alone, fears public speaking, and easily blushes. The person experiences excessive concern about and expectations of humiliation and embarrassment. *Simple phobia* is the diagnosis for a person who has developed a fear of a specific object or situation. The fear commonly focuses on an animal, reptile, rodent, or insect, or on a situation such as claustrophobia (fear of confining places) or acrophobia (fear of heights).

Treatment Plan

The treatment of the phobic patient involves several parameters. First, it must provide for immediate intervention and stabilization. The panic must be controlled; the anxiety, relieved; and the avoidance, gently challenged. Second, referral must be established. The phobic condition commonly requires long-term treatment. Third, medication must be considered. Minor tranquilizers, if employed only for short periods, can be effective. Imipramine (Tofranil) 50 mg three times daily has proven itself in treating the phobic, depressed patient (11).

Immediate Emergency Department Therapy

The ED physician provides immediate therapy to the phobic patient in a number of ways. The patient is reassured by the physical examination and the physician's attitude. The interview with the physician opens new opportunities for the patient. The diagnosis offers comfort. Finally, the referral supplies the promise of further treatment and hope.

Reassurance is the most important form of immediate therapy the ED physician can offer. Reassurance results from a firm, confident attitude and approach and a thorough physical examination which enables the physician to assure the patient of good physical health.

The interview is therapeutic. The physician's questions challenge the patient's avoidance. The patient discovers that it is possible to talk about these subjects and gain relief.

The diagnosis and the referral provide immediate therapy. The patient finds relief in having a *known* condition with a recognized treatment. The referral verifies the promise of therapy and hope.

CARE AFTER THE EMERGENCY

Mrs Burnheart makes a number of discoveries as a result of the EMTs' intervention and the ED evaluation. She finds she does not die when she goes out. She is in good physical health. She learns people take her "ridiculous problem" seriously. She feels her family cares about her. Her family also gains insight into the situation and welcomes the help.

The patient starts in a day treatment program. Her husband brings her there each day and picks her up. She spends five weeks in the program and finds upon leaving that she can talk with people again and can survive outside the home.

In conjunction with the day treatment, and continuing afterwards, Mrs Burnheart begins weekly sessions with a psychiatrist. She remains in treatment for one and one-half years. By the termination of the therapy she has taken several college courses, has started a part-time job, and drives her car alone.

Through therapy Mrs Burnheart gains insights into her symptoms and learns new ways to handle her conflicts. She comes to accept her feelings toward her mother and develops a better relationship. She confronts her husband and expresses sadness over the last child's going to school (12). She takes the risk and returns to her own formal education.

The phobic patient requires referral. As with Mrs Burnheart, the EMTs' intervention and the ED evaluation provide the turning point. The phobic patient often needs long-term treatment. Hospitalization, day treatment, and individual therapy compose the major referrals.

Hospitalization

Phobic patients rarely require hospitalization. Indeed, frequently they oppose it. There are three indications for hospitalizing patients with phobia. First, if the patient is at risk to attempt suicide, then the physician must arrange for hospitalization. Second, if the patient experiences total incapacitation due to the phobias, then inpatient treatment provides the most rapid method to restore function (13). Third, if the patient comes to the ED only after extreme difficulty and refuses all outpatient therapy, then hospitalization offers the only method of treatment.

Day Treatment

Day treatment is the therapy of choice for the immediate ED referral for the significantly agoraphobic patient. It provides a number of important features: location, structure, social support, and family relief.

Day treatment gives phobic patients a place to go. They must leave the home every day. Going to treatment becomes their job. Daily it halts the withdrawal and interrupts the avoidance pattern.

The daily program gives the patient's life a structure. The job analogy remains appropriate. Mrs Burnheart's job is the day treatment program. It provides her with tasks and organization.

Day treatment furnishes the patient with a social support system. Staff and other patients are with the patient. They can help to diffuse the anxiety and offer a discussion forum.

Day treatment offers the family some relief. By the time of the crisis, Mrs Burnheart's family has become exhausted by the symptoms. They have grown tired of supplying her with companions and have felt the burden and pain of her anxiety. Day treatment gives them "a break."

Home treatment only serves to reinforce the patient's avoidance. If it is undertaken it must be programmed as a method to help the patient out of the house. The worker must proceed on a gradual desensitizing schedule that permits the patient ultimately to leave the home. The goal of home intervention must be to achieve treatment out of the house.

Outpatient Psychotherapy

Outpatient therapy is the treatment of choice for the phobic patient. It includes three modalities: insight-oriented psychotherapy, behavior therapy, and medication. The treatment may combine all three, or one method may predominate.

Insight-oriented therapy stresses reassurance, linkage of symptoms to events and emotions, childhood experiences, and personal growth. The therapist assures the patient that talking diminishes symptoms. The therapist then attempts to help the patient understand the meaning of the symptoms. Mrs Burnheart comes to understand the cause of her phobia. The therapist also assists the patient in examining childhood events which contribute to the current behavior. Mrs Burnheart had retreated to her bedroom when the family quarrelled. Finally, the therapist strives to promote growth in many areas: family, career, and school.

Behavior therapy stresses methods to deal with the presenting symptoms (14). It is most effective with simple phobia, for example, claustrophobia. It involves relaxation exercises, desensitization, and rehearsal. Through relaxation exercises the patient learns to control anxiety and tension. Then, when the person confronts the phobic object, he or she can be in command of mental and physical responses. In desensitization programs, the patient gradually comes to deal with the dreaded object. The person who fears snakes may at first see a snake at thirty feet for a few seconds. At each desensitizing session the patient moves closer to it. Rehearsal provides the patient with a way of working through a feared event before the actual encounter. Behavioral techniques also offer the patient reassurances. Behavioral methods are part of the EMTs' intervention.

In certain situations, medications are valuable in the treatment of phobic patients. The antidepressant imipramine (Tofranil) has demonstrated its effectiveness. The dose employed is between 150 and 300 mg daily.

REFERENCES

1. Fine A: *The Development of Freud's Thought*. New York, Jason Aranson Inc, 1973.
2. MacKinnon RA, Michels R: *The Psychiatric Interview in Clinical Practice*. Philadelphia, WB Saunders, 1971.

3. Waites TF: Hyperventilation—chronic and acute. *Arch Intern Med* 138:1700-1701, 1978.

4. Deutsch H: *Neuroses and Character Types.* New York, International Universities Press, 1965.

5. Slater P: *The Pursuit of Loneliness.* Boston, Beacon Press, 1970.

6. Miller TP: The child who refuses to attend school. *Am J Psychiatry* 118:398-404, 1966.

7. Eisenberg L: School phobia: A study of the communication of anxiety. *Am J Psychiatry* 114:712-718, 1958.

8. Pittman FS, Langsley DG, DeYoung LD: Work and school phobias: A family approach to treatment. *Am J Psychiatry* 124:1535-1541, 1968.

9. Quitkin FM, Rifkin A, Kaplan J, et al: Phobic anxiety syndrome complicated by drug dependence and addiction, in Klein DF, Gittelman-Klein R (eds): *Progress in Psychiatric Drug Treatment.* New York, Brunner/Mazel, 1975, pp 550-556.

10. *Diagnostic and Statistical Manual of Mental Disorders,* ed 3. Washington DC, American Psychiatric Association, 1980.

11. Klein DF: Importance of psychiatric diagnosis in prediction of clinical drug effect. *Arch Gen Psychiatry* 16:118-126, 1967.

12. Soreff S: The last child to school. *Primary Care* 4:355-365, 1977.

13. Cumming J, Cumming E: *Ego & Milieu.* New York, Atherton Press, 1970.

14. Friedman P, Goldstein J: Phobic reactions, in Arieti S, Brody EB (eds): *American Handbook of Psychiatry,* ed 2. New York, Basic Books, 1974, vol 3, pp 110-140.

7

The Lonely Patient

THE PATIENT

Each person lives in his or her own world. Most people fill their lives with people, activities, and events, but there are some who find only loneliness. Lonely people dwell in prisons made by themselves, their families, and their environments. They experience existence as empty and the world as vacant. The loneliness on occasion becomes so oppressive that they seek help.

Sandra Poulin is alone at home this Tuesday night. She feels uncomfortable, lonely, sad, and bewildered. At 29 years of age she has a good bookkeeping job. Although through that position she has made several acquaintances, she resists any offers of friendship. She does not date. She has a pet cat and attends church infrequently. On earlier occasions when she has felt alone, she has called a "hot line" emergency telephone service and has talked with one particular volunteer.

This Tuesday she feels particularly isolated and distressed. Her widowed mother, who lives nearby, has gone on a group tour of Europe. Her volunteer telephone contact is not on duty. Earlier in the evening her cat has run away. However, after an hour of frantic searching, she finds the pet. She feels very much alone. She wants to do something about it this time. At her ambivalent request, a hot line worker calls the local rescue unit.

The unit responds promptly. The EMTs are perplexed by the situation. Miss Poulin seems "okay." She does not look "crazy," nor does she appear to be in any acute distress. In addition, she expresses dismay over their presence in her house. She feels some comfort in talking with one member of the team, alone. Hesitantly she manages to tell her story. Reluctantly she agrees to accompany them to the ED to repeat her story, adding, "But that is all I will do."

Loneliness is a bewildering, pervasive, and protracted experience for the patient and those close to the patient. It presents a perplexing picture filled with paradoxes, pathos, and pride. It embodies the noble American virtues expounded by Thoreau (1) and the terror described by Admiral Byrd (2). Loneliness comes to dominate patients' lives by coloring their mood, altering their perceptions, and affecting their behavior.

The Patient's Mood

The mood of loneliness is an admixture of many contradictory feelings. Gray colors the affect. Depression and anxiety, tinged with anger, accompany loneliness. It also includes longing, pride, and alienation.

Gray describes the mood of loneliness. In contrast to the blue of depression, the black of grief, and the red of rage, the color of loneliness is bland and persistent gray. The mood of loneliness is featureless and toneless (3).

Depression accompanies loneliness. This depression has a distinctive quality. It is more a chronic, existential dilemma than an acute reaction. It is a melancholic mood. More regret than pain characterizes this depression.

Anxiety also accompanies loneliness. The anxiety has a long-term, smoldering quality. Thus only a slightly elevated level of anxiety is enough for Miss Poulin finally to do something. Social situations frequently heighten this anxiety. Also, in circumstances where lonely people feel they have no control, their anxiety increases.

Lonely patients demonstrate a paradoxical anger. They feel anger when their life space is invaded, but they also express annoyance about being left alone. This paradox places the patient in a most bewildering emotional predicament.

Lonely patients are characterized by longing. Despite their occasional protestations that they can manage alone, they secretly yearn for human contact. They want relationships but, at the time, interaction causes them anxiety. This longing accounts for the ambivalence of Sandra Poulin's call for help.

Loneliness also carries with it a sense of pride. Individualism has long been an American tradition and myth (4). Slater brilliantly articulates this cultural phenomenon in *The Pursuit of Loneliness* (5). Because individualism has been so idealized, lonely people feel a subtle sense of pride. They have done it all on their own; they are self-sufficient.

Lonely patients feel alienated from society. They do not see themselves as part of society. Nor do they believe others care about them. This alienation engenders a negative, pessimistic affect in the patients. It also accounts for their thinly veiled hostility toward people who intrude into their life space.

The Patient's Perceptions

Control, limited intimacy, negativism, and individualism are the key perceptual features of the lonely person. Each of these qualities perpetuates the mood and justifies the subsequent behavior.

Lonely people care a great deal about control. They want to control their environments, their lives, and, to some extent, other people. They believe that if they do not exercise control, they are controlled. Loss of control is perceived as a phophecy of personal catastrophe.

Lonely people believe in limited intimacy or none at all. Personal relationships are threatening: they compete with the patient's control. Consequently, any intimacy is limited. The limited or nonexistent intimacy belies a basic difficulty with trust. The lonely patient experiences many problems in trusting people.

The lonely patient has a deep-seated expectation of failure and doom. This nihilistic view leads the patient to avoid any obligations or personal risks.

As discussed earlier in connection with pride, lonely patients have put their faith in individualism. They consider themselves indeed noble, uncompromising, independent, and unassailable.

The Patient's Behavior

The lonely person's mood and perceptions translate into a number of behaviors. These include withdrawal, limited communication, solitary habits, reliance on pets, and inconspicuous dressing.

Withdrawal characterizes lonely patients' behavior. They practice avoidance. They drop out of all but required organizations. They maintain no social contacts. They avoid personal obligations. They isolate themselves at home and at work. If they visit the ED, they often come at night to avoid the crowds.

Lonely patients employ means of communication that control and limit intimacy. They often do well over the telephone or in a letter. Miss Poulin feels much more secure in her relationship over the telephone with the volunteer than she does in a face to face situation.

Lonely patients undertake a number of activities alone. These include eating and using alcohol. In both eating and drinking, the solitude predisposes to abusive overindulgence because of the absence of any interpersonal checks. Drinking or eating alone can also result in feelings of guilt.

The lonely patient often relies on pets for companionship and responsiveness. The crisis with Miss Poulin in part commences when she temporarily loses her cat.

The gray color of the lonely patient's mood is reflected in the person's apparel. Lonely people dress drably. People do not notice them.

THE CAUSES OF LONELINESS

Loneliness as a psychiatric problem results from intrapsychic, interpersonal, and biologic changes. The intrapsychic and interpersonal factors compose the major causes, although in certain situations the biologic factor predominates. Often the intrapsychic and interpersonal elements blend.

Intrapsychic Causes of Loneliness

For lonely people, inner reality becomes the only reality. Their intrapsychic life becomes their whole life (6). An extensive fantasy life, extreme sensitivity, fear of rejection, self-condemnation, secrecy, and the requirement for control constitute the principle intrapsychic causes of loneliness.

Often, the patient lives in a fantasy world.

> A 16-year-old girl developed a unique verbal relationship with her two stuffed animals, Pinky and Joey. During the year preceding her ED admission, she had taken to discussing her school and family difficulties with these dolls. She imagined that they offered her advice and consoled her. Gradually she ceased her activities outside the home and then her activities outside the bedroom. She depended more and more upon her "friends." This fantasy world seemed to her far safer than school and home.

Sometimes a patient develops an elaborate imaginary relationship with a famous television personality; the relationship then becomes the focus of the patient's life. A rich, involved, extensive fantasy life ultimately excludes the rest of the world. It becomes at one time both the cause and the result of loneliness.

Excessive fear of criticism leads to loneliness. Highly sensitive people go to great extremes to avoid criticism. Such sensitive people perceive many neutral comments as insults and attacks. As a result they withdraw from society. This maneuver protects them but renders them lonely.

Fear of rejection is a companion to fear of criticism. The patients so dread any rejection by anybody that they avoid everyone. These people reject others before they themselves can possibly be rejected. The isolation is protective but perpetuates the loneliness.

Frequently, lonely patients consider themselves "bad," "no good," "damned," or like "Saturday's child." Consequently they believe they are not worthy of joining with others. In the extreme, patients manifest delusions of contaminating those about them. One schizophrenic patient claimed the interviewer risked destruction by being with him.

Secrets produce loneliness. Not infrequently, the lonely person leads a secret life; the secret may be a homosexual relationship, solitary drinking, or certain fetishes. Patients believe disclosure would cause embarrassment and disgrace. They maintain their secrecy by living very privately, and they are isolated in the process.

Lonely patients wish to control their entire surroundings — people, events, and things. It proves to be quite difficult, so the patients retreat to more restricted situations that they can control. They withdraw into their homes, limit their relationships, and regiment their lives. Their houses often appear immaculate and their possessions meticulously organized. They have gained a certain measure of control and ability to predict what will happen around them.

Interpersonal Causes of Loneliness

Loneliness follows in the wake of interpersonal changes. The interpersonal causes are more immediate and identifiable than the intrapsychic factors. The significant interpersonal alterations include loss, conflict, disease, and impending death.

Losses produce loneliness. Significant losses include death, divorce, separation, and a child's departure. Each of these events leaves someone without someone. The absence becomes defeating; the empty bed, intolerable; and the silence, oppressive.

Family conflicts isolate individuals within the household and cause loneliness.

> A 12-year-old boy, an only child, felt alone at home. His parents continually fought, both verbally and physically. They often threatened divorce. He believed loyalty to one meant betrayal of the other. So he withdrew. Most of his time at home he spent in his room. He avoided family life whenever he could and occasionally considered running away from home. He felt very lonely.

A domineering spouse leads to domestic loneliness. In this situation one spouse feels threatened if he or she develops any outside contacts. One woman seen in the ED feared for her life if her husband found out she went there. He stated he would kill her if she left the house.

Illnesses and dying are tremendously isolating, lonely, and private experiences. Disease can cause withdrawal and regression by its attendant discomfort and pain. As Satran writes, "The critically ill and those near death may experience intense loneliness" (4,p282). In addition, people withdraw from the patient. They have other things to do. Indeed, the patient in the midst of a busy hospital may be one of the most lonely of all people.

Biologic Causes of Loneliness

The biologic causes of loneliness are of two types. In the first, because of an illness or medication the patient cannot interact satisfactorily with the social environment. In the second, the physical environment produces loneliness.

Any mental status alteration that diminishes patients' ability to involve themselves with their surroundings leads to loneliness. Organic mental disorders produce this isolation (7).

Disorders that cloud the sensorium can be particularly restricting to the patient's social life. The minor tranquilizers cause disorientation and lack of sensory input in elderly people. This medication effect causes elderly patients to feel even more withdrawn.

Environmental factors cause loneliness. Where one lives and the opportunities for getting out are important ingredients of life. Sensory deprivation can occur in the city.

An elderly widow living on the top floor of a tenement house experiences great fear and loneliness. She is afraid to go out at night because of the street gangs. Friends become reluctant to visit her "unsafe" neighborhood. Her children live at some distance and "have their own lives." She has little money to purchase transportation.

THE REACTIONS OF OTHERS

The reactions of others to the lonely patient follow a particular sequence. First, others are bewildered by the patient and try to help. Then they become frustrated. Finally they give up and avoid the patient.

People are initially bewildered by the lonely patient. They often start by asking, "Why don't you go out and meet someone?" The patient's reluctance and fears seem insignificant to them. "So you will encounter a few rejecting people—everyone does!" The patient remains unconvinced and does not change. The others persist in their recommendations: they cannot fathom the isolation. They offer further suggestions and alternatives, all to no avail. The patient perceives these recommendations as criticisms.

The lonely person's friends soon become frustrated. Their good wishes have not changed the situation. They feel rejected and hurt. They get annoyed with the patient. They lose their patience and begin to express anger. The patient takes their annoyance as rejection and retreats even further.

Finally, the others avoid the patient. They stop suggesting and visiting. They withdraw. The isolated patient produces an avoiding relationship. Loneliness begets mutual withdrawal and further loneliness.

THE INITIATION OF THE EMERGENCY

A number of events, threats, and conditions persuade a lonely person to seek help. The events range from subtle to obvious and include absences, losses, intrusions, and heightened conflicts. The threats are threats of self-destruction. The conditions involve existential considerations and the patient's tolerance of the loneliness.

An absence or loss precipitates a crisis in a lonely person. Sandra Poulin becomes acutely anxious and seeks immediate help when her mother is not available and the loss of her pet is threatened. The lonely person has very few social relationships. When one of those is interrupted, the patient's contacts are drastically diminished. One 33-year-old woman comes to the ED each time her mother goes away from the home for a trip. The younger woman admits herself to the hospital to decrease the isolation and the terror of being home alone.

An intrusion threatens the lonely patient's life. A visitor can so disrupt the patient's living space, routine, and control as to cause a crisis. The patient has achieved a sense of mastery over the environment. An intruder challenges all that has been gained. The patient can retreat no further than to stay home, but now even the home is invaded. On the other hand, the visitor may initiate help after viewing the isolation of the patient.

Heightened family conflict drives the withdrawn person into panic. When it is no longer possible to tolerate the altercations and the violence, the patient is forced to acknowledge that isolating oneself at home is not a satisfactory solution. It then becomes necessary to seek help outside the home.

Loneliness leads to thoughts and plans of suicide. The thought of suicide in and of itself is often enough to propel the patient to seek help. One patient reported he knew his situation was desperate when he "actually considered suicide." The people who are still in social contact with the patient may also initiate the crisis when they perceive the patient's self-destructive threats and behavior.

Ultimately, the crush of loneliness drives a person for help (3). The isolation becomes intolerable; the self-imposed prison and exile grow too oppressive. To an extent this situation represents an existential crisis. The person confronts existential loneliness. As Buber wrote, "At times the man, shuddering at the alienation between *I* and the world, comes to reflect that something is to be done" (8,p70).

THE EMTs' RESPONSE TO THE EMERGENCY

Patience, respect, gentleness, and self-awareness should characterize the EMTs' response to the lonely person's crisis. The EMTs must strive to appear nonthreatening and nonprovocative. The lonely patient requires an unhurried, measured response. This situation particularly calls for the EMTs to monitor their personal reactions to the patient. The interactions with Sandra Poulin are slow and difficult, but because the EMTs do not hurry her, they succeed.

The EMTs' response follows a deliberate routine. The intervention begins with a handshake and a personal and professional introduction. It proceeds with an early and careful explanation for their presence and a description of their plans. An EMT must accompany the patient throughout the transport.

The EMTs follow two specific techniques in intervening with a lonely person in crisis. First, only one EMT works with the patient at a time. Preferably, the same EMT stays with the patient throughout the intervention. Second, that involved EMT maintains a distance from the patient. Moving too close provokes further anxiety.

The EMTs must recognize and then control their own feelings toward the patient. The EMTs often experience a sequence of reactions: bewilderment, frustration, and avoidance. As a result, they underestimate the depth and seriousness of the patient's problem. Instead, they offer "home style advice" and may not transport the patient. In the end they, too, avoid the patient. This error can be prevented by a recognition of the frustration involved and of the need for the EMTs' professional response at all times.

THE EMERGENCY DEPARTMENT EVALUATION

The ED visit is a critical phase in the lonely person's crisis. The staff has a triple rsponsibility: to guide the patient gently through the ED; to gain the patient's confidence and cooperation during the evaluation; and to enlist the patient's participation in the referral process. The ED evaluation includes the reception, the physical examination, the chief complaint, the psychiatric evaluation, and the mental status examination.

The Reception

The Ed staff must continue the gentle, patient, and respectful treatment begun by the EMTs. A measured, slightly personal, but not challenging approach is best during the ED intervention. As in the EMTs' phase of the emergency, the patient should not be required to interact with more than one staff member. The staff person should begin with an introduction which includes a handshake, a formal name, and an identification of one's professional role.

Asking for help seems to lonely patients like a tenuous, risky proposition. They feel vulnerable and are continually tempted to withdraw. A staff member's remaining with the patient and maintaining a respectful personal space between them ensures the patient's staying in the ED. This approach extends to the interview. The physician must see the patient alone before talking with any other people who may have accompanied the person to the ED.

The judicious use of delay can actually aid the lonely patient. The woman who came to the ED each time her mother left her alone benefitted from the interactions in the waiting room. In fact, if staff treated her too promptly, she felt unsatisfied. She needed time in the ED milieu to master her loneliness.

As with other kinds of patients, ED staff must recognize and monitor their reactions toward the lonely patient. Staff, like other people, tend to respond to the lonely person with the sequence of puzzlement, frustration, and avoidance. Indeed, by being aware of their feelings toward the patient, the ED personnel can grasp the family's reactions.

Through a deliberately paced intervention, the staff gains the patient's confidence and participation. The patient's involvement is necessary in order to achieve a thorough evaluation and to secure an appropriate referral.

Physical Examination

The physical examination consists of pulse, blood pressure, and temperature measurements. Unless indicated, a further examination initially may serve only to increase the patient's apprehension.

Chief Complaint

The chief complaint highlights and encapsulates the plight of the lonely patient. It offers clues to the current crisis and suggests routes for intervention. Common chief complaints include "I can't take it any more"; "It's too lonely, I can't go home again"; "I'm lonely"; "I need somebody"; "I have no one"; and "No one cares."

Psychiatric Evaluation

Certain aspects of the psychiatric evaluation are especially useful. The interviewer must inquire particularly about the history of present illness, social history, developmental history, history of psychiatric therapy, medical history, and medication use.

The history of present illness (HPI) supplies clues to the origin of the present crisis. It addresses the question, Why did this emergency happen when it did? Despite the chronicity of the problem, the HPI highlights the critical dynamics and parameters of the patient's immediate life. For Miss Poulin, the absence of her mother and the threatened loss of her cat create the crisis. The HPI also provides insights into Miss Poulin's character.

The social history supplies the interviewer with critical information. The social history reveals where the patient lives, under what conditions, and with whom. It includes information about support systems—friends, coworkers, relatives, and pets. The interviewer also explores what sustains this person in the community. In essence, the social history deals with work, school, activities, and hobbies.

The developmental history often suggests a lifelong pattern of loneliness. Isolated people usually were solitary during childhood. They may recall family pressure to maintain isolation (9). Some families hold the attitude "we against the world" and promote seclusion.

Many lonely patients have previously been in psychiatric treatment. A history of the therapy serves two purposes. First, it documents the length and extent of the problem. Second, it supplies information about which therapies have been effective and which have not. Lonely patients commonly report good experiences with individual therapy but difficulty with group therapy.

A medical history and medication inventory search for organic factors promoting loneliness. Serious, chronic, and terminal illnesses isolate the patient. Certain medications, including minor tranquilizers in the elderly, cause clouded mental status and produce withdrawal.

Mental Status Examination

The interviewer should pay particular attention to the following parts of the mental status examination: appearance, affect, thought content, suicidal ideation, homicidal intent, and insight.

The lonely person's appearance suggests the diagnosis. The bland, drab garb portrays the patient's gray, lonely, isolated feelings. These patients present themselves unappealingly.

The person's affect suggests the patient's underlying emotional experience of loneliness. The greater the depth of the patient's depression or anxiety, the more acute pain the patient feels. Anger is an affect noted in lonely patients. They also long to be with someone. Frequently they display flat affect. In some cases they express pride about their stoic individualism.

The physician's exploration of the patient's thought content offers information concerning preoccupations, delusions, and hallucinations. Often the lonely person is preoccupied with certain things to the exclusion of the rest of life. Some patients develop delusions of mythical relationships. Under extreme situations lonely patients hallucinate (10).

Loneliness leads to suicide. The lonely person frequently carries inside the knowledge of a way out. Under certain circumstances the suicide threat increases and the patient actively considers it. No mental status examination is complete without an inquiry about both suicide and homicide.

Patients' insight into their problems helps to determine appropriate referrals. The fact that the patient recognizes loneliness as a problem presents an opportunity for therapy. Frequently patients have achieved insight from years of self-evaluation. This ability to share that intimate personal knowledge with someone in the ED marks a turning point and a reversal of the seclusion.

DIAGNOSIS, TREATMENT PLAN, AND IMMEDIATE EMERGENCY DEPARTMENT THERAPY

The information gained in the evaluation sets the scene for a diagnosis and a treatment plan. The evaluation process itself provides the patient with immediate therapy.

Diagnosis

An acute situational diagnosis coupled with a personality description best describes the lonely patient most frequently encountered in the ED. Adjustment disorder with depressed mood, with anxious mood, or with mixed emotional features characterizes the transitory disturbance which brings the patient to the ED. Asocial, schizotypal, unstable, or avoidant personality disorder describes the patient's underlying personality (11). Neither the adjustment disorder nor the personality disorder alone accounts for the emergency. The disturbance by itself, for example, the absence of one's mother, for most people would not lead to an ED admission. However, in the asocial, schizotypal, unstable, or avoidant personality, it is enough.

There are major distinctions among these four personality disorders. Patients with asocial personality have no close friendships, desire little social involvement, and feel indifferent to people's reactions to them. Patients with schizotypal personality, a latent form of schizophrenia, display magical thinking and ideas of reference. They struggle with perceptual distortions. People with unstable personality demonstrate marked oscillations in their interpersonal relationships, mood, and identity. They vacillate between intense longing and strong desires to withdraw. In avoidant personality, patients show excessive social withdrawal, hypersensitivity, and shyness. They want social involvement but are afraid of it.

Miss Poulin has an adjustment disorder with mixed emotional features. She also manifests an avoidant personality disorder.

The schizophrenic patient (12), the depressed patient, and the patient with an organic mental disorder also experience loneliness. This book includes chapters devoted to each.

Treatment Plan

The treatment plan for the lonely patient requires an effective contact with the patient in the ED and individual outpatient psychotherapy. These patients frequently avoid hospitalization and feel uncomfortable in therapy groups.

Immediate Emergency Department Therapy

The psychiatric evaluation interview in the ED is therapy. Sullivan (13) stresses this concept. The ED interview is usually the first time the patient has talked about himself or herself with anyone. The interviewer has been handed an unparalleled opportunity to deal with the whole patient rather than with just the facade. If this encounter succeeds the patient comes away discovering that self-disclosure is not only safe but also beneficial. An effective interview prepares the patient for engaging in psychotherapy.

CARE AFTER THE EMERGENCY

> Miss Poulin, much to her own astonishment, feels "okay" after the ED interview. "It was not so bad as I thought," she notes, "although it was difficult at times." She clearly does not wish hospitalization because she has to take care of her cat and go to work the next day. She accepts the idea of individual outpatient psychotherapy sessions.
>
> She commences weekly individual sessions. There she hesitantly talks about herself, her fears of rejection, her extremely high standards of behavior, and her reliance upon her mother. Gradually she undertakes ventures into the social arena. She joins a church group. Later, she invites an acquaintance from work to be her friend. She benefits from the respect and openness of her therapist.

Treatment options after the patient is seen in the ED include inpatient treatment, day treatment, telephone follow-up, home visits, and outpatient therapies. Individual psychotherapy is the treatment of choice for growth experience for the lonely patient.

Hospitalization must be short-term. The dangers of complete isolation and suicide are indications for inpatient treatment. But most lonely patients resist this therapy. The "crowds" on the unit scare them. They fear the loss of autonomy. Similarly, day treatment is threatening to lonely patients.

Frequently, lonely patients rely on telephone therapy. They prefer the relatively anonymous situation to face to face contacts. In certain circumstances—for the isolated rural patient, the physically restricted individual, or the limited elderly person—the telephone provides the only way to "get out." Daily telephone checks often sustain the patient. The telephone is a powerful therapeutic, interpersonal tool (14).

Home visits, if the patient permits, are another route to break down the isolation. For a severely withdrawn patient, home visits begin the process of helping the person back into the community.

Individual psychotherapy is, however, the treatment of choice. Within the shelter of a one to one relationship the patient experiences acceptance and experiments with interpersonal skills. The therapist gently moves the patient toward the community and reverses, with therapeutic support, the patient's withdrawal.

REFERENCES

1. Thoreau HD: *Walden.* Pennsylvania, Franklin Center, The Franklin Library, 1976.
2. Byrd RE: *Alone.* New York, Avon Books, 1968.
3. Sullivan HS: *The Interpersonal Theory of Psychiatry.* New York, WW Norton & Co, 1953.
4. Satran G: Notes on loneliness. *J Am Acad Psychoanal* 6:281–300, 1978.
5. Slater P: *The Pursuit of Loneliness.* Boston, Beacon Press, 1970.
6. Laing RD: *The Divided Self.* Baltimore, Penguin Books, 1970.
7. Rohde P: The withdrawn patient. *Practitioner* 220:223–227, 1978.
8. Buber M: *I and Thou.* New York, Charles Scribner & Sons, 1958.
9. Barnett J: On the dynamics of interpersonal isolation. *J Am Acad Psychoanal* 6:59–70, 1978.
10. Solomon P, Leiderman H, Mendelson J, et al: Sensory deprivation. *Am J Psychiatry* 114:357–363, 1957.
11. *Diagnostic and Statistical Manual of Mental Disorders,* ed 3. Washington, DC, American Psychiatric Association, 1980.
12. Schwartz DM, Grinker RR, Harrow M, et al: Six clinical features of schizophrenia. *J Nerv Ment Dis* 166:831–838, 1978.
13. Sullivan HS: *The Psychiatric Interview.* New York, WW Norton & Co, 1954.
14. MacKinnon RA, Michels R: *The Psychiatric Interview in Clinical Practice.* Philadelphia, WB Saunders Co, 1971.

8

The Paranoid, Violent Patient

Of all psychiatric emergency patients, the paranoid, violent person is the most dangerous — the greatest threat to the family, the biggest challenge to the EMTs, and the most important responsibility for the ED staff.

THE PATIENT

The paranoid patient dwells in the world of the perpetual enemy. The walls have ears; the woods have eyes; danger dwells everywhere; and no place is safe. While claiming to be innocent, the patient maintains vigilance against a dreaded assailant.

Mark Perkins, age 35, threatens to kill his wife. She flees and at a neighbor's home telephones 911. The two children, ages nine and seven years, remain terrified in their rooms as their father downstairs drinks, rails against their mother, shouts obscenities, proclaims his righteousness, rummages about for an old gun, mutters about suicide, and blames her boss for the whole situation.

The crisis began a year ago when Mrs Perkins, for financial reasons, began part-time work as a secretary for an automobile agency. Mr Perkins only reluctantly agreed and felt betrayed by her absence from the house. He has always perceived himself as inadequate as a husband and wage earner; her job confirms his failures. He does not like his job as a truck driver and worries about his health. After she begins employment, he drinks more, keeps his wife at a distance, has an upper GI study, and wonders about his wife's fidelity. Because she has increased difficulty relating to him, she starts to confide in her employer.

Mark Perkins believes his wife and her boss are conspiring against him. This private, quiet, sensitive, suspicious, solitary man knows they

are the source of his trouble. He has struggled through school, has suf-
fered through his parents' quarrels and eventual divorce, has been
humiliated by his father, has experienced identity difficulty in his ado-
lescence, and has felt unloved as a child.
   The crisis erupts when his wife announces her plan to work full-time.
This convinces him she and the employer are having an affair. He reacts
with rage, threatening to kill her and her boss.

   The paranoid patient displays marked mood disturbances, major perceptual
alterations, and significant behavioral disruptions.

The Patient's Mood

The paranoid patient displays a number of focused, conflicting emotions. These
include feelings of anger, fear, depression, grandiosity, and innocence.
   The mood disturbance of the paranoid patient is focused. The person's emotions develop from particular events and become directed toward certain specific
objects. Unlike the anxious patient, who experiences diffuse discomfort that arises
for unknown reasons, the paranoid person displays feelings based on specific injustices and aimed toward precise targets. Mr Perkins's anger develops when his
wife goes to work and is directed toward her and her employer.
   Paranoid patients feel angry (1). They resent their lot in life and are embittered
by their observations that others have better positions than they. They have "a
chip on the shoulder." Anger becomes their major emotional experience. Mr Perkins hates his wife and her boss.
   Fear dominates the paranoid person's life. These patients fear plots against
themselves, physical disease, loss of autonomy, humiliation, physical injury,
attacks upon themselves, and people.
   They experience the conflicting emotions of depression and grandiosity. Their
losses, humiliations, and accumulated injustices generate sadness and melancholy.
On the other hand, paranoid patients sense themselves to be superior to everyone
else. Although saddened by his wife's behavior, Mr Perkins feels himself morally
superior to her employer.
   Finally, paranoid patients feel remarkably innocent. In the midst of the storm
they create, they portray themselves as righteous. They are puzzled by others'
emotions and pride themselves on their own calmness.

The Patient's Perceptions

A unique constellation of perceptual characteristics composes the central feature
of the paranoid patient (2). These include projective thinking, distrust, egocentricity, the demand for independence, hypochondria, feelings of inferiority, and delu-

sions. Collectively these qualities determine the patient's mood and govern behavior.

Projective thinking is the cardinal perceptual mechanism of paranoid people (3). This mechanism requires two mental steps. First, the patients deny any feelings in themselves. They do not hate or resent anyone; nor do they envy anyone. Second, they attribute these reactions to others. The others hate and resent them. Patients convert the people in the environment into enemies. Mark Perkins views his wife's boss as plotting against him.

The paranoid person mistrusts people. Suspiciousness permeates paranoid thinking. The patient doubts all motivations. Erikson (4) views basic trust as the first and most fundamental step in healthy psychosexual development. Without trust, people must rely solely on themselves and must maintain constant vigil.

Egocentricity characterizes paranoid patient's thinking. They view themselves as the center of the universe; as the key, unique individual in the global scheme; and as the focal point of their environment. As Cooper (1978) notes, this egocentricity finds expression in the patients' grandiosity. Mark Perkins can comprehend his wife's employment only as an insult to his fiscal capabilities.

Paranoid patients demand, cherish, and protect their independence. They fear any limitation on it and any intrusion into it. To acknowledge that they need someone threatens their independence. To rely on someone requires trust.

Paranoid people worry about their health. If they do acknowledge "something is wrong," they look to a physical cause. They accept a medical explanation in preference to an emotional one. Mark Perkins has an upper GI study.

Beneath the egocentricity, paranoid patients harbor a self-image of inferiority. They defend themselves against their inadequacy with grandiosity. When they do become aware of their deficiencies, depression breaks through.

Paranoid people develop delusions. The delusions represent the conclusions drawn from projective thinking, distrust, and egocentricity. Patients envision plots to discredit and destroy them. On a global scale, they see the FBI, CIA, or Communists in league against them. The delusions also serve to verify and amplify the patient's importance.

The Patient's Behavior

Paranoid patient's perceptions and mood translate into their behavior in a number of ways. Their world views find expression in seclusion, avoidance, and independence. They search for medical causes for their discomforts. They may come for psychiatric help. When stressed, they erupt with suicidal and homicidal behavior. Violence becomes the ultimate expression of their system of thinking.

Paranoid patients become seclusive, avoid close relationships, and assert their independence. They do not readily share their ideas and feelings. They work and live privately. They prefer to spend time alone, decline social events, and limit their personal relationships. They deprive themselves of situations in which they would get any feedback about their ideas. Because of similar dynamics, they emphasize their independence. They resent intrusions and dislike being dependent on anyone. Mark Perkins has lost contact with his wife, children, and friends.

Paranoid people often search for a physical cause for their distress. They go from physician to physician looking for a diagnosis. They try diets and various preparations and will not accept "nothing physically wrong" as an answer. When delusional, the patients believe someone has poisoned them.

Paranoid patients with insight seek help. They voluntarily come to an ED or to a psychotherapist for assistance. They realize their behavior, especially the violence, is not usual for them. Lion and colleagues (6) observed that violent patients often come on their own to an ED.

As depression surfaces, the paranoid person may turn to self-destructive activity. Mr Perkins threatens suicide as he perceives the loss of his wife.

Many paranoid patients ultimately strike out at those in the environment. They fight the intruders. Since others are plotting against the patient, it becomes necessary to kill them first. Menninger (7) describes how the paranoid person maintains identity by fighting for it. The patient searches for a weapon or stockpiles guns and ammunition. Mr Perkins fights back.

THE CAUSES OF PARANOIA

Intrapsychic, interpersonal, and biologic factors cause the development of paranoia and predispose to the subsequent violent behavior. Intrapsychic mechanisms produce a paranoid view; interpersonal conditions lead to suspiciousness; and the biologic factors contribute to instability. The ultimate crisis often reflects the interplay of these three underlying causes.

Intrapsychic Causes of Paranoia

Intrapsychic factors contribute in several ways. First, paranoid patients' perceptions dispose them to creating and becoming involved in difficult situations. Second, their psychodynamics set up conflicts with the social environment. Third, developmental events influence the evolution of personality and correlate with later violent behavior.

Projective thinking, distrust, egocentricity, and feelings of inferiority create for these patients a world of internal vigilance and external hostility. By ascribing their resentment to others, they limit their world and encounter danger everywhere. Mark Perkins sees his wife and her employer as enemies. Distrust promotes his withdrawal and contributes to his anger. Egocentricity further isolates him and antagonizes others. Inferiority produces a long-term feeling of unhappiness, dissatisfaction, and injustice.

Delusions are the ultimate intrapsychic cause of paranoid behavior. In the delusion the patient has a tangible enemy; this justifies distrust and also means the patient is important. The CIA considers the person of such significance that they actually send spies.

The paranoid patient wrestles with certain psychodynamic conflicts which generate internal and external difficulties. These involve psychosexual identity issues, independence, and aloneness.

The psychosexual issue takes several forms. On one level, the paranoid person lacks a clear sexual identity (8). As a result patients become preoccupied with their sexuality—for the man, his masculinity; and for the woman, her femininity. Patients view certain events as threatening to their self-image. On another level, Freud (9) and Fenichel (10) assert a homosexual dynamic in the development of paranoia. A man loves another man. He converts this unacceptable feeling to hate. He hates that man. Then, through projection, that man hates him.

Independence plays a major role in the dynamics of paranoid people. They demand and assert autonomy. They fight any attempt to abridge or limit their freedom.

Paranoid people are solitary people. As a consequence they have limited peer contact and little opportunity to check their views with others. Mr Perkins is a quiet, suspicious "loner," isolated within the family and within the community.

Two factors contribute to the development of a paranoid personality and have been shown to correlate with violent behavior: parental deprivation and exposure to violence. Early maternal and paternal deprivation lead to basic distrust. Additionally, the parents of the paranoid person often have been brutal toward their child. Ideally, parent functions as the protector and lover of the infant. A child who lacks this parenting does not develop basic trust. Similarly, early exposure to violence not only does not promote trust but also gives the child permission to use violence (11).

Additionally the triad of childhood enuresis, pyromania, and sadistic treatment of animals has been cited by Lion et al (6) and Halleck (8) as associated with adult violence. Justice and colleagues (12) find violence more highly correlated with a history of fighting, temper tantrums, school problems, and truancy.

Interpersonal Causes of Paranoia

A number of interpersonal factors promote paranoid thinking and produce violence. These include loss, intrusion, frustration, a dehumanization experience, certain social settings, and family dynamics.

A personal loss can activate projective reasoning and produce violence. As Fox (13) describes, a soldier frequently responds to the combat death of a buddy with vengeance and aggression. Rejection by a friend or lover results in feelings of betrayal, thoughts of blame, and belligerent behavior. A 35-year-old father visited his critically ill 7-year-old son in an intensive care unit. The child had just had cardiac surgery. The father threatened to kill the surgeon if the boy died. A loss which challenges the person's psychosexual identity intensifies the rage reaction. The alleged affair of Mark Perkins's wife threatens his marriage and his masculinity.

Paranoid people resent intrusions. They pride themselves on their independence and their distance. If someone violates their personal space, they become uncomfortable. An 18-year-old college freshman resented his roommate. He had wanted a single room. He complained that his roommate studied the wrong way and interfered with his life. In no way could the roommate appease him. They had a brief wrestling match about what time to have the alarm clock go off. Eventually the roommate moved out.

Interpersonal frustration sets the stage for an eventual crisis in a number of settings. When paranoid people encounter defeat, they become resentful and belligerent. When they feel shamed and humiliated, they become particularly prone toward retaliation.

Dehumanization promotes violence. The patient comes to view other people as less than human; to see them as animals, subhumans, or aliens; and to stereotype them. Dehumanization occurs in a variety of very stressful interpersonal relationships, including combat, labor strife, student uprisings, and police conflicts. Violence becomes much more acceptable after dehumanization has taken place, since the person actually does not perceive that his assault is on *real* people.

Certain social institutions and settings foster violence. In the global sense, the rootless and the oppressed find themselves on the attack. American society accepts and sanctions violence through the media, especially television and movies. Certain subcultural groups such as gangs reward violence.

The family is the primary arena for violence. Harbin (14) found that at least 50 percent of all homicides occur within the family or between lovers. The family, through its intense relationships, immense power to frustrate, and ability to define one's sexual identity, is not only a major maturation institution but also the recipient of violence.

Biologic Causes of Paranoia

Biologic factors produce paranoid thinking and contribute to violent behavior. Prominent factors include alcohol, abused substances, medications, genetic influences, delirium, sexual dysfunctions, and seizure disorders.

Alcohol is a major activator of paranoid thinking and potentiator of violent behavior. Alcohol intoxication is the most common biologic cause of psychiatric emergencies involving aggression. Acute intoxication can produce an acute paranoid episode. A 24-year-old man, after consuming two six-packs of beer, left his date when she refused to dance with him. He accused her of having affairs and sleeping around. Later, when sober, he apologized to her for his "stupid" behavior. Chronic ethyl alcohol use can lead to paranoia (15). A person, usually with a poor heterosexual adaption, after years of alcohol abuse develops jealousy and infidelity delusions about his or her spouse. A 48-year-old man drank a fifth of Scotch each night. He slowly evolved a theory of his wife's infidelity and became convinced of her affair. Acute intoxication causes aggressive behavior. Pathological intoxication (alcohol idiosyncratic intoxication) is an extreme of alcohol-induced violence (16). In this situation a person, usually young, consumes a small amount of alcohol — an amount far below the intoxication level — and then erupts with violence. Later the person has no recollection of the activities that took place. Alcohol lowers the patient's inhibitions toward anger and aggression. Mark Perkins's rage grows as his alcohol consumption increases.

Certain abused substances have been associated with paranoia and violence. Of the stimulants, amphetamines especially produce projective thinking and aggression (11). Amphetamines in all three phases — intoxication, chronic use, and withdrawal — trigger violence. Patients report "feeling paranoid" while on "uppers." a 16-year-old girl used to carry a hunting knife when she used "speed." She looked for a fight. LSD and PCP have been known to produce aggressive episodes and even murder (17). Paradoxically, Manschreck and Petri (18) report barbiturates can also produce aggression.

Numerous medications produce paranoid thinking and aggressiveness. L-dihydroxyphenylalanine (L-dopa) causes paranoid episodes in patients being treated for Parkinson's disease (19). Tricyclic antidepressants can trigger hostile behavior, as reported by Rampling (20).

A 28-year-old social worker experienced a "depression." Her physician prescribed imipramine (Tofranil) 25 mg three times a day. She then believed she had venereal disease and feared giving it to her son and husband. As her delusion grew, her depression deepened. Her physician increased the Tofranil to 50 mg three times daily. The patient decided to save her husband from the social humiliation of having the venereal disease discovered. She struck him on the head with a rolling pin while he slept.

When the paranoid, violent person has a weapon, destructiveness increases greatly. Weapons promote the chances that the victims of aggression will be injured, maimed, or killed.

A 38-year-old man believed the Communists were after him. He saw evidences of their plot. He had had an episode of paranoid thought disorder one year before and had required inpatient treatment. He had stopped his Thorazine two months before. As he perceived them closing

in upon him, he retreated to his home. There he had stockpiled a small
arsenal of guns. He started firing from his house; one bullet struck and
killed a passerby. The availability of guns converted this man's delusion
into a homicide.

Genetic influences contribute to violence. Although studies are in conflict, Grant
(11) and Halleck (8) note that people with XYY chromosomes have a high incidence of aggressive behavior. Moreover, violence does appear to run in some
families.

Delirium and organic mental disorders result in aggression. As patients with
diminished integrative capacity struggle to comprehend the environment, they
develop a paranoid outlook and strike out at those about them. Instead of recognizing the loss of his glasses, an 84-year-old man became abusive to those about
him, accusing them of stealing the glasses.

Loss of sexual ability causes a violent response in some people. Whatever the
cause of the loss, they respond with rage. This loss challenges and undermines
sexual identity. Mr Perkins grows more resentful of his working wife. As a result
he cannot perform sexually with her. He becomes enraged by his impotence.

Temporal lobe epilepsy, psychomotor epilepsy, can produce aggressive behavior (21). The seizure involves the temporal area and limbic system. Its four characteristics are an aura, activation of the autonomic nervous system, automation,
and amnesia. The patient perceives the coming of the seizure through an aura.
This can take the form of an epigastric sensation, déjà vu (a feeling of familiarity
with a new situation), or hallucination. As with other kinds of seizures, the autonomic nervous system becomes activated and produces pupillary changes and
incontinence. The patient then exhibits automatic behavior, which consists of stereotyped, expressionless, staring behavior. Finally, the patient has amnesia for the
proceedings.

THE REACTIONS OF OTHERS

The family and friends strongly react to the paranoid, violent patient. They
respond initially with concern and guilt, then with pain and anger, and finally with
flight and avoidance. They ask for help for the patient and for themselves.

Frequently, families faced with a paranoid member react with concern and
blame. They accept and believe the patient's statements that people are plotting
against him or her. They see the person as an innocent victim. They acknowledge
their contribution to the crisis. Initially Mrs Perkins thinks her working has caused
the entire problem and even considers quitting her job. But as her husband's
accusations accumulate, she realizes it is much more *his* problem and distortion.

As the patient's paranoia mounts and behavior becomes more violent, family members and friends experience pain and anger. Paranoid people, through their resentments, threats, blame, and egocentricity, hurt those closest to them. Not infrequently, they have assaulted family members on several occasions before the psychiatric emergencey. The significant others find their relations with the patients fraught with mental and physical pain, and they respond with their own anger. Paranoid patients manage to elicit the responses they claim to fear most from others. Family and friends *do* turn against them and hate them.

Ultimately, family and friends flee and avoid the patient. As Mrs Perkins does, they run for their lives. They see the anger, they hear the threats, and they observe the violence. They no longer have any interest in understanding the person. On subsequent occasions they choose to avoid the patient. The paranoid person's seclusive, isolating behavior leads other people to withdraw. A 61-year-old retired furniture salesman with an alcohol problem and a long history of blame and violence toward his wife (now ex-wife) and children bitterly complains, "No one comes to visit me anymore." His wife divorced him. His children hate him, fear him, and frankly avoid him.

Despite the threats and violence, many families and friends remain devoted and appropriately concerned, and they seek help. Quite frequently the family initiates the psychiatric intervention. Mrs Perkins does call 911 in response to her husband's rage. She recognizes he has a problem and needs help.

THE INITIATION OF THE EMERGENCY

Under certain circumstances the paranoid, violent patient comes to the EMTs' and ED's attention. These situations include the family's request for help, the patient's homicidal behavior, suicidal behavior, a moment of sudden clarification, and the patient's seeking assistance.

Often the family reaches its limit of tolerance and requests intervention. They feel threatened, concerned and terrorized. Either they persuade the patient to come to the ED with them or they call for help. Frequently it is only when the family takes a strong stand that the patient obtains assistance. A 28-year-old executive used to drink and beat his wife on weekends. The wife suffered through the relationship for several years until she confided in a friend. Through the friend she discovered that not all husbands strike their wives. She then threatened to leave her husband if he did not stop and get help. He went to an ED for a referral for therapy.

Homicide — the threat or the attempt — activates the crisis. A paranoid person can blame others for decades, but actually threatening or attempting to kill someone creates an emergency. Mr Perkins has accused his wife all year of indiscretions, but when he tries to assault her, she goes for help.

Becoming suicidal, either with threats or attempts, activates the psychiatric emergency. A 61-year-old divorced, egocentric, hypochondriacal, and grandiose retired salesman became acutely depressed when his children ceased to pay any attention to him. When they did not send him "even a Father's Day card," he contemplated suicide. His family physician recommended psychiatric consultation at the ED.

Sudden clarification is a unique form of emergency among paranoid patients. It occurs when the patient suddenly puts together a series of disconnected observations into a coherent, often dangerous, delusion. Mr Perkins does not like his wife's working. He had found her at the telephone one day, talking to her boss. She seems less available sexually to him. She goes to her job fifteen minutes early one day. Then she wants to work full-time. Suddenly he concludes that she is having an affair with her boss. Everything is clarified.

It is not unusual for paranoid, aggressive patients themselves to seek help. They recognize their aggressive potential and want aid to control it. A 29-year-old housewife came to the ED because she feared hurting her 5-year-old son. She frequently quarrelled with her husband. She recognized her resentment toward *his* son as inappropriate but did not understand its origin.

THE EMTs' RESPONSE TO THE EMERGENCY

The police and the EMT unit promptly answer Mrs Perkins's frantic call. They encounter an angry, vindictive, menacing Mark Perkins. He blames his wife for their presence. Since, fortunately, he has not located his gun, the EMTs take command of the situation with the police forming the backdrop. Jim Jones, the senior member of the EMT unit, introduces himself. Then, sitting at a distance of eight feet from Mr Perkins, he explains the purpose of their intervention and their transport plan.

Mr Perkins launches into a series of unfavorable comments about his wife and her boss, which he follows with accusations and threats. Jim Jones engages Mr Perkins in a discussion of the situation; the presence of the other EMTs and the police assures that Mr Perkins does not leave. Jim Jones rapidly secures permission for the two children upstairs to join their mother at a neighbor's house. Mark Perkins tries to explain the situation to Jim Jones. During the conversation, when Jim moves a little closer to Mr Perkins, Mark voices threats to kill the boss.

After considerable discussion Mark Perkins agrees to go with Jim Jones to talk with the doctor. They proceed to the hospital with the other EMTs seated at a distance in the rescue vehicle. Mr Jones asks Mrs Perkins to come to the ED in another vehicle.

The paranoid, violent patient requires a responsible, commanding EMT response. Proper technique is mandatory throughout the intervention (22). The EMTs' approach must include prompt response, identification, engagement of the patient, and command of the situation.

Speed is an essential ingredient in the EMTs' response. It saves lives. The EMTs' presence provides protection for potential and actual victims of violence; the EMTs function as a buffer between the patient and others. By their promptness the EMTs also signify their concern and responsibility for the situation.

Early, clear, and repeated identification of themselves is another important part of the EMTs' intervention. Personnel must use their formal names and their professional titles. Their names, their greeting, and their handshake emphasize the person to person contact. By introducing themselves the EMTs begin to reverse the dehumanization. The more the patient sees the EMT as a person, the less likely he or she will be to attack. The introduction serves also to eliminate misidentification. In the patient's delusion or delirium the EMTs may be mistaken for enemy agents. EMTs must remind the patient periodically of their identity in order to separate themselves from the imagined foes.

Following their introduction, EMTs must establish a distant engagement of the patient. Jim Jones demonstrates this technique. He makes contact with the patient; he talks and listens, But he remains physically distant. One must respect the paranoid patient's body buffer zone (23).

The EMTs must assume responsible command of the situation. Doing this requires both an attitude toward the violent patient and a number of techniques. Violence is a temporary phenomenon which with proper intervention the patient can move beyond. Techniques include leadership, adequate numbers of personnel, recognition of one's personal reactions, a stated plan, removal of weapons, appropriate use of people, a distant family involvement, continuous accompaniment of the patient, and the transmission of information.

Leadership is a key factor in the EMTs' intervention. An effective approach requires that one person be in command. This person remains clearly identifiable to both the patient and the other EMTs. Jim Jones, by his experience and techniques, quickly becomes identified by the patient and the others as the person in charge.

All intervention with the violent patient revolves around having the proper number of back-up people. Having too few personnel leads to wrestling contests between the patient and the EMTs, and elopements. A cardinal precept is to display force before it is employed. As a corollary, before EMTs use force they must have enough force to employ. The greater the number of personnel, the faster and more easily the EMTs will establish command of the situation.

EMTs experience a host of reactions toward violent patients (24). They feel anger, fear, and vengeance. They also want to flee and avoid these patients. EMTs are helped by realizing that the patient's anger is not directed at them personally. EMTs must develop a professional, trained, helping posture toward violent patients.

A stated plan becomes an article of faith in the intervention. Telling patients what to expect not only prepares them for the intervention sequence but also provides them with an implement for trusting. Paranoid patients observe in infinite detail the EMTs' adherence to the stated plan. When the plan is immaculately followed, the patient starts to trust.

EMTs must remove all weapons. These include pills, which could be used to overdose; liquor, which increases the patient's intoxication; and knives and guns, which could be used to assault others. EMTs must observe several further points: (1) avoid taking a knife directly from a patient—have the patient place the weapon on a table, and then remove it from the table; (2) if the patient has a gun, call the police; and (3) under certain circumstances the patient requires a personal search for weapons.

A police officer has a definite role in the approach to the paranoid, violent patient. The presence of the police dramatically provides the patient with clear limits. A police officer is the only person skilled in dealing with an armed patient.

The EMTs must secure the participation of the family, but at a distance. Since the family members are the most common target for violence, the EMTs must protect them. Family involvement is important as a source of information and as an aid in the referral process.

An EMT must be with the patient at all times. Continuous accompaniment continues the person to person engagement, prevents the patient from striking out at others, and also prevents elopement.

The transmission of the EMTs' information to the ED staff greatly enhances the patient's treatment. First, the EMTs can alert the ED to expect the arrival of a potentially violent patient (25). EMTs have valuable observations concerning the patient, the patient's behavior, and the home situation. A 25-year-old man threatened to kill his wife. The EMTs brought him and his wife to the ED. The patient told the ED personnel, "Everything is fine." The EMTs reported that he had aimed a gun at his wife and had a large hand gun arsenal in his house. Based on the EMTs' information, the ED physician elected to admit this patient to the hospital.

THE EMERGENCY DEPARTMENT EVALUATION

The EMT unit arrives at the ED with Mr Perkins during the change of shift. Because the radioed information of their coming has been "lost," and because of the simultaneous admission of an automobile accident victim, Mr Perkins has to wait to be seen. During this interval several of the EMTs leave and Mark Perkins's anger resurfaces. When the intern enters the examination room, the patient lunges for him. The doctor retreats and summons hospital security personnel. Then, under the intern's direction, the ED staff and the security personnel confront and restrain Mr Perkins.

Throughout the evaluation Mr Perkins remains enraged, threatening, and dangerous. The physician has to obtain much of the history from the patient's wife. Mark Perkins adamantly refuses help and still wants to "get" his wife and her boss. He threatens to kill his wife if she commits him to a psychiatric hospital. Ultimately the physician and the patient's wife arrange for his involuntary hospitalization.

The ED intervention with the paranoid, violent patient marks the critical turning point in the course of the emergency. The ED staff not only must advance the patient control established by the EMTs but also must determine the proper referral to treat the patient and to protect the intended victims. The ED approach must include an effective reception, a physical examination, an elicitation of the chief complaint, a psychiatric evaluation, and a mental status examination.

The Reception

The reception phase of the ED evaluation is the most important step in the intervention. All further evaluation and referral depends on controling the patient and the situation. Effective intervention consists of a prompt reception, staff indentification, respect for the patient, the parrying of the anger, removal of weapons, patient isolation, physician leadership, adequate number of staff, recognition of staff attitudes, family participation, and constant supervision of the patient.

The reception for the violent patient must be swift, focused, and organized. It establishes the required control. Delays permit the patient's aggression to escalate and allow critical personnel to disperse. Police and EMTs serve to control the patient during this decisive transition phase from the community to an ED admission.

ED staff must identify themselves and address the patient by the patient's formal name. By introducing themselves by both their formal names and their professional titles, staff members underscore for the patient their *humanness* and reinforce their *helping* role. They rely upon their professional titles to declare their therapeutic aims. Through their identification, the uniforms, and their professional conduct, they distinguish themselves from the patient's delusions, misinterpretations, and delirium. By addressing the patient formally, the ED staff reinforces the person's adult, independent role.

The ED personnel must treat the paranoid patient with dignity. They demonstrate their respect not only by their identification of themselves but also by giving the patient an explanation for each step in the ED evaluation. They avoid lies.

Most important, they must strive not to humiliate the patient. Through their continued interest in the person's welfare, they can promote a therapeutic alliance even with the most difficult patient.

Parrying the anger and aggression is one particularly useful technique for staff dealing with an aggressive patient. In this approach the physician reminds the patient that the doctor is not the object of the patient's anger. By helping patients distinguish between the cause of their rage and the physician's treatment role, the physician begins to forge a therapeutic alliance.

The ED staff must demand the turning over of *all* weapons. No treatment can be rendered to an armed patient. These implements include knives, scissors, pills, bottles, razors, and guns. The staff must also halt any alcohol consumption or pill taking. A 68-year-old man sat in the quiet room swearing, threatening, and drinking. Some staff believed that if they took away his bottle he would get worse. Finally, they confronted the patient and asked for his pint. He reluctantly surrendered it, quieted down, and then fell asleep.

Violent patients must be treated in isolation. They must be engaged away from the "eye" of the ED. In seclusion the staff can control the patients' aggression and limit those at whom it is directed. In the isolation room the staff must remove possible weapons. Violent patients can also employ ashtrays as very effective, harmful missiles.

The physician must take and demonstrate command of the situation. He or she must at a distance confront and engage the patient. The physician must muster the forces, deploy them, and direct them. This role includes giving the orders to the rest of the ED staff and to security personnel.

The physician must employ personnel in sufficient numbers to control and restrain the patient. Even the most violent patients usually scan the environment to see the forces aligned against them. The greater the number, the more diminished the aggression. As an effective technique the physician displays the personnel before employing them.

The physician must recognize his or her own reactions to the violent patient and then respond in a controlled manner. Physicians in this situation often experience anxiety, fear, anger, and helplessness. Alternately, they may feel they alone can help the patient. They believe the patient would never hurt them (26). The ED doctor seems shocked that Mr Perkins tries to attack him. The physician controls violence with a calm assertiveness and adequate personnel.

The family must be kept involved in the evaluation but at a distance. They provide critical historical data and observations and play a major role in the referral process. Mrs Perkins has to take a strong stand and commit her husband for treatment.

ED staff or security personnel must be with the patient at all times. They prevent elopement. They protect others from the rage. They preclude the patient's hurting himself.

Physical Examination

The ED physician faces a critical clinical decision concerning the extent of the physical examination. Clearly biologic factors contribute to the crisis (27). The vital signs—pulse, temperature, and blood pressure—provide very valuable information and baseline data. Yet the physician must weigh the gains from the physical examination against further patient arousal. On one hand, the physical closeness and contact of the examination often panic and increase the aggressiveness of the violent patient. On the other, paranoid patients, anxious to find a medical reason for their problems, welcome the physical investigation. Two concepts are most useful in this situation. First, the physician does better to delay the complete physical examination while the patient is violent. Second, when the physician does undertake to perform the examination, it is essential to plan it carefully with the patient first. The reasons for the examination must be explained in order to preclude any misinterpretation by the patient.

Chief Complaint

The chief complaint reveals the many facets and dimensions of the crisis. It reflects the basic projective mechanism: "I'm fine," "My wife should be here," or "*They* said I should come for help." The chief complaint may highlight the patient's aggressiveness: "I want to kill my wife," "I'm going to get those fellows," or "I will avenge!" It sometimes demonstrates the patient's insights: "I want help to control my anger," "I think of killing my wife and I know something is wrong," or "I struck my child too hard." It may suggest the delusional basis of the crisis: "The CIA is after me," or "Please, protect me from the Mafia." The physician records Mr Perkins's chief complaint as "I want to get my wife and her boss; it's all their fault."

Psychiatric Evaluation

The physician must emphasize certain portions of the psychiatric evaluation. These aspects include the history of present illness (HPI), social history, psychiatric history, history of alcohol and abused substances, developmental history, criminal and violence history, and medical history.

The HPI depicts the recent events and explains the current crisis. By obtaining the HPI the physician explores stresses, conflicts, and pressures, and seeks to learn why the crisis occurred at this time. Through directed and specific inquiry, the physician develops a picture of the crisis and its emergence.

The social history explores where and with whom the patient resides. Certain neighborhoods seem to breed aggression, distrust, and violence. High levels of unemployment, drug and alcohol abuse, and family disruptions promote violence.

Where people live in cramped quarters, exposed to aggressive, intoxicated people, they tend toward explosive episodes. The social history helps the physician to understand the patient's living situation, to comprehend the patient's interpersonal context, and to appreciate the type of environment to which the patient will ultimately return.

The psychiatric history provides information about the patient's mental health treatment and medications. Not infrequently paranoid, violent patients have psychiatric histories (28). They have been seen in the ED for psychiatric problems, have been in psychiatric hospitals, have received outpatient treatment, and have taken psychotropic medications.

The physician must inquire about the patient's use of alcohol and abused substances. This part of the psychiatric history is particularly significant since these substances highly correlate with paranoia and violence.

A developmental history reveals many significant events which contribute to a mistrusting and aggressive personality. A family background featuring deprivation, brutality, violence, altercations, assault, alcoholism, rape, and incest produces paranoid people. Bed wetting, fire setting, and cruelty toward animals correlate with violence (29). A history of school problems, truancy, fighting, and temper tantrums also has been linked with aggressiveness.

The physician must explore the patient's history of criminal activity and violence. Steadman et al (30) report that the violent patient will often have been involved with the criminal justice system. According to Halleck (8), a history of violence is the single item most highly correlated with future aggressiveness. The physician must specifically inquire about previous violent episodes. When did they occur? Where? What happened: threats, assaults, or homicide? What was the patient's reaction to the violence? How similar are those episodes to the current crisis? A history of past violence strongly predicts future aggressive behavior.

Finally, the physician must obtain a medical and medication history, since many diseases and pharmacological preparations precipitate paranoid, violent episodes.

Mental Status Examination

The physician next focuses on the mental status examination. Particularly important aspects of the examination for the paranoid, violent patient include his appearance, affect, thought content, homicidal plans, suicidal thoughts, judgment, insight, and sensorium.

Patients' *appearance* often portrays their paranoia. Suspicious patients keep their social distance and avoid direct eye contact. They wear sunglasses and look elsewhere when conversing with the interviewer. They scan the environment, check for exits, demand only one person in the room with them at a time, and sit with their backs against the wall. Aggressive patients appear threatening, hostile, and combative. Their kinesics say, "Watch it". Their overall demeanor connotes assault.

Anger dominates the paranoid patient's affect. The interviewer senses the rage and frustration. The patient feels wronged by everyone and wants vengeance. The paranoid patient also feels shame and depression.

Paranoid, violent patients' thought content reveals a great deal of information about their unique mental processes. Their stream of conversation reflects blame and demonstrates erratic impulsiveness (31). These patients abruptly change the subject. They have delusions; they have hallucinations, usually auditory. They report hearing people talking about them and accusing them. Their thoughts acquire a referential quality: they see everyone as interested in them and imagine that newspaper articles are directed toward them. Their thought content demonstrates their egocentricity.

The physician must make a detailed exploration into the patient's homicidal plans. It is essential to ask if the patient has any thoughts of killing anyone and to find out how specific the thoughts are. Next, the physician asks whether the patient has plans to kill someone. Often the patient harbors nonspecific ideas about murder; other patients present a well thought out scheme to purchase a gun, kill the person, and then cleverly dispose of the body. Mr Perkins is evolving a plan to kill his wife.

The physician must also assess the patient's suicidal potential. The patient may wish above all to save face and may see suicide as the means to this end. Here again, the physician must make a very detailed inquiry about thoughts and plans of suicide.

The physician must evaluate the patient's judgment: how has the person handled the situation? The paranoid, violent person frequently demonstrates poor judgment as evidenced by distorted, projective thinking and impulsive behavior. The HPI provides major clues about the patient's judgment.

The amount of insight the patient has influences the development of the crisis and the referral. Not infrequently, the potentially violent patient demonstrates a great deal of insight.

The physician must assess the patient's sensorium. Points to be evaluated are orientation to person, place, and time; and immediate, recent, and distant recall.

DIAGNOSIS, TREATMENT PLAN, AND IMMEDIATE EMERGENCY DEPARTMENT THERAPY

The ED physician must use the information gained during the evaluation, the results of laboratory studies, observations made during the intervention, and the experiences of the family and EMTs to reach a diagnosis, determine a treatment plan, and decide on the immediate therapy.

Diagnosis

The psychiatrist the ED physician calls in for consultation diagnoses Mr Mark Perkins as having a paranoid disorder in a paranoid personality. He bases this diagnosis on Mr Perkins's persistent delusions and threats, even as he sobers, and his long history of suspiciousness and distrust.

A wide variety of diagnoses apply to paranoid, violent patients. The diagnostic categories include paranoid disorder, paranoid personality disorder, paranoid schizophrenia, mania, the alcohol induced state, the substances precipitated state, organic mental disorder, and psychomotor epilepsy (16).

The paranoid disorder features a central delusion or delusions of jealousy with little impairment of function. Mark Perkins focuses his life about his wife's infidelity, although he is able to work. Other criteria include the absence of schizophrenic symptoms, absence of manic syndrome or depression syndrome, the duration of the illness of at least one week, and absence of organic mental disorder. Paranoid and schizoid personality disorders, as well as migration and deafness, predispose to this condition.

Suspiciousness, mistrust of persons, and hypersensitivity characterize the patient with a paranoid personality disorder. This person has a long history of expecting trickery and remains highly vigilant at all times. The diagnostic criteria involve three areas. First, the mistrust and suspicion must include at least four of the following: (1) expectation of fraud; (2) high level of vigilance; (3) defensiveness; (4) denying all personal blame even where appropriate; (5) doubting of others' loyalty; (6) searching to reaffirm one's bias to the exclusion of missing the total picture; and (7) looking constantly for special messages and secret motives. Second, the patient exhibits hypersensitivity with at least two of the following: (1) affective "coldness"; (2) emphasis upon the objective and rational; (3) the absence of humor; and (4) the lack of tenderness. Finally, the patient does not demonstrate characteristics of schizophrenia.

Paranoid schizophrenic patients meet all the criteria of schizophrenia (see Chapter 11) and in addition have a major delusive focus. As schizophrenic patients, they exhibit profound disturbances of affects, thoughts, and their integration. As paranoid patients they develop one or more major delusional systems: persecution, grandiosity, or jealousness. Further, these patients' hallucinations may have a persecutory or grandiose quality.

A patient in a manic episode can demonstrate paranoid ideation and violence (32). A delusion has become the focus of the person's life. The other qualities of mania—pressured speech, grandiosity, and irritability—are also present. The history reveals periods of highs and lows and often includes a family member with a similar pattern. A depression frequently follows the paranoid episode.

Alcohol consumption results in paranoia and violence in a number of ways. In alcohol idiosyncratic intoxication (pathological intoxication), the patient rapidly goes into an aggressive episode after ingesting a small amount of alcohol. Later there is amnesia for the entire sequence. In alcohol intoxication (well documented on college campuses, in saloons, and at office parties), the patient overindulges in spirits and displays offensive, belligerent, and grandiose behavior. In alcohol withdrawal and alcohol withdrawal delirium (delirium tremens), the patient after stopping drinking can display irritability, hyperactivity, and aggressiveness. In the former, the symptoms occur shortly after the patient ceases intake; in the latter, the patient has stopped three to five days before the onset of gross disturbances.

A number of substances, when ingested, inhaled, or administered intravenously cause paranoid, violent behavior. These substances include amphetamines, barbiturates, cannabis, cocaine, lysergic acid diethylamide (LSD), and phencyclidine (PCP). Each has been responsible for delusional thinking in certain patients.

Delirium, an organic mental disorder, produces a paranoid, violent patient (33). Psychomotor epilepsy occasionally is first demonstrated by a violent episode (34). Patients feel an aura before the event. They go through stereotyped behavior. They show autonomic nervous system disturbances such as incontinence. They have amnesia for the entire episode. An electroencephalogram with nasopharyngeal leads often demonstrates a spike in the temporal lobe area.

Treatment Plan

The physician in developing a treatment plan must take into account two objectives. The first is to provide immediate therapy. The second is to establish an effective referral. In many cases the paranoid, violent patient requires hospitalization. Often this must be done involuntarily. Inpatient treatment not only helps the patient but also protects others, especially families. A recent court finding was that if a physician releases a patient who has made threats, that physician has a responsibility to inform the intended victims (35). In the *Tarasoff* case, a patient killed a college student. He had told his therapist the name of the young woman. The California courts ruled that the therapist should have informed the young woman.

Immediate Emergency Department Therapy

The ED physician and staff achieve a number of objectives in the treatment of the paranoid, violent patient. They stop the violence. They administer the appropriate medications, reinforce alternatives to aggression, and give the patient time to reorganize. Finally, they establish a referral.

The ED staff must stop the violence. The patient comes to them "out of control"; demonstrating impulsiveness, aggression, and belligerence; threatening harm; and seeming very menacing. In this situation the ED does in fact function in the capacity of social control as well as medical care (36). It is not unusual for violent patients, after confronting a large and controlling ED staff, to then sit down and discuss the problem. The ED, by establishing its command of the situation, permits the patient to talk. A 32-year-old "tough guy" came to the ED with the police after he threatened to beat up a roommate. He initially challenged the ED staff and demanded to leave. Once he was made aware of the forces aligned there, as well as the physician's insistence that he stay, he told his story with a great deal of relief.

Medications are quite effective in controlling violent patients. Haloperidol (Haldol) 2 to 5 mg intramuscularly every half hour has been highly effective (37). Chlorpromazine (Thorazine) 50 to 100 mg has "taken the edge" off potentially violent patients who want help to control their aggression. Paraldehyde PO helps acutely agitated alcoholic patients experiencing withdrawal.

In the ED the physician and staff demonstrate alternatives to violence. They show by example the benefits of talking about problems. They confront difficult topics without flight or aggression. They reward the patient's verbal expression by listening.

Time in the ED helps violent, paranoid patients through their crises. After the initial prompt intervention, patients often require time to "get themselves together." A 28-year-old man came to the ED acutely intoxicated and wanting to kill his wife, who planned to divorce him. After five hours in the ED, two sessions with a psychiatrist, a long visit with his mother and sister, and a communion with his priest, he felt better, wanted the divorce, and went to stay with his parents.

Finally, the ED has the responsibility to set up an effective referral.

When the ED has done effective, immediate therapy, the patient recognizes it. As Lion et al (6) point out, that patient will return to the ED the next time rather than acting violently. Trust will have been established.

CARE AFTER THE EMERGENCY

Mark Perkins follows a stormy course after the ED intervention. He enters a psychiatric hospital involuntarily. He claims during the early period of his admission that his wife, not he, should be there and that he still wants to kill her. In the commitment hearing the judge rules that Mr Perkins must remain in the hospital involuntarily for treatment for sixty days.

Mr Perkins resents the hospital, the staff, and the therapy. He refuses medication and portrays himself as a martyr. A young staff psychiatrist works with him. Initially, Mark Perkins uses the sessions to complain about everything. The psychiatrist slowly wades into discussions about emotions; Mr Perkins denies all feelings. Gradually, grudgingly, the patient begins to look forward to his sessions. With sadness he reviews his childhood and his fear of abandonment. He links this fear with feelings of abandonment brought on by his wife's working.

His wife visits him. At first she remains afraid. But as she demonstrates her loyalty, he starts again to believe her. He eventually signs into the hospital and fully participates in the program.

Upon discharge, a psychiatrist sees Mr Perkins in weekly sessions. He continues to gain insight into his development, his family, and himself. He finally realizes that when he feels depressed he becomes paranoid. He had experienced a loss when his wife worked. In response he had become suspicious of her and then developed a jealous rage.

The therapeutic course for paranoid, violent patients involves two major treatments: hospitalizaion and outpatient psychotherapy. The ED physician, in arranging a referral, must weigh not only the patient's therapy but also the family's and the community's safety. The ED physician and staff must regard violence as a temporary phenomenon. Once the episode has been controlled, the patient can reintegrate and benefit from therapy.

Hospitalization

Under a number of circumstances, hospitalization is the treatment of choice: dangerousness to others or self, continuing rage, mania, and incapacitation. If the risk of homicide or suicide is high the physician must arrange for inpatient treatment, involuntary if necessary. The physician has the responsibility to protect the intended victim as well as the patient. If the rage continues, hospitalization becomes necessary. If the patient experiences a manic episode, inpatient treatment provides the best place to control behavior, to perform the required laboratory studies, to begin the appropriate medications (lithium carbonate), and to monitor its effects. If the paranoid condition has produced a total inability to function, the hospitalization can be very effective.

Outpatient Psychotherapy

Outpatient psychotherapy is the treatment of choice under certain conditions. Outpatient therapy is appropriate for patients who have insight and want therapy. In addition, the patients must feel they can control their violence. The family must remain supportive and not feel threatened by the patient.

Therapy Principles

The psychiatrist, in treating the paranoid, violent patient over any length of time, must follow a number of specific techniques. These maneuvers apply regardless of setting. They include an interested, distant relationship; fixed appointments;

constant emphasis upon discussion of feelings; the use of appropriate medications; and a respectful, trusting, working alliance.

The therapist must maintain an interested, distant relationship to the patient. The therapist demonstrates concern for the patient through both questions and listening. It is necessary also to keep an interpersonal space and to avoid any physical contact and any jokes. The therapist must not sit too close to the patient, and should permit the patient the greatest autonomy possible.

The therapist must establish a fixed appointment schedule. For example, on an inpatient unit the psychiatrist might see the patient every Monday, Wednesday, and Friday at 10 AM for 45 minutes, and for outpatient therapy they might have sessions every Tuesday at 3 PM; this kind of routine gives the patient a schedule and creates a structure where mutual trust can develop.

The therapist emphasizes the patient's feelings. Mark Perkins denies any emotions, although he acknowledges that his wife hates him. His psychiatrist continually asks him, "How do you feel about that?" Slowly, Mr Perkins becomes aware of his feelings.

A number of psychotropic medications are especially effective for paranoid, violent patients. Antipsychotic preparations have demonstrated their ability to diminish aggressiveness. These drugs include haloperidol (Haldol) 5 to 10 mg four times a day, thioridazine hydrochloride (Mellaril) 50 to 100 mg four times daily, chlorpromazine hydrochloride (Thorazine) 25 to 100 mg four times daily, and trifluoperazine hydrochloride (Stelazine) 2 to 5 mg three times daily. Lithium carbonate controls mania and prevents manic episodes. The usual dosage is 300 mg three times a day, with the therapeutic fasting blood level between 0.5 and 1.0 mg/100 ml. Some studies indicate that lithium carbonate also decreases violence (38). Chlordiazepoxide hydrochloride (Librium) 25 mg four times daily and paraldehyde 10 to 30 ml PO every four hours are effective for violence accompanying alcohol withdrawal (39). Anticonvulsant drugs — phenytoin (Dilantin), mephenytoin (Mesantoin), ethotoin (Peganone), methsuximide (Celontin), primidone (Mysoline), and phenobarbital — control psychomotor seizures (40).

Finally, the basis of therapy must be the achievement of mutual respect and trust between the patient and the therapist.

REFERENCES

1. MacKinnon RA, Michels R: *The Psychiatric Interview in Clinical Practice.* Philadelphia, WB Saunders Co, 1971.

2. Swanson DW, Bohnert PJ, Smith JA: *The Paranoid.* Boston, Little Brown & Co, 1970.

3. Freud A: *The Ego and the Mechanisms of Defense.* New York, International Universities Press, 1946.

4. Erikson EH: *Childhood and Society,* ed 2. New York, WW Norton & Co, 1963.

124 MANAGEMENT OF THE PSYCHIATRIC EMERGENCY

5. Cooper AF: The suspicious patient. *Practitioner* 220:270-275, 1978.
6. Lion JR, Bach-Y-Rita G, Ervin FR: Violent patients in the emergency room. *Am J Psychiatry* 125:1706-1711, 1969.
7. Menninger K: *The Vital Balance.* New York, Viking Press, 1967.
8. Halleck SL: Psychodynamic aspects of violence. *Bull Am Acad Psychiatry Law* 4:328-335, 1976.
9. Freud S: *Three Case Histories.* New York, Collier Books, 1972.
10. Fenichel O: *The Psychoanalytic Theory of Neurosis.* New York, WW Norton & Co, 1945.
11. Grant DA: A model of violence. *Aust NZ J Psychiatry* 12:123-126, 1978.
12. Justice B, Justice R, Kraft IA: Early warning signs of violence: Is a triad enough? *Am J Psychiatry* 131:457-459, 1974.
13. Fox RP: Narcissistic rage and the problem of combat aggression. *Arch Gen Psychiatry* 31:807-811, 1974.
14. Harbin HT: Episodic dyscontrol and family dynamics. *Am J Psychiatry* 134:1113-1116, 1977.
15. Kolb LC: *Modern Clinical Psychiatry,* ed 8. Philadelphia, WB Saunders Co, 1973.
16. *Diagnostic and Statistical Manual of Mental Disorders,* ed 3. Washington DC, American Psychiatric Association, 1980.
17. Fauman MA, Fauman BJ: Violence associated with phencyclidine abuse. *Am J Psychiatry* 136:1584-1586, 1979.
18. Manschreck TC, Petri M: The paranoid syndrome. *Lancet* 1:251-253, 1978.
19. Goodwin FK: Behavioral effects of L-dopa in man, in Shader RI (ed): *Psychiatric Complications of Medical Drugs.* New York, Raven Press, 1972, pp 149-174.
20. Rampling D: Aggression: A paradoxical response to tricyclic antidepressants. *Am J Psychiatry* 135:117-118, 1978.
21. Blumer D: Temporal lobe epilepsy and its psychiatric significance, in Benson DF, Blumer D (eds): *Psychiatric Aspects of Neurologic Disease.* New York, Grune & Stratton, 1975, pp 171-198.
22. Guirguis EF: Management of disturbed patients: An alternative to the use of mechanical restraints. *J Clin Psychiatry* 39:295-303, 1978.
23. Hall ET: *The Hidden Dimension.* Garden City, Doubleday & Co, 1966.
24. Lion JR, Pasternak SA: Countertransference reactions to violent patients. *Am J Psychiatry* 130:207-210, 1973.
25. Edelman SE: Managing the violent patient in a community mental health center. *Hosp Community Psychiatry* 29:460-462, 1978.
26. Whitman RM, Armao BB, Dent OB: Assault on the therapist. *Am J Psychiatry* 133:426-429, 1976.
27. Hall RCW, Popkin MK, Devaul RA, et al: Physical illness presenting as psychiatric disease. *Arch Gen Psychiatry* 35:1315-1320, 1978.
28. Grunberg F, Klinger BI, Grumet BR: Homicide and community-based psychiatry. *J Nerv Ment Dis* 166:868-874, 1978.
29. Hellman DS, Blackman H: Enuresis, firesetting and cruelty to animals: A triad predictive of adult crime. *Am J Psychiatry* 122:1431-1435, 1966.
30. Steadman HJ, Cocozza JJ, Melick E: Explaining the increased arrest rate among mental patients: The changing clientele of state hospitals. *Am J Psychiatry* 135:816-820, 1978.
31. Satten J, Menninger K, Rosen I, et al: Murder without apparent motives: A study in personality disorganization. *Am J Psychiatry* 117:48-53, 1960.

32. Fry WF: Paranoid episodes in manic-depressive psychoses. *Am J Psychiatry* 135:974-976, 1978.

33. Koranyi EK: Morbidity and rate of undiagnosed physical illnesses in a psychiatric clinic population. *Arch Gen Psychiatry* 36:414-419, 1979.

34. Lawall J: Psychiatric presentation of seizure disorders. *Am J Psychiatry* 133:321-323, 1976.

35. Gureritz H: Tarasoff: Protective privilege versus public peril. *Am J Psychiatry* 134:289-292, 1977.

36. Morrice JKW: Emergency psychiatry. *Br J Psychiatry* 114:485-491, 1968.

37. Donlon PT, Hopkin J, Tupin JP: Overview: Efficacy and safety of the rapid neuroleptization method with injectable haloperidol. *Am J Psychiatry* 136:273-278, 1979.

38. Tupin JP: Management of violent patients, in Shader RI (ed): *Manual of Psychiatric Therapeutics.* Boston, Little Brown & Co, 1978, pp 125-136.

39. Greenblatt DJ, Shader RI: Treatment of the alcohol withdrawal syndrome, in Shader RI (ed): *Manual of Psychiatric Therapeutics.* Boston, Little, Brown & Co, 1978, pp 211-235.

40. Glaser GH: Epilepsy: Neuropsychological aspects, In Arieti S (ed): *American Handbook of Psychiatry,* ed 2. New York, Basic Book Inc, 1975, vol 4, pp 314-355.

9

The Disoriented Patient

THE PATIENT

The disoriented patient travels in a once familiar world as a stranger, at sea where once was land. Muddled, the person attempts to comprehend and cope with a changing internal universe (1).

> At 71 years of age Joe Clark feels strangely remote from life. He strikes out at his wife for no reason, spontaneously cries for a few minutes, loses his way while taking a walk in the neighborhood, rambles in his discourse, dresses shabbily, constantly reminisces about the war, becomes confused at night, fails to recognize Mrs Clark occasionally, forgets things, leaves the stove on, and makes up stories.
>
> Mr Clark retired from accounting six years ago. At the time he had noticed he made "stupid" errors. Since then he has developed further difficulty in doing even simple calculations. He has also lost interest in many activities: bridge, movies, and friends. However, if pushed by his wife, he participates. In his youth he practiced thrift; now he has become a miser.
>
> He has enjoyed excellent health throughout his life, although during a recent hospitalization for prostate surgery he became combative and accused the staff of stealing from him. The behavior ended when he returned home.
>
> Mrs Clark's apprehension grows as her husband's behavior deteriorates. He is oblivious of her concern. She wants help but fears losing him. Then within one week he gets lost, stays up all night, hallucinates, and becomes belligerently agitated. She calls the rescue unit.
>
> They respond and find a man placidly seated in the living room watching television. Mr Clark wonders who they are while Mrs Clark explains the situation to them. Mr Clark walks into the kitchen and begins to cry. He abruptly stops sobbing and asks who these people are.

126

The EMTs bring Mr and Mrs Clark to the hospital. Although skeptical about what can be done, they want to help Mrs Clark.
Mr Clark is disoriented. He has an organic mental disorder. It influences his mood, alters his perceptions, and changes his behavior.

The Patient's Mood

The disoriented patient experiences a variety of fluctuating emotions. Fluctuation characterizes these moods, which range from depression to anxiety, from a blunted quality to catastrophic rage, from anger and suspicion to serenity, and from intensity to shallowness.

The disoriented patient often rapidly changes moods. The transition from laughter to tears occurs unexpectedly, suddenly, without provocation. Inexplicably, Mr Clark sobs, feels despondent, and gives up for several minutes. Abruptly, he resumes his activity.

Disoriented patients feel depressed. They experience a sadness and melancholy borne of many losses. They have lost some of their mental accuracy, memory, and intellectual sharpness. Jobs, friends, opportunities, and experiences have gone by. The future seems dim. Joe Clark grieves about his diminished mental ability, mourns the end of his career, and views his future with concern.

Disoriented patients experience anxiety and apprehension borne of a diminished comprehension and command of the situation. The familiar has become confused and obscure; the unfamiliar, overwhelming and frightening. They feel anxious because they cannot figure things out. Even simple tasks challenge them and make them feel uncomfortable.

Frequently, disoriented patients exhibit blunted affect. They become dull, feel emotionally impoverished, and act lifeless. The diminished mental capacity leads to blandness, remoteness, and hollowness to their personalities. Their emotional withdrawal reflects this quality. Mr Clark feels and acts like a shadow of his former self.

Catastrophic rage ensues when the patient encounters a task he or she cannot perform (2). The patient has sustained severe brain damage and confronts a project which at one time would have been quite feasible. The response is rage and overwhelming anxiety. The rage reflects and amplifies the frustration which the person cannot verbally express.

A 24-year-old man suffered severe brain damage in an automobile accident. After his hospitalization he returned to his parents' home. One day he received a postcard from an old friend. The picture showed a place he had been two years before the accident. As he attempted to retrieve the memory, he became overwhelmed with anger, fear, and anxiety. He wrecked his room. Later he had no recall of the episode.

Occasionally the patient responds with anger, frustrated by the inability to perform mental tasks. Mr Clark feels annoyed by his diminished capacity. He is angry at himself and the task.

In other instances, patients display suspiciousness. They blame family and friends for their losses. Oblivious of the reasons for their own deficiencies, disoriented people see others as the cause. When Mr Clark misplaces his glasses at home and forgets where he has put them, he blames his wife.

Sometimes patients discover serenity in disorientation. They feel calm and at peace. They accept their limitations and adjust to the situation. An 84-year-old widow did fine in her apartment. She felt serene and comfortable. She handled her forgetfulness by making lists and took care of her diminished mental faculties by keeping everything organized, scheduled, and the *same* as always.

The Patient's Perceptions

The disoriented patient demonstrates pronounced perceptual alterations which vary greatly from one time to another. The affected perceptions include the thought processes, obsessions, hallucinations, illusions, delusions, and confabulations. Additional changes involve insight, orientation, and recall.

One of the more remarkable qualities of the disoriented patient is the perceptional variation from one time to another. At one time the patient speaks coherently, logically, and intelligently, demonstrating a good command of information and recall. Then a short time later the same person's discourse is disorganized and incomprehensible. These variations can occur quite dramatically and drastically within a short time.

Disoriented patients' thoughts display a number of features. These patients become circumstantial, taking forever and using much verbiage to answer a question. Disoriented people may be tangential, never replying to the actual inquiry. Or, conversely, they may exhibit a paucity of discourse, answering with few words and using a very limited vocabulary. They become almost caricatures of themselves; one man called out, "Hope, sonny!" in all situations. Disoriented patients develop either a very narrow, concrete mental approach or overly abstract thought processes. They focus on one idea or issue at a time. They develop obsessions, for example, preoccupation with bowel functions. Disoriented patients express themselves expansively, illogically, and incoherently.

The disoriented patient has hallucinations, especially visual ones. Withdrawing alcoholic patients are notorious for seeing snakes and pink elephants. Hallucinations can also be auditory, tactile, or olfactory. Hallucinations seem real, and patients react to them. In the week before ED admission, Mr Clark sees two men in his house.

Illusions are common among disoriented patients. Diminished vision, lighting, mental ability, and hearing lead to these experiences. One patient cried out, "A snake on the floor!" When he turned on the light, he discovered the snake to be a cane.

Disoriented patients develop delusions. Common delusions are that one's spouse is unfaithful and that one is the intended victim of some plot. Delusions represent a solution to forgetfulness and a manifestation of suspiciousness.

The patient confabulates. As Mercer and colleagues (3) suggest, in confabulation the patient fabricates a story in reply to a question he or she cannot answer. Mr Clark weaves great tales in response to any number of questions. He does not intentionally lie; he simply fills his mental gaps with stories.

The disorientation frequently impairs the patient's insight. Disoriented people practice denial and see nothing wrong with themselves and their behavior. They are no longer effective observers of their own behavior and their impact on others. Mr Clark remains genuinely oblivious of his limitations and his effect upon his wife.

The three spheres of orientation—person, place, and time—become affected. The person first loses appreciation of time: hour, day, date, month, and year. Later, if the condition persists and worsens, the patient experiences difficulty with place. Mr Clark has no concept of time and becomes lost when he walks too far from home. The inability to recall one's name (disorientation as to person) reflects a very severe form of organic impairment. Mr Clark does know his name.

Disorientation alters the patient's memory. The patient usually loses recent recall first. Ability to remember daily events and those within the week deteriorates. Only in severe impairment does the patient experience difficulty with distant memory. Joe Clark talks for hours about the war but cannot recall meals. He forgets who the EMTs are.

The Patient's Behavior

Disoriented patients display a number of behavioral disturbances. These patients exhibit problems with dress, activity level, self-destructiveness, violence, judgment, and adaptation to change.

Mr Clark wears old, dull, uncoordinated clothes. His shirt has several cigarette holes in it. Frequently he forgets to zip his fly.

Disoriented patients' activity level demonstrates one of two extremes. Some patients become hyperactive. They pace all the time; they must be on the go; they constantly undertake new projects, often finishing few. Other patients become very sedentary. They sit for hours, sleep much of the time, withdraw from relatives and friends, and begin no projects.

Disorientation places people at risk for intentional or accidental self-destruction. Some patients kill themselves because of their diminished ability and their depression. A 60-year-old university professor committed suicide after his memory began to deteriorate. In his note he said his knowledge was his only contribution to the world; without that, he saw no reason for living. Disoriented people also endanger themselves accidentally, through poor judgment. They walk on the road late at night or leave the gas on.

Disoriented patients sometimes become violent because of their anger, delusions, illusions, and hallucinations. Their internal restraints have become diminished. Mr Clark strikes out at his wife.

Disoriented patients exercise poor judgment. This trait results from their forgetfulness. They leave cigarettes burning; they fail to turn off the stove; they wander too far from home; they walk into traffic; they do not care what they wear.

Disoriented patients encounter difficulty in the evening. Diminished sensory capability, decreased capacity for integration, and reduced light contribute to distorted perception of the environment. Patients become confused, have illusions, and feel frightened. This phenomenon has been called "sundowning." Mr Clark has difficulty at night. He becomes distressed, disturbed, and disruptive.

Disoriented patients tolerate change very poorly. They do best in a structured, familiar environment. An alteration in the routine or a change of location challenges them. They cannot integrate and adjust rapidly. As a result they become anxious or angry. Mr Clark becomes delusional and angry in the hospital; he improves as soon as he returns home.

THE CAUSES OF DISORIENTATION

Biologic factors cause disorientation, and intrapsychic qualities and interpersonal conditions act as contributing factors.

Intrapsychic Factors in Disorientation

Personality factors contribute to disorientation in two ways. First, the organic processes tend to exaggerate and amplify personality characteristics. Second, individual features influence the way each person handles mental changes. These factors work together to constitute the intrapsychic influence.

The underlying organic factors which cause disorientation amplify and highlight the patient's premorbid personality. Often patients become almost caricatures of themselves. The quiet, introspective person changes into a withdrawn hermit. Extroverts erupt with almost manic behavior, inappropriately introducing themselves everywhere and telling jokes on all occasions. Mildly distrustful people emerge as jealous paranoids. Obsessive-compulsive people preoccupy themselves with order, cleanliness, and control. Mr Clark in his youth exhibited concern about money. He believed, "Watch the pennies and the dollars will take care of themselves." As he ages he develops an obsession about money. He never has enough, he complains about all expenses, and he counts his money each day.

Patients' personalities affect the ways they react to mental changes. Obsessive-compulsive people frequently respond to diminished capacity by becoming depressed. They no longer feel in control of their faculties. Hard-driving patients attempt to compensate by undertaking projects that do not require mental precision. Flexible, tolerant people learn to accept the limitations and adjust to them. Lipowski (4) notes that those who are dependent on the environment for their basic orientation frequently encounter difficulty and distress when they sustain organic mental disturbance.

Interpersonal Factors in Disorientation

Under extreme conditions, interpersonal factors cause disorientation; generally they instead contribute to the patient's response to organic causes.

Two extreme interpersonal conditions cause disorientation: excessive stimulation and no stimulation. In the first, too many people with too many conflicts and demands bombard the person. They cause lack of sleep and constantly vie for attention. In certain confined living situations, such as crowded tenements, the patient can experience confusion and feel lost. In the other extreme, the absence of interpersonal contacts results in disorientation. Severe sensory deprivation causes an acute loss of orientation. Solomon et al (5) report that the longer the deprivation persists, the more profound the disorientation becomes.

Biologic Causes of Disorientation

Biologic factors cause disorientation and produce organic mental disorders. The following list makes evident the fact that a great variety of biologic factors cause disorientation. It should also be clear from the nature of the listed items that it is appropriate for disoriented patients to be treated in an ED. The *italicized* causes are potentially reversible.

I. Neurologic causes of disorientation
   A. Degenerative encephalopathies
      1. Presenile dementia
         Alzheimer's disease
         Pick's disease
      2. Senile dementia
   B. The epilepsies
      1. *Postictal states*
      2. *Psychomotor seizures*
      3. *Petit mal status epilepticus*
      4. *Electroconvulsive therapy (ECT)*

C. Demyelinating disease
   1. *Multiple sclerosis*
D. Mechanical disturbance
   1. *Normal pressure hydrocephalus*
E. Huntington's disease
F. *Parkinson's disease*
G. Cerebrovascular disorders
   1. *Infarction*
   2. *Hemorrhage*
      a. Subarachnoid
      b. *Epidural*
      c. *Subdural*
      d. *Intracerebral*
   3. *Diffuse cerebral atherosclerosis*
II. Medical causes of disorientation
   A. Cardiovascular disorders
      1. *Arrhythmia*
      2. *Congestive heart failure*
      3. *Hypertensive encephalopathy*
      4. *Shock*
   B. Endocrine disorders
      1. Adrenal dysfunctions
         Hypoadrenalism
         Cushing's disease
         Pheochromocytoma
      2. Pancreas dysfunctions
         Diabetes mellitus
         Hypoglycemia
      3. Parathyroid dysfunctions
         Hypoparathyroidism
         Hyperparathyroidism
      4. *Pituitary hypofunction*
      5. Thyroid dysfunctions
         Myxedema
         Thyrotoxicosis
      6. *Eclampsia*

C. Fluid and electrolyte imbalances
   1. Fluids
      Dehydration
      Water intoxication
   2. Electrolytes
      Hypernatremia and hyponatremia
      Hypercalcemia and hypocalcemia
      Hyperkalemia and hypokalemia
      Hypermagnesemia and hypomagnesemia
D. Hematologic disorders
   1. Anemias
      Vitamin B₁₂ deficiency
      Other anemias
   2. *Polycythemia*
E. Infectious disorders
   1. *Encephalitis*
      a. Subacute sclerosing panencephalitis (SSPE) due to
         1. Measles
         2. Rubella
      b. Progressive multifocal leukoencephalopathy (PML)
      c. Jakob-Creutzfeldt syndrome
      d. *Herpes simplex*
   2. *Malaria*
   3. *Meningitis*
      a. *Bacterial*
      b. *Viral*
      c. *Fungal*
   4. *Pneumonia*
   5. *Septicemia*
   6. *General paresis*
   7. *Typhoid fever*
   8. *Cerebral abscess*
F. Metabolic disorders
   1. *Hepatic failure*
   2. *Renal failure*
   3. *Wilson's disease*

G. Oncologic influences

   1. Primary tumor

      a. *CNS tumor*

      b. *Tumors elsewhere, especially of lung, causing remote effects*

   2. Metastatic disease from:
   Lung
   Kidney
   Breast
   Thyroid
   Stomach
   Prostate

H. Pulmonary disorders

   1. *Chronic obstructive pulmonary disease*

   2. *Respiratory arrest*

I. Collagen disease

   1. *Systemic lupus erythematosus*

III. Surgery

   A. Cardiac surgery

IV. Head trauma

V. Environmental factors

   A. *Electrical shock*

   B. *Hyperthermia*

   C. *Hypothermia*

VI. Substance use

   A. Intoxication

      1. *Alcohol*

      2. Sedatives, including
      Barbiturates
      Benzodiazepines
      Bromides

      3. *Opiates*

      4. *Cocaine*

      5. *Amphetamines*

      6. *Phencyclidine (PCP)*

      7. Hallucinogens
      Lysergic acid diethylamide (LSD)
      Mescaline

      8. *Cannabis*

B. Chronic abuse
   1. *Alcohol*
C. Withdrawal syndrome
   1. *Alcohol*
   2. *Sedatives, including*
      Barbiturates
      Benzodiazepines
      Bromides
   3. *Amphetamines*
VII. Medications
   A. *Anticholinergics*
   B. *Anticonvulsants*
   C. *Digitalis*
   D. *Quinidine*
   E. *Salicylates*
   F. Antiparkinsonian drugs
      1. L-*dopa*
      2. *Extrapyramidal drugs, for example, trihexphenidyl hydrochloride (Artane)*
   G. *Penicillin*
   H. *Steroids*
   I. *Bromides*
   J. *Scopolamine*
   K. *Antimarial drugs*
   L. *Anti-inflammation drugs*
   M. Psychotropic medications
      1. *Lithium carbonate*
      2. Antidepressants, including
         Tricyclic antidepressants
         MAO inhibitors
   N. *Antineoplastic drugs*
   O. *Ergotamines*
   P. *Cimetidine*
VIII. Poisons
   A. *Methyl alcohol*
   B. *Ethylene glycol*
   C. *Organic solvents*

D. *Carbon monoxide*
E. *Heavy metals*
   Lead
   Mercury
F. *Organophosphorus insecticides*
IX. Psychiatric problems (pseudodementia)
   A. *Dissociative reactions*
      1. *Conversion reaction*
      2. *Ganser's syndrome*
      3. *Fugue state*
   B. *Depression*

THE REACTIONS OF OTHERS

The disoriented patient generates varied reactions in family and friends. They respond to the patient's gradually deteriorating mental status with depression, anger, bewilderment, denial, overprotection, fear, abandonment, concern, or a mixture of these. Their reactions often precipitate the psychiatric crisis, contribute to the evaluation and treatment, and influence the referral.

The family becomes depressed by the living loss of the loved one. The person's condition has progressively removed him or her from them, and they are deprived because of that loss. They recall the patient's prior personality, good times, and family fun; they see the person's diminished future. The spouse feels sad about the lack of companionship; the children miss the patient's emotional availability as a parent and grandparent. Mrs Clark experiences a depression as her husband deteriorates. His dementia erodes her hopes and plans.

Family and friends feel anger toward the patient. They respond with anger to the loss of their relationship. Additionally, the person's forgetfulness, poor judgment, exaggerated personality traits, lability of affect, and lack of comprehension annoy them. They complain of having to repeat themselves all the time or of having to "baby sit." They resent the evening disturbances.

The patient's mood lability and perceptional alterations cause bewilderment to both family and friends. They experience great difficulty in adjusting to the unpredictability. At one time of day the person acts appropriately, demonstrates good comprehension, and responds warmly; at another time he or she becomes belligerent, forgets recent events, and withdraws.

In some cases, the family responds with denial; in others, it reacts by infantalizing the patient. In the former reaction the family simply refuses to recognize the patient's changes. They deny having any problems and conduct family business as usual. In the latter response the family smothers the patient. They do *every-*

thing for the person, deprive the patient of any autonomy, and treat him or her like a child.

Families sometimes react with fear. This fear has two meanings. First, family members may actually become frightened by the patient. The moods, violence, and unpredictabilities make them afraid. Certainly Mrs Clark has reason to fear physical abuse from her husband. Second, families fear the loss of the patient. They do not want their family member placed in a nursing home or hospital. They desire the person's presence at home regardless of mental condition. Mrs Clark clearly wants to be with her husband. She is afraid that getting help will lead to his placement in an old people's home.

In other circumstances, the family feels unable to care for the patient and wants him or her out of the home. They are overwhelmed and burdened by the disorientation. The patient requires too much time, acts too inappropriately, and exceeds all reasonable family capabilities. They seek and, on occasion, demand hospitalization or nursing home placement.

But most often the family reacts with concern. They recognize a problem exists and seek assistance. They want to help the patient. But they also want aid in controlling the behavior.

THE INITIATION OF THE EMERGENCY

A number of events produce EMT and ED intervention with disoriented patients. Although the basic organic mental disorder may have been evolving for days or decades, certain of the patient's actions or the family's responses call for immediate assistance. The patient generates the crisis by becoming violent or self-destructive, by feeling distressed about the symptoms, and by getting lost. The family asks for help when they sense the person needs medical attention, when they can no longer tolerate the behavior, or when they feel inadequate to provide care. Generally, the more rapid the evolution of the disorientation, the more quickly the family seeks help. This chapter focuses upon the slowly developing organic mental disorder. Chapter 13, the Patient Reacting to Alcohol or Abused Substances, discusses rapidly emerging disorientation.

The patient's violent behavior triggers a crisis. In confusion and frustration, the disoriented person attacks others. These combative episodes are rarely organized. A careful history frequently reveals that the patient only *threatened* violence, raising a cane or shouting obscenities. Mr Clark strikes out at his wife.

The patient's self-destructive threats and behavior precipitate the crisis. Often the patient recognizes the mental decline, feels depressed, foresees no improvement, and attempts suicide. Disoriented people also engage in unintentional self-destructive activity: walking in traffic, leaving the stove on, or neglecting to take prescribed medication.

In other situations, patients with insight become alarmed by their symptoms. They recognize that crying all the time, anxiety, insomnia, pacing, and becoming too easily fatigued are signals of a problem. They are aware of their loss of memory and want help with it. They know that they do not know.

Not infrequently, the patient comes to the EMTs' and ED's attention by getting lost. At that point the police find a confused, unidentified person who has wandered too far from home or has become disoriented while shopping.

The majority of emergencies arise because the family or friends seek help. The patients frequently remain oblivious of the inappropriateness of their own statement and actions.

The family seeks medical attention. They recognize loss of memory and disorientation as signals of an underlying medical problem. They want a medical evaluation and examination of their loved one. They look for a diagnosis and a treatment plan.

Or they can no longer tolerate the behavior. The violence, inappropriate statements, dress, and behavior, and the disruptions have made living with the person impossible. The family feels too much stress and distress.

Finally, the family members recognize the limits of their ability to sustain the patient. The need for constant attention, supervision, and structure becomes too much for them. They cannot leave the patient alone even for a short time. Despite their love and concern, they cannot manage any more. They seek an alternative placement.

THE EMTs' RESPONSE TO THE EMERGENCY

The disoriented patient requires an organized and structured EMT response. In the face of a "confused" patient, the EMTs provide a firm, controlling approach and have the responsibility to impose order on the situation. The EMTs' approach must include a prompt response, early and frequent personal identification, a command of the situation, removal of dangerous implements, a stated and reiterated intervention plan, an appreciation of their own attitudes, structure, involvement of the family, and constant accompaniment of the patient.

The EMTs must respond promptly. Their presence checks the disorientation. A rapid intervention establishes their interest in the person and family and sets the tone for the remaining sequence.

The EMTs must identify themselves and periodically remind the patient of their identification. They use both their formal names and professional titles. They must address the patient by his or her formal name. By doing this they underscore the person's adult role and check the tendency to infantalize the patient. More important, they must continually reintroduce themselves and in this fashion can correct any of the patient's misconceptions about the reason for their presence. The disoriented patient forgets their names. By the time Mr Clark reaches the kitchen he has forgotten their names.

Early in the intervention the EMTs must establish their control of the situation. They must emphasize that the patient requires attention and that they will provide it. By their vocal tones and activities, they display command of the situation.

They must remove any dangerous implements. The disoriented patient often strikes out randomly to express anger and frustration. The EMTs must take away potential weapons: canes, knitting needles, scissors, and so forth.

The EMTs must state and reiterate the intervention plan. The stated plan reassures the patient and, most of all, the family. The EMTs must periodically remind the patient of the plan.

EMTs must be aware of their own attitudes. They may believe they have nothing to offer. The problems encountered by the patient and family may seem like natural aspects of aging. If the EMTs see the patient's condition as irreversible, they feel impotent. They do not feel they can offer anything to Mr and Mrs Clark. They must put forward a firm, professional, helping approach.

They must impose structure on the situation. They do this through their presence and their intervention plan. But most importantly, they can establish a physical structure with limits. The rescue vehicle provides boundaries and the structure; it furnishes an orientation.

The family must be involved in the intervention. They provide the historical and medical information. Often they are the only reliable source of that information. They can stay with the patient. They must accompany the patient and the EMTs to the ED. Mrs Clark is the most important source of information concerning her husband.

Finally, someone must accompany the patient at all times. The disoriented patient has a high risk of wandering off. In confusion the person will walk away and into danger: traffic or the woods. Additionally, the companion provides continual orientation, reassurance, and direction for the patient.

THE EMERGENCY DEPARTMENT EVALUATION

The ED is uniquely suited to provide comprehensive evaluation of disoriented patients. It has the capability to investigate both the medical and psychiatric dimensions of the crisis, to address each, and to set up proper referrals. The ED approach encompasses the reception, the physical examination, the chief complaint, the psychiatric evaluation, and the mental status examination.

The Reception

The reception sets the stage and ensures the medical and psychiatric evaluation (6). During the reception, ED staff must establish their control of the situation, provide limits and structure for the patient, and take responsibility for the person. The reception involves a prompt response, staff identification, clearly delineated structure, controlled sensory input, recognition of personnel attitudes, family participation, and constant supervision.

The disoriented patient needs a prompt ED reception for several reasons. By the staff's rapid intervention they establish their command and control of the situation. By this response, they preclude the patient's wandering about the ED. A 55-year-old, disoriented man walked from cubicle to cubicle, introducing himself to other patients and thoroughly disrupting the ED.

The reception commences with an introduction and identification of staff and an orientation of the patient. Staff must use both formal names and professional titles. They must address the patient by formal name and avoid infantilizing, diminutive first names. In the reception the staff also orients the patient by reminding the person of his or her own name and explaining where the patient is and what time it is.

The staff establishes a structure for the patient and family in a number of ways. They advance a treatment plan and then periodically reiterate it. They orient the patient frequently. They employ a quiet room away from the turmoil of the rest of the ED. This room provides boundaries and limits for the patient.

Staff must control the sensory stimulation the patient receives. The patient has difficulty comprehending and integrating the ED experience. The strangeness, newness, confusion, noise, and rapid pace of the ED increase discomfort and anxiety for the disoriented patient. A quiet room and a limited number of staff interacting with the patient help to control the sensory input.

Staff must recognize their own attitudes toward the disoriented patient and then display a professional posture. Staff occasionally demonstrate irritation with patients who have chronic organic mental disorders. They express annoyance about the presence of such a patient in an acute treatment facility and doubt, also, that they have anything to offer. They view the patient as being "dumped" and resent the family. The disoriented person frustrates their efforts by slow replies or by inappropriate answers to their questions. The patient's inability to recall details hampers their history taking. In the face of the patient's rambling discourse and loss of memory, the staff must display a firm, professional approach.

The family's participation must be secured. They can furnish key medical and psychiatric information. In fact, under some circumstances the family and friends may be the only sources of data. They can stay with the patient and become involved in the referral process. Mrs Clark calls for assistance. She also supplies key historical data and plays a major role in the referral.

Finally, staff or family must be with the patient at all times. This prevents wandering about or leaving the ED. It checks any self-destructive behavior. The accompanying person can continually orient the patient and provide companionship. The disoriented patient can be overwhelmed by the strange ED environment and can react catastrophically. Having someone present and interpreting the milieu to the patient at all times prevents this reaction.

Physical Examination

The disoriented patient requires a physical examination. It commences with pulse, blood pressure, and temperature but includes a complete neurologic and medical examination. Denny-Brown (7), Scheinberg and associates (8), and Van Allen (9) provide excellent guides to this critical physical examination. Laboratory studies must be performed: skull films, urinalysis, hematocrit, hemoglobin, white blood cell count, electrolytes, blood gases, serum glucose, BUN, spinal fluid analysis, electrocardiogram, and chest film.

In the neurologic and medical examination, the physician must pay particular attention to the number of facets. In the neurologic section the physician must note the state of the pupils and their reactivity, visualize the fundus, and observe the eye movements for nystagmus. The reflexes must be assessed, especially the snout, palmomental, and Babinski reflexes and checked for asymmetry. The medical examination must emphasize the cardiac, pulmonary, and abdominal areas.

Chief Complaint

The chief complaint characterizes the patient, the crisis, and the family's reactions. The patient reveals much by saying, "I don't know why I'm here," "Who are you?" and "I want to go home." Some patients demonstrate insight by reporting, "I'm losing my memory," or "I get confused easily." The chief complaint depicts the crisis: "I'm lost," or "My family wants me here." Or it depicts the family's dynamics: "We pay taxes, you must help him," "We cannot cope," "Please help us," or "He tried to kill me."

Psychiatric Evaluation

The ED physician must gain a complete psychiatric and medical history from the patient, the family, and the patient's physician. The doctor and hospital chart furnish essential information. The physician, in developing the evaluation, focuses on the history of present illness (HPI); social history; family history; psychiatric history, including use of psychotropic medication; occupational background; history of alcohol and substance use; and medical history, emphasizing diseases, surgery, trauma, and medications.

The HPI explains and amplifies recent events. It highlights acute changes, the patient's current behavior, and the family's responses. It aims to answer the basic question of why the emergency occurred now rather than at another time. The crisis provides insights about the patient, the patient's dynamics, the medical problem, and the family's interaction. These insights are especially significant in view of the chronic course that the disoriented patient follows. Mr Clark has had a long history of difficulty but only after the combination of his getting lost, staying up at night, and striking out does his wife call for help.

The social history furnishes data about where the patient lives and with whom. An 84-year-old man lived alone. In his disorientation he left lighted cigarettes about the apartment and forgot to turn off the stove. His apartment was in a large cluster of wooden tenements. His behavior constituted a danger to himself and the neighborhood. The ED physician arranged for hospitalization.

The family history offers information concerning familial patterns of disease. A number of diseases which cause organic mental disorders are inherited, for example, Huntington's disease.

The physician pays attention to the psychiatric history, emphasizing medications. In delineating the differential diagnosis between organic disease and a function illness such as depression, the physician focuses on history of psychiatric treatment, hospitalization, and medication. Not infrequently, the patient currently takes a psychotropic preparation.

The physician must investigate the patient's occupational background. In today's highly technological civilization people are exposed to a variety of toxic materials on the job. Lead and mercury can cause signs and symptoms of organic mental disorder.

Alcohol and abused substances contribute to or cause the patient's disorientation. Disorientation occurs during acute intoxication (with alcohol, PCP, LSD, and barbiturates), as a result of chronic use (of alcohol), and during the withdrawal phase (of abuse of alcohol and barbiturates). The physician must vigorously pursue a history of alcohol and substance use. It is necessary to inquire specifically into the amount consumed and for what period, and whether there have been recent changes in intake.

The physician must develop a complete medical evaluation, including inquiry into current diseases, recent surgery, trauma, and medication. Neurologic and medical diseases cause disorientation. Cardiac surgery has been highly correlated with disorientation. Head trauma, especially if subdural hematoma results, alters the mental status. Medications precipitate disorientation.

Mental Status Examination

The mental status examination is the most important psychiatric tool for assessing the disoriented patient, pointing toward an organic diagnosis, and documenting the patient's state *at that moment*. Since the behavior of the disoriented patient usually changes from time to time, the examination records it at the time of evaluation and serves as a reference point for later comparisons. In assessing the patient's mental status, the physician must evaluate appearance, affect, thought content, suicidal thoughts, plans for homicide, judgment, insight, intellect, and above all the sensorium. Assessment findings must be accurately and completely documented.

The disoriented patient's appearance often furnishes the diagnosis. These patients are disheveled, unshaven, and unkempt. Frequently they have cigarette holes in their unbuttoned shirts. They wear ill-fitting, uncoordinated apparel. They pace or sit motionless and without eye contact.

Disoriented patients' affect is labile and shallow. Their mood rapidly changes from depression to indifference to silliness, without apparent cause. Their emotions seem superficial, hollow, and plastic. The interviewer experiences difficulty sensing the patient's feelings.

The thought content furnishes diagnostic clues in its alterations and organization, and through its delusions, obsessions, hallucinations, and illusions. The disoriented patient's level of coherence and consciousness changes during the interview. At certain points the patient's conversation flows coherently; at other points it rambles illogically. Disoriented people may have delusions. They may become preoccupied by certain concerns, especially their health. They experience hallucinations, usually visual ones. They distort the environment by having illusions.

The physician must ask about suicide and homicide. The patient caught up in disorientation can become self-destructive and combative.

The physician must assess the patient's judgment. This can be done through the HPI and family's report.

The physician must explore the patient's insight into his or her condition. Disoriented patients often possess little insight.

An estimation of the patient's intelligence provides another comparison point. The organic disease erodes the patient's intelligence and diminishes mental capabilities. Mr Clark has prided himself on his accounting ability; now he has difficulty performing simple calculations.

The physician must emphasize the sensorium examination: orientation, recall, calculations, and proverbs. The patient's orientation to person, place, and time must be assessed. The physician asks about time of day, day of week, date, month, and year, and inquires about where and who the patient thinks he or she is.

The physician evaluates recall in three dimensions: immediate, recent, and distant. Immediate recall is tested by asking the patient to remember three test words (table, red, and 63 Broadway) for one minute. Recent recollection pertains to events of the last several days; distant recall has to do with past experiences such as high school. In the HPI, the patient reveals loss of recent recall. Recent and immediate memory losses are the hallmarks of organic mental disorder.

The physician uses mathematics to further delineate the patient's mental status by asking the person to subtract 7 serially from 100 (100 minus 7 equals 93, 7 from 93 equals 86, and so on down to 2). Most people can do this subtraction with only one or two mistakes. The test measures the patient's ability to handle a number of complex problems.

Finally, the physician asks the patient to interpret proverbs. The disoriented patient either gives "concrete," literal replies or cannot handle the subject at all. When the physician asks Mr Clark what is meant by "People who live in glass houses should not throw stones," he replies, "They will break the window." Disoriented patients lose their abstracting ability. They cannot expound on proverbs; they instead can express only the most narrow, specific interpretation of them.

DIAGNOSIS, TREATMENT PLAN, AND IMMEDIATE EMERGENCY DEPARTMENT THERAPY

The evaluation culminates in a diagnosis, determines the treatment plan, and indicates what kind of immediate ED therapy is appropriate.

Diagnosis

The ED physician diagnoses Mr Clark as having progressive idiopathic dementia of senile onset and with depressive features. He bases his diagnosis on the history obtained from Mrs Clark, the physical examination, laboratory studies, and Mr Clark's mental status.

The history indicates a gradually developing change in his mental condition and behavior. He does not have a record of hypertension, diabetes, or heart failure. He takes no medications and only occasionally consumes alcohol. Except for recent prostate surgery, he has not been hospitalized for 50 years.

The neurologic examination reveals no focal abnormality, papilledema, or asymmetry. The cardiovascular examination demonstrates a normal pulse, blood pressure, and rhythm. The lungs are clear. Laboratory studies showed no evidence of anemia, electrolyte disturbance,

*renal or hepatic failure, or glucose abnormality. The physician reads Mr
Clark's ECG as within normal limits.*

*The significant mental status findings include the patient's disheveled
appearance, labile but generally depressed affect, rambling discourse
with visual hallucinations, poor judgment and insight, diminished intellectual ability, disorientation to time, loss of recent recall, difficulty with
calculations, and concrete interpretation of proverbs.*

For the diagnosis of progressive idiopathic dementia to be made, specific criteria
must be met (10). First, the assessment data must fit the criteria for dementia.
That is, the patient must demonstrate (1) deterioration of intellectual abilities; (2)
memory impairment; (3) impaired abstract reasoning, or poor judgment or
impulse control, or altered personality; and (4) no intoxication or delirium; in
addition (5) tests must reveal a physical causative factor or, in the absence of a
physical cause, all other psychiatric etiologies must be eliminated. Second, the
condition must have begun insidiously and followed a uniformly progressive course
of deterioration. Third, specific other causes of dementia must have been eliminated by history, examination, and tests.

Treatment Plan

The evaluation and the family reactions determine the treatment plan for the
disoriented patient. The evaluation indicates areas to investigate further in order
to reach a confirmed diagnosis, and it also identifies target symptoms to treat.
The family's response to the patient suggests reasonable referral possibilities.

The treatment plan encompasses the immediate ED therapy, treatment of
underlying physical conditions, diminution of symptoms by making alterations in
the patient's life and medications, and referral.

Immediate Emergency Department Therapy

The ED intervention for the disoriented patient provides immediate therapy in a
number of areas. It controls the patient's behavior. It commences the identification
of the etiology. It allows the patient to feel helped and supplies support to the
family. It arranges the proper referral.

The ED intervention controls the behavior. By supplying structure, the staff
take command of the situation and halt the disruptive activities. Personnel challenge the patient's disorientation by helping him or her become oriented. This
approach suggests to family members that the patient can be controlled and
assisted.

ED intervention launches the investigation to find the underlying cause of the
person's disorientation. Through the history, physical examination, and laboratory

studies, the search for the causes commences. The patient and family find reassurance through the investigative approach.

Patients can gain immediate relief from the evaluation. They feel people pay attention to them. Their disruptions in a sense reflect their wish for people to care about them. They may feel isolated, depressed, and forgotten. Mr Clark sees himself as useless and unimportant. The interview process emphasized his significance.

The family benefits from the evaluation. They can finally tell their story and feel someone listens. Mrs Clark is overjoyed when the ED physician indicates that her husband can be treated and that his behavior can improve.

Finally, the ED intervention arranges for the referral. This referral includes further laboratory studies, psychotherapy, medication, and help for the patient at home or placement in the appropriate facility.

CARE AFTER THE EMERGENCY

Mrs Clark wants her husband at home. Despite the physician's suggestion of a nursing home, she wishes only to have help in keeping him at home. Together Mrs Clark and the physician organize his home care program.

That program has several aspects. Mrs Clark will establish a regular, fixed, daily schedule. She will place a large calendar in the kitchen and keep a night light on. She will continue to encourage her husband to go out. The ED social worker arranges for a mental health worker to visit the Clarks twice a week. In addition to the worker's seeing Mr Clark, the visit will free Mrs Clark to get away for a couple of hours. The social worker also sets up an appointment to a senior citizens' center. Once a week the patient can get together there with others. The ED physician refers Mr Clark to a family physician, since Mr Clark does not have a doctor. The physician also prescribes doxepin (Sinequan) 10 mg three times daily and haloperidol (Haldol) 2 mg at bedtime.

Mrs Clark appreciates the evaluation and treatment program. Mr Clark smiles, not knowing why, and goes along with the program. He improves at home on this regimen.

Four factors determine the appropriate referral for the disoriented patient. The reversibility of the underlying cause influences the referral decision. Where the cause of the disorientation is potentially reversible, the physician must employ vigorous treatment. The patient with digitalis toxicity requires hospitalization. The severity of the symptoms and the behavior dictate the referral. A violent, assaultive, disoriented patient requires restraint and institutional controls. The reaction of the family directs the patient referral. Mrs Clark's strong desire to care for her husband makes home treatment feasible. Some families demand institutional placement. The availability of resources influences the referral. The family has to wait until a nursing home bed becomes available.

A number of referral options are available for disoriented patients. These include hospitalization, nursing home placement, day treatment programs, home visits, and outpatient psychotherapy.

Hospitalization becomes the treatment of choice under several circumstances. The violent, combative, potentially homicidal, disoriented patient needs hospitalization. The suicidal disoriented patient also requires hospitalization. The patient with a medically or surgically treatable cause to the disorientation benefits from inpatient intervention. Occasionally, where no family alternatives exist, and the patient displays severe disorientation, acute care hospitalization is the only option.

Boarding homes and nursing homes frequently provide the most effective long-term care for the disoriented patient. They supervise the patient; orient him or her; and provide structure, socialization, and food.

A variety of day treatment experiences help to sustain disoriented patients in the community. These include church groups, senior citizens' groups, day treatment programs, and activity groups. They serve two functions. First, they offer patients a social outlet, a place to go. Second, it provides relief for the family. While the patient attends the program the family members are free to do other things.

Home visits benefit the patient greatly. They furnish social experience at home. The visits become a focus in an isolated life, and they help patients and families see that someone cares. Mr Clark looks forward to the visits of the mental health worker and appreciates the interest and interaction.

Patients gain from outpatient psychotherapy. They can use it to resolve conflicts about aging and diminished capacity. Therapy breaks down isolation and permits patients to talk about themselves. It also provides for monitoring and adjusting medications.

A number of principles apply to the treatment of disoriented patients in all referral settings. These involve structure, attention to physical condition, orientation, optimum stimulation, and medications.

Structure sustains disoriented patients. Staff or family must strive to develop a daily schedule and then adhere to it. A posted program helps patients to orient themselves.

Disoriented patients require careful monitoring of their physical condition. Frequently they neglect their own health and ignore changes. Medical alterations affect the disoriented and cause further deterioration. The ED physician arranges for Mr Clark to be followed by a family doctor.

People in the patient's environment must periodically orient him or her. Staff and family often overlook the memory problems. They assume the person remembers. To forestall the patient's anxiety and embarrassment, other people must reintroduce themselves and provide gentle reminders about the date and place. The disoriented patient requires a specific level of stimulation. Too much input escalates anxiety, confusion, and distress. Alternatively, too little sensory input promotes disorientation. The understimulated person withdraws and further loses interest in society.

Psychotropic medications benefit the disoriented patient when used appropriately and in correct dosage (11). Elderly patients require smaller doses of these medications, experience many of the side effects, and have greater difficulty metabolizing the drugs (12). The agitated patient requires thioridazine (Mellaril) 10 to 25 mg three times a day or haloperidol (Haldol) 1 to 2 mg three times daily. Minor tranquilizers cloud the patient's consciousness and produce further disorientation. A low dosage of doxepin (Sinequan), 10 mg three times daily or 25 mg at bedtime, is effective for depressed patients. If a patient becomes preoccupied with certain ideas, trifluoperazine (Stelazine) 1 mg twice or three times daily interrupts the obsessions. For sleep, chloral hydrate 250 to 1000 mg at bedtime or diphenhydramine hydrochloride (Benadryl) 25 to 50 mg at bedtime is effective.

REFERENCES

1. Pitt B: The muddled patient. *Practitioner* 220:199-202, 1978.
2. Goldstein K: *After-effects of Brain Injuries in War.* New York, Grune & Stratton, 1942.
3. Mercer B, Wapner W, Gardner H, et al: A study of confabulation. *Arch Neurol* 34:429-433, 1977.
4. Lipowski Z: Organic brain syndromes: Overview and classification, in Benson DF, Blumer D (eds): *Psychiatric Aspects of Neurologic Disease.* New York, Grune & Stratton, 1975, pp 11-35.
5. Solomon P, Leiderman PH, Mendelson J, et al: Sensory deprivation. *Am J Psychiatry* 114:357-363, 1957.
6. MacKinnon RA, Michels R: *The Psychiatric Interview in Clinical Practice.* Philadelphia, WB Saunders Co, 1971.
7. Denny-Brown D: *Handbook of Neurological Examination and Case Recording.* Cambridge, Harvard University Press, 1972.
8. Scheinberg LC, Taylor JM, Schaumburg HH: *Neurology Handbook.* Flushing NY, Medical Examination Publishing Co, 1972.
9. Van Allen MW: *Pictorial Manual of Neurologic Tests.* Chicago, Year Book Medical Publishers, 1969.
10. *Diagnostic and Statistical Manual of Mental Disorders,* ed 3. Washington DC, American Psychiatric Association, 1980.
11. Salzman C, Van der Kolk B, Shader RI: in Shader RI (ed): *Manual of Psychiatric Therapeutics.* Boston, Little Brown & Co, 1978, pp 171-184.
12. Beattie BC, Sellers EM: Psychoactive drug use in the elderly: The pharmocokinetics. *Psychosomatics* 20:474-479, 1979.

10

The Suicidal Patient

Thousands of Americans attempt suicide in an effort to solve their struggles and conflicts. Over 25,000 succeed annually (1). Suicide—the threat and the act—consitutes a major psychiatric emergency.

THE PATIENT

Sally Stoller sits alone with a bottle of aspirin tablets and starts to ingest them. She has not been sleeping or eating well, has been drinking more, and has been depressed. She has just telephoned her boyfriend, whom she had recently broken up with, to say good-bye. Her father committed suicide when she was 12 years old. She saw a physician four weeks ago for headaches, and last week she talked to a girl friend about killing herself.

Miss Stoller, a Protestant, attends graduate school as a chemistry major and lives alone. She went to a psychotherapist for 10 sessions during her freshman year at college because she felt "down" and could find no meaning in life. She believes the world will be better off without her.

When she does not answer the telephone, her boyfriend calls the police and the rescue unit. Both arrive at the same time as he does. Despite her developing lethargy, she asks them to leave. As they confer she takes out a razor blade. They remove both the pills and the blade. At their insistence she accompanies them to the ED.

Suicidal patients demonstrate a wide spectrum of moods, perceptions, and behaviors. This variety stands in contrast to the unified description of depressed and anxious patients. For each patient, threatening, attempting, and completing suicide represents a unique constellation of characteristics, motives, and stresses.

149

The Patient's Mood

One of several emotions dominates the suicidal person's mood: depression, fear, anger, or calm. Each mood reaches an extraordinary intensity. The patient experiences the affect with an unrelenting, overwhelming pain that makes suicide seem the *only* alternative.

The suicidal patient most commonly feels deeply depressed; the depression is characterized by despair and desperation and dominated by feelings of hopelessness and helplessness. The future ceases to matter; life has no meaning. Sally Stoller feels hopelessness and desperation.

Other suicidal patients experience intense fear. Fear, panic, and anxiety are extremely stressful and intolerable emotions from which patients seek any means of escape.

> A 58-year-old man suffered from advanced chronic obstructive pulmonary disease (COPD) and encountered extreme dyspnea on trips to the bathroom. Additionally, he had a cardiac condition necessitating surgery. The thought of an operation terrified him. He committed suicide with a handgun the day before his scheduled hospital admission. His current discomfort was difficult, but the dread of surgery made his life unbearable.

Some patients feel angry and use suicide to obtain revenge. Frequently they want a lover, parent, child, or friend to be hurt by their death. They fantasy their families expressing regrets at the graveside. They leave notes proclaiming their rage. They adopt an "I'll show them" attitude. In one sense Sally Stoller wants to get back at her boyfriend, to show him what he did to her, and to make him feel bad.

In some instances the patient experiences a remarkable calm before attempting suicide. To them suicide represents a solution, an end to strife, and an escape from both mental and physical pain. One 30-year-old man struggled with a severe depressive illness for several months. He had manic-depressive disease. During that time his physician used antidepressants and electroconvulsive therapy (ECT) without success. Suddenly the patient appeared different. He felt better and became calm. Two days later, while on pass from the inpatient unit, he hanged himself. His note said, "I have found a way out of the pain."

The Patient's Perceptions

Several types of perceptual experiences contribute to the suicidal patient's mental picture. These include nihilistic delusions, extreme guilt, seeking of spiritual reunion, wanting just punishment, and self-destructive hallucinations. These perceptions often reach the delusional level and reflect major psychopathology.

Some patients develop delusions that they are intensely evil. They view themselves as a source of corruption and pestilence which must be removed. One schizophrenic young man asked his mother for a gun to shoot himself because "I am so bad." He believed the world would be saved by his death.

An extreme sense of guilt propels some people into suicidal behavior. They consider themselves undesirably burdensome to loved ones. Both depressed patients and chronically, physically ill patients find dependence and help intolerable. Sally Stoller does not want to be a burden to society, her mother, or her friends any longer.

Some patients enter into a suicidal act in the hope of achieving reunion with a dead loved one. They believe that through their death they can rejoin a lost spouse, lover, or parent.

Sometimes people attempt to kill themselves as punishment for some wrongdoing. A 48-year-old police officer attempted to hang himself. Earlier that day his service revolver had accidentally discharged, killing his wife. He cited the Biblical saying "An eye for an eye" as the reason for his death. In other situations a patient may inflate a slight indiscretion into a cause for suicide. A 24-year-old, very sensitive woman wanted to kill herself after making a minor bookkeeping error at work. She believed her employer would fire her for permanently marring the company name.

Finally, some patients receive messages about self-destruction. These messages generally take the form of auditory hallucinations. The patient notes that the "voices command me to die" or "I was told to kill myself." In other situations patients envision their own death and act out "the scene."

The Patient's Behavior

Suicidal patients demonstrate a range of behavior. At one extreme, they attempt self-destruction impulsively; at the other, they meticulously plan their death. In the middle area patients ambivalently approach death. At the extremes, the probability of succeeding increases.

The impulsive people act on the emotions of the moment, use available implements, and, if they survive, often regret their behavior. They react to acute loss, alcohol, or the street drugs. They take available medications, use a gun only if one is readily accessible, or cut themselves if a knife is at hand. Later, upon reflection, such a person may say, "I did a silly thing." A 16-year-old girl found out her "steady" had "dumped" her for another girl. She ran into the bathroom and took five aspirin. She felt sick, vomited, and went downstairs and told her parents. Later, she did not want him "anyway" and felt ashamed.

At the other extreme, patients meticulously orchestrate their own death. They plan suicide. They stockpile pills. They purchase a gun and ammunition. They learn how to attach the exhaust pipe to the inside of the car, or they investigate the least painful way to die. If these patients do not succeed in killing themselves, they become angry and disappointed and plan to try again. A 50-year-old businessman fills several prescriptions for barbiturates at different pharmacies, goes to a distant town, registers under an assumed name at a hotel, and takes all the pills. He tells his family he is on a business trip. His office does not expect to hear from him for two days.

Most suicidal patients fit somewhere between these extremes. They telegraph messages to family and friends about their distress. They visit physicians' offices. They take pills when they know someone might discover them before they die. They want to die; they also want help; they just do not really know (2). Sally Stoller sends her distress signal to her physician, her friend, and her boyfriend.

THE CAUSES OF SUICIDAL BEHAVIOR

Intrapsychic, interpersonal, and biologic factors cause, contribute to, or correlate with suicidal behavior in several ways. They precipitate a suicidal act. They predispose the patient to employ self-destructive behavior when under stress. They diminish the patient's controls and allow suicidal drives to surface. They correlate statistically and clinically to suicide attempts and completions.

Intrapsychic Causes of Suicidal Behavior

The decision to kill oneself involves a number of intrapsychic factors. Certain childhood experiences predispose one to consider suicide. Attitudes toward self, life, and control influence one to reflect upon and enact self-destruction. Particular hallucinations propel individuals toward suicide. Religion correlates with suicidal behavior.

A suicide in the family affects all the surviving members. As Dubin (3) observed, children especially feel the impact of a parent's suicide. Such an event predisposes them later in their lives to consider suicide. Self-destruction has been established as one of the family's mechanisms to cope with stress. If the patient identified closely with the suicidal relative, he or she may feel a compulsion to repeat the behavior. Her father's suicide greatly influences Sally Stoller. She wonders whether she might be just like him.

Extremely negative self-images and self-concepts promote suicidal behavior. Patients then consider themselves unredeemable sinners, deformed, imperfect, inadequate, or worthless.

Some people attempt and complete suicide because they cannot find any meaning to life. They see no mission, no order, and no purpose. As Viktor Frankl

(4,p20) cites, the reason for suicide is that "life seemed meaningless." Sally Stoller struggles to find a reason for her life. In college she sought therapy to help her find it. In graduate school she is lost.

Control is a major issue for suicidal people. They must be in command of their lives, their environments, and their destinies. If circumstances trap them, then suicide is one area in which they still can be in control. Nietzsche (5,p91) noted, "The thought of suicide is a great consolation: by means of it one gets successfully through many a bad night." The 58-year-old man with severe COPD found himself trapped by illness, imprisoned by physical limitations, and terrified by the impending operation. He felt he controlled only one thing—his death.

Hallucinations influence some patients to take their lives. Most commonly these people, who have either a thought disorder or a drug reaction, experience auditory hallucinations telling them to commit suicide. The voices accuse the patients of wrongdoing and command them to die. Patients report hearing "voices in my head" ordering them to cut themselves, jump out a window, or run into an oncoming vehicle. Other patients see scenes of their own death or of dead people beckoning them.

Protestants have a much higher rate of suicide than do Catholics or Jews (3).

Interpersonal Causes of Suicidal Behavior

Interpersonal factors constitute the major determinants of suicidal behavior. The two principal factors involve disturbed relationships and significant losses. Additionally, one's occupation and living situation correlate with suicide attempts and completions.

The patient uses suicide both to escape from and to influence a disturbed, conflicting relationship. In the former situation, an intolerable, stressful relationship causes one to consider suicide as a way out. A person may, for example, feel trapped by his boss, dominated by his girl friend, unappreciated by his wife, or oppressed by his parents. In the other situation, the patient's suicidal behavior provides a powerful message to the other party. These patients want the significant others to recognize the patients' distress and to know about the depression or anger.

Losses precipitate suicide attempts and completions. Widowed people have a higher rate of suicide than married people (6). The death reflects the depression and for some the wish to join the departed. Other losses include divorces, children's leaving home, surgery, and outcomes of political elections. Loss produces depression; depression leads to suicide. Sally Stoller responds to loss of her boyfriend by taking an overdose.

Certain professions and occupations have excessive suicide rates. Blachly and colleagues (7) report that physicians, dentists, and attorneys kill themselves at alarmingly high rates. According to Frankl (4), suicide is the second commonest cause of death in the college student population. Heiman (8) notes that law officers have a high suicide rate. The unemployed are overrepresented in self-destructive incidents.

A stressful living situation leads a person to attempt suicide. Prison is an extremely painful social environment. Smialek and Spitz (9) point out that prisoners kill themselves at an extremely high rate. The successful suicide rate among people who live alone is also high.

Biologic Causes of Suicidal Behavior

Biologic factors correlate with self-destructive behavior. These factors include alcohol, drugs, illness, and organicity, sex, and age.

Alcohol becomes involved in suicidal behavior in a number of ways (1). Patients attempt suicide because of alcoholism. The economic and social decline initiated by drinking leads to depression and suicide. Depression is deepened by continuing use of alcohol as losses become more intense and defeats greater. Alcohol seems to bring out suicidal thoughts and behavior that are successfully avoided when one is sober. Numerous suicidal people attempt suicide only while intoxicated. Sally Stoller has been drinking more since her romance broke up. The drinking has increased her depression, distorted her judgment, and accelerated her wish to die.

Abused substances contribute to self-destructive behavior. They provide a readily available route to death. Excessive intravenous heroin or cocaine ranks as a frequent cause of death in the drug-using population. Coming off amphetamines produces depression. Both LSD and PCP cause "bad trips," psychosis, and self-destructive behavior.

Some patients respond to medical illness with suicide. This reaction occurs most frequently in chronic, unrelenting, disabling, painful diseases. High suicide rates have been noted among patients with cancer, COPD, and spinal cord injuries. Abram and associates (10) report that patients on hemodialysis have a suicide rate 400 times that of the general population.

Organic brain impairment contributes to suicidal behavior. It deepens the depression. It produces confusion by which the patient frequently "accidentally" ingests too many pills. It impairs judgment and clouds the future.

Other biologic correlates of suicide include sex and age. Women exceed men in suicide attempts, but men surpass women in completed suicides. The rate of completed suicides increases with age. The older the patient, the more likely he or she is to actually succeed in the suicide attempt.

THE REACTIONS OF OTHERS

The patient's suicide messages and attempt produce a variety of responses in family members and friends. They feel anger and guilt. Some avoid the patient.

Others make light of the threat or the attempt. Still others offer encouragement to repeat the attempt. Many find themselves confused. Most show concern and intervene. Their reactions affect and often determine the outcome of the patient's suicidal behavior.

Family members and friends express anger at the suicidal patient. They become enraged, infuriated, and affronted by the suggestion of suicide and certainly by the attempt. As Slater (11) observed, suicide challenges them personally and their value system. They see suicide as a rejection of them, as an abandonment of everything, and as a repudiation of society. "How can you do this to me — to us?"

Other feel guilt. They see themselves as being to blame and they focus on their contributions and failures. They wonder whether "we drove him to it." Painfully they review recent and distant events to find a cause and to fault themselves. Sally Stoller's boyfriend feels guilty because of the breakup and blames himself for the overdose.

Others withdraw from the patient. They are stressed by the threats and the attempt. They handle their stress by avoiding the patient. They declare themselves not responsible for "whatever happens."

Some people make light of the threats and the attempts. They counter with the myths about suicide: "People who kill themselves do not talk about it" and "If she really wanted to die, she would have taken more pills or used a gun."

Still others actually encourage the patient to commit suicide. They subtly support the behavior by introducing guns into the home or keeping excessive amounts of medications available to a depressed patient. In some instances they actively participate in the suicide plan. A 65-year-old woman had metastatic breast cancer. She spent her days in intense pain. She could not eat or sleep; she lost weight and wanted to die. Her son, at her request, left a large quantity of pain pills by her bedside. The following night she took a fatal overdose.

In many instances the family or friends feel confused by the suicidal patient. Conflicting emotions overwhelm and paralyze them. They feel anger, guilt, and concern. They want at the same time both to flee and to help.

Most family members and friends respond with concern and intervene. They recognize the patient's threats of suicide as distress signals. They take the message seriously and urge the patient to seek help. They see a suicide attempt as a major manifestation of a psychiatric problem. They demand that the person get help. Sally Stoller's boyfriend hears the true message of good-bye and he calls for help.

THE INITIATION OF THE EMERGENCY

Although the patient's suicide threats and attempts commence the crisis, one of three events actually brings the suicidal person to EMTs' and the ED's attention.

The patient may realize the need for help and seek it. The family and friends may recognize the seriousness of the situation and demand that the patient obtain assistance. Or a chance discovery by others interrupts the attempt and they summon aid.

Frequently patients' own suicidal thoughts, plans, or attempt jar them into recognition of the problem and motivate them to find help. One 50-year-old woman came to the ED visibly upset and depressed. She knew she needed help when "for the first time in my life I thought of killing myself." Some patients seek the ED to control suicidal impulses or call the ED after consuming pills. Some awake from an overdose or look at their cut wrists, realize what they have just done, and come to the ED. Their own suicidal behavior catapults them into seeking help.

In other situations the family and friends recognize the gravity of the suicidal message or attempt and insist that the person obtain help. They will not tolerate suicidal behavior; they demonstrate concern for the patient, and often they see the necessity for help more clearly than does the patient. Sally Stoller's boyfriend calls for assistance; his response initiates the intervention sequence.

Many times circumstances and chance play a part in the commencement of the intervention. A family member returns home early, discovers the comatose patient, and summons a rescue unit. A passerby notices someone lingering by the side of a bridge, befriends that person, listens, and then takes the person to the ED. In each situation a chance discovery interrupts the self-destruction and leads to intervention.

THE EMTs' RESPONSE TO THE EMERGENCY

The EMTs' response to the suicidal person must be prompt, organized, affirmative, and decisive. It must counter and confront the chaos, the patient's behavior, and the family's confusion. The suicidal patient requires maximum EMT skill, performance, and training. Improper technique promotes patient deterioration and can result in death. The EMTs initially respond to Sally Stoller sluggishly, haphazardly, and inefficiently. After she attempts to cut her wrist, the EMTs employ a firm, organized approach. This proves decisive. The EMT intervention for the suicidal patient demands a prompt response, identification of themselves, physical attention to the patient, a stated plan, removal of dangerous implements, recognition of their own attitudes, an affirmative approach, and constant accompaniment.

The EMTs' response must be prompt. Delays lead to increased morbidity and mortality. Rapid intervention interrupts further medication ingestion or poisonous gas inhalation and prevents the patient from leaving. Promptness sets the tone for the entire approach.

The EMTs commence the intervention by identifying themselves. They must use their names and emphasize their professional titles and role. Their insignias and uniforms symbolize professional, trained involvement. In a sense, they represent society's prohibition against suicide.

Immediately the EMTs must address the physical needs of the patient. These include stopping the bleeding, assisting with breathing, and establishing an intravenous infusion line (IV). The medical problems must be addressed first in the intervention sequence.

The rescue unit personnel must inform the patient and the family of the plan. In contrast to other types of patients in crisis, suicidal patients must be given few options. The plan must be definite and firm.

EMTs must remove any injurious implements. They must take away medications, glass objects, knives, and guns. Where indicated, they may search the patient for implements of self-destruction. Patients have been known to hurt themselves during the intervention. Sally Stoller attempts to cut herself with a razor while the EMTs confer. EMTs must bring with them to the ED any medicine bottles from which the patient may have ingested medications. Identification of ingested substances aids in proper medical management.

EMTs' attitudes affect their responses. They share many of the family's views about suicide. They feel anger toward the patient, take the attempt lightly, or have little sympathy for the patient. As a result of these attitudes, they could render less than professional intervention. The suicidal patient requires a professional approach.

The EMTs must employ an affirmative attitude toward these patients. People attempt suicide because of depression, despair, demoralization, and desperation. Self-destructive behavior is a strong statement that life is not worth living. The EMTs' posture and response must be positive. They must act on the side of life and living.

EMTs must accompany the patient throughout the intervention and the transport. Continuous accompaniment provides patients with contact throughout the crisis and prevents them from further hurting themselves. It also precludes patients' premature departure from assistance. Suicidal patients must not be left alone.

THE EMERGENCY DEPARTMENT EVALUATION

The ED evaluation and treatment of the suicidal patient must be decisive. It represents the turning point in the crisis. The staff must effectively intervene, prevent the suicide, instill hope, cause a change in the patient's life, and involve the person in further therapy. The ED approach includes the reception, physical examination, chief complaint, psychiatric evaluation, and mental status examination.

The Reception

The ED reception of the suicidal patient constitutes one of the most critical transition points in the intervention sequence. Effective reception hinges upon prompt attention, staff identification, firm control, patient protection, constant supervision, awareness of staff attitudes, use of EMTs' information, family involvement, and an affirmation of hope.

The suicidal patient requires prompt medical and psychiatric attention. Ingested medications must be removed (with ipecac) or absorbed (with charcoal); bleeding must be controlled; respiration supported. Speed is essential. The ED psychiatric evaluation must be insisted upon and premature departure must be prevented.

Staff must introduce and identify themselves. They must use their names and their professional titles. Their uniforms, their professional roles, and their milieu symbolize help.

The physician's approach must be one of firm control. The patient and family must be shown that the physician has command of the situation. The physician achieves this by a rapid response, a professional attitude, demonstrated leadership, and proper deployment of security workers.

Effective ED treatment requires protection and constant supervision of the patient. Staff must remove any dangerous implements from the patient. These include pills, glass, knives, and guns. Patients can hurt themselves *in* the ED. Staff or family must remain with the patient at all times. This reduces isolation and loneliness, prevents self-injury, and impedes elopement.

ED staff must be aware of their own attitudes toward the suicidal patient, and then they must act professionally. Staff feelings toward suicide reflect the anger noted earlier. Indeed, since ED personnel see many suicidal patients, they may develop callous, hostile responses to these patients. Staff must recognize that the suicidal act is a major manifestation of depression.

The physician must utilize the EMTs' information. Their observations of the patient's residence, their report of the circumstances of the act, and their experiences with the patient provide essential data for the evaluation. EMTs supply the pill containers. They note the presence of firearms at the patient's home.

The physician must secure involvement of the family for several reasons. First, they supply information concerning the patient and the attempt. Second, their reactions to the threat or attempt must be assessed. Those responding with indifference or encouragement offer a lethal environment for the patient to return to. Third, the family can stay with the patient. Fourth, the family members provide referral assistance. In certain cases they must help in the commitment process.

Finally, and this aspect of the reception is paramount, the physician and the entire ED staff must portray an affirmative attitude. They must offer the patient hope and help through their interactions.

Physical Examination

The first priority is to save life. All ED management must emphasize appropriate medical and surgical intervention, then psychiatric evaluation. Both phases of this sequence are critical.

A number of principles apply to the medical-surgical approaches to the suicidal patient. First, speed is paramount. Second, medicine has reached the sophisticated level where specific overdoses require specific interventions. Physostigmine has emerged as the drug of choice in treating tricyclic antidepressant overdoses (12); naloxone hydrochloride (Narcan) is a narcotic antagonist used to counteract opiate overdoses. Third, the suicide patient warrants a complete physical examination. A young man lacerated his wrists. The ED physician sutured these. The patient complained of leg pain. Further examination revealed he had also cut his thighs. Fourth, patients occasionally attempt suicide in more than one way simultaneously. Sally Stoller takes pills and also attempts to cut herself. The patient who attempts suicide with a vehicle may have also taken an overdose. Fifth, a nurse or physician must be with the patient throughout the entire course of ED treatment. Patients undergoing medical or surgical intervention can try to injure themselves further during therapy.

Chief Complaint

The patient's chief complaint describes the crisis, reveals its dynamics, and portrays the person's reaction to it. "I took some pills," "I want to kill myself," or "They stopped me from hanging myself," depicts the suicidal nature of the emergency. "I did it to get back at him," "I hope they're happy now," or "Now they'll see how much I am hurting" suggests dynamics behind the attempt. "I wish I'd succeeded," "I am not sure about living," or "I did a foolish thing" shows the patient's reaction to the attempt.

Psychiatric Evaluation

The physician must undertake an organized approach to discover what happened and why it occurred. Particularly relevant parts of the evaluation are the history of present illness (HPI), social history, family history, religion, work history, psychiatric history, alcohol and drug use history, medical history, and history of medication use.

The HPI furnishes critical information about the nature of the suicide threat and attempt. The physician must elicit and pursue in great detail the events surrounding a suicide attempt. He or she must proceed with a series of questions: Where were you when you took the pills? Were you alone? Did you take all the pills? Had you planned to take them? When was someone expected home? What did you do immediately after the overdose? If the person you called had not been home, what had you planned to do? One especially productive question for the physician to ask is, "What did you think your suicide would accomplish?" This inquiry approach avoids the use of *why* did you do it, which the patient finds offensive, and yields a great deal of information. The details help to determine the extent and severity of the attempt.

The social history describes the patient's living situation, provides information concerning the dynamics of the attempt, and describes the environment to which the patient might have to return. A patient living alone has a high risk of completing the suicidal act. Sally Stoller resides by herself. If her boyfriend does not respond, no one else will discover her in time.

A family history of suicide is a very significant factor. Previous suicide in the family correlates highly with suicide attempts and completions. Shepherd and Barraclough (13) note that this factor increases in importance if a parent committed suicide when the patient was younger than 13 years old. Exposure to a family suicide has a lifelong impact upon the patient. Sally Stoller is all too familiar with suicide. Her father committed suicide.

The physician must inquire about the patient's religion and belief system. Protestants have a high suicide rate; Catholics, a low rate. In many instances, the patient's beliefs preclude suicide. To these patients suicide is a sin. In other situations, the patient's philosophical and ethical ideals condone and, under certain circumstances, demand suicide.

The physician must explore the patient's work history. Unemployment correlates with suicide, as does job termination. Occupational stresses cause depression and feelings of entrapment. A 43-year-old man, a nurse, abused drugs. His supervisor caught him stealing from the narcotic supply and terminated his employment. That night he took a massive overdose. Only chance discovery and summons of aid by a neighbor saved his life.

An inquiry into the patient's psychiatric history yields critical information. Former psychiatric patients can kill themselves. It is notable that in the majority of these situations the patient has seen a physician within a month of attempting suicide (14). Often the suicidal patient is currently in treatment. Winokov and Tsuang (15) report that suicide correlates highly with a history and diagnosis of mania, depression, or schizophrenia. Avery and Winokur (16) further note that the patient with a recent history of treated depression remains at a high risk to attempt suicide. Psychiatric patients often require and take medications. These preparations provide a method of suicide. The physician must elicit a complete list of medications, dosages, and quantities on hand. The pills or the container brought by the EMTs can be most useful.

The physician must also make inquiry into alcohol and drug use. Alcoholism correlates highly with suicidal behavior. Drugs play a role. Both alcohol and other drugs cause depression and furnish the means to commit suicide.

The physician must investigate the patient's medical history and medication use. Chronic, debilitating, and painful disease correlates with suicide attempts and completions. Even patients with nonfatal illnesses may distort physicians' statements and believe their condition is terminal. Additionally, the doctor must make inquiry into the medication the patient takes. Certain preparations, including digitalis and insulin, produce fatal results if used to excess.

Mental Status Examination

The physician must undertake a complete mental inventory of the suicidal patient. This provides a psychiatric picture of the patient at the moment of evaluation and offers clues about probable behavior. The physician must emphasize affect, thought content, suicidal thoughts and plans, homicidal thoughts and plans, judgment, insight, and sensorium.

The physician must pay particular attention to the patient's mood. The suicidal patient experiences intense depression or anxiety. The interviewer comes away deeply affected, sensing the patient's anguish. The physician must recognize his or her own reaction as evidence of the patient's pain and suicide potential. Equally discomforting for the physician is the calm patient. A patient quietly relaxed while discussing suicide should cause concern. This tranquility often reflects a definite resolve to kill oneself.

Thought content relates to suicidal potential in many ways. Patients' concepts predispose them to kill themselves. Depressive ideas such as "They would be better off with me dead"; bizarre notions such as "By death I will enter stage seven of the higher level of reason"; or paranoid concepts like "They want me to kill myself" all lead to suicidal behavior. Delusions promote self-destructive activities: "My death will save the world." Hallucinations can set up a suicide.

The physician must specifically inquire about suicidal thoughts and plans. It is mandatory to ask patients whether they think about hurting themselves. When a patient answers affirmatively, the physician must pursue the topic. Does the patient have an occasional suicidal thought or a preoccupation? The physician must next ask about suicide plans in order to discover how detailed and specific the plans are. The more refined, organized, and prepared the plan is, the greater is the danger of suicide. A patient with vague, occasional thoughts of suicide represents a lower risk than a person who calculates the number of pills required or plans to purchase a revolver.

Additionally, the physician must ask about previous suicidal thoughts and attempts and must explore the circumstances of each, the patient's reactions to them, and the family's responses. All too often patients who kill themselves have histories of suicide threats and attempts. Sally Stoller has a history of overdose.

The physician must explore the patient's thoughts and plans about homicide. If suicide represents anger turned inward, then homicide is aggression directed outward. Self-murder and murder become interlaced. A depressed mother believed the world was so bad the she resolved to kill her children and then herself. She would not leave them on this evil planet. In another situation EMTs brought an intoxicated, depressed man to the ED because he wanted to kill himself. During his ED evaluation he dramatically changed his mind and wanted to kill his brother. The risk of suicide involves the danger of homicide.

The physician must assess the patient's judgment. How has the patient handled the stresses? Indeed, the suicide attempt represents problems with judgment. The HPI furnishes further evidence of the patient's method of dealing with the crisis.

Insight is also an important issue. How much does the patient understand his or her behavior? The patient who says, "I did a silly thing" has some insight into the actions. Occasionally a patient also recognizes the manipulative quality or vengeful component of the suicidal behavior.

The physician must examine the patient's sensorium—orientation, recall, calculations, and obstructions. The mental status examination provides a record of the mental status of the patient at the time of the examination. Especially when an overdose is involved, that mental status may change; the patient becomes either more lethargic or more alert. The assessment of sensorium provides a reference point by which to monitor the patient.

DIAGNOSIS, TREATMENT PLAN, AND IMMEDIATE EMERGENCY DEPARTMENT THERAPY

The ED intervention must produce a diagnosis and an implemented treatment plan, and it must provide immediate therapy. The physician must strive for an accurate diagnosis, since proper treatment depends upon it. The physician must develop a precise treatment plan, implement it, and render therapy. Suicidal threats and actions necessitate a firm, organized, directed, and exact ED approach toward diagnosis, immediate therapy, and referral.

Diagnosis

The physician diagnoses Sally Stoller as having an adjustment disorder with depressed mood. He views her behavior as a reaction to the rupture of her relationship with her boyfriend. He also makes a secondary diagnosis—episodic affective disorder, major depressive disorder, recurrent—since she has experienced a significant depression, has had a prior episode, and has a family history of depressions.

Adjustment disorder with depressed mood is a diagnosis in both the general psychiatric emergency population and the suicidal patient category. A reaction to an identifiable life event constitutes the prominent feature of this diagnosis. The intensity ranges from mild to severe. The criteria for making this diagnosis are (1) the patient's behavior is a reaction to some clearly identifiable stress; (2) that reaction is marked by either impaired function or an excess of expected symptoms; (3) the response is not reflective of underlying psychiatric illness; (4) the reaction is not typical of other recognized diagnostic categories; and (5) the disorder remits upon cessation of the stress.

Suidical threats, attempts, and completions occur in a large variety of diagnostic categories. Affective disorders carry high suicide rates, with the depressive groups (both major depressive disorder, single episode or recurrent; and bipolar affective disorder) especially prominent (17). Mania is also associated with suicide. Patients emerging from deep depression and heading toward a manic state are particularly at risk to kill themselves. The schizophrenic disorders also correlate with suicidal behavior. Schizophrenic patients attempt suicide in response to the delusions, disorganization, or hallucinations that characterize their disease or in reaction to the chronicity of the illness. Paranoid people carry a suicide risk. Patients who cannot project their anger onto others turn it against themselves; they become depressed and then they consider suicide. In the delirium associated with substance abuse and organic mental disorder, the patient can become suicidal. Patients with personality disorders become suicidal when stressed. The person with an antisocial personality attempts suicide when caught and confined.

Treatment Plan

Three major concepts must guide the physician in developing a treatment plan for the suicidal patient: change, responsibility, and a definite, implemented referral. These three considerations reflect the unique situation of the suicidal patient.

The key concept in the intervention is change. If the patient does not feel a change after the EMTs' transport, the ED's therapy, the follow-up treatment, and the family's involvement, there is an extremely high risk that the patient will complete the suicide. The change takes many forms. Patients may come to feel that the attempt was foolish; they may feel the family really does care; they may gain insight into the suicidal behavior from psychotherapy; they may discover from the EMTs' and the ED's response that people want to help; or they may "see the light at the end of the tunnel" after they begin taking antidepressants. In each case *something* in the person's life is changed. The physician must secure a change before sending the patient out. If Miss Stoller returns to her apartment without any feeling of change, she will succeed in her suicide attempt.

The physician has responsibilty for the suicidal patient. In few areas of medicine does the state mandate patient restraint and treatment. A patient who has a myocardial infarction or a fractured extremity and declines treatment remains free to leave the ED. Yet the physician has the prerogative to impose control and render assistance to suicidal patients and can commit them to prevent suicide.

The physician must implement a definite referral. The suicidal patient requires an organized, secured referral. The plan must not be left to chance. The physician either must refer the patient to a hospital and secure safe transportation to that hospital or must arrange for a definite outpatient appointment. If the family plans to take the patient home, they must be with him or her at all times and must remove weapons from the home.

Immediate Emergency Department Therapy

The immediate therapy provided in the ED must save the life, instill hope, reverse the helplessness, develop an alternative to suicide, and establish the referral. These themes must underscore all ED activity with the suicidal patient.

The patient's life must be saved. This is of course the cardinal mission of the ED. All appropriate medical-surgical treatments must be employed. Their use carries with it the implication of the patient's worth. The removal of weapons and the prevention of elopement makes evident the staff's determination to halt the suicidal behavior. It is obvious to the patient that they want to help.

The ED therapy must instill hope and begin to restore morale. The ED's reception, the staff's attitude, and the physician's interview create the feeling that something can be done. All of these emphasize the patient's worth and value. If the family and friends respond with concern, they become sources of future help. The whole process trumpets that the patient has a future.

The ED therapy must reverse the patients' helplessness. Patients become involved in the interview. They talk about their plight and share their depression. Their participation begins the process of getting help and helping themselves.

The physician and the patient must begin to develop alternatives to suicide. By the time patients threaten and attempt suicide, they have limited their options to one—death. Starting in the ED, they commence the search for another approach. The development of an alternative to death constitutes the required change in the patient and the patient's situation.

Finally, the ED must establish a definite referral for the suicidal patient, either a secured hospital admission or a scheduled outpatient appointment. This referral emphasizes hope and help.

CARE AFTER THE EMERGENCY

The ED physician administers ipecac to Miss Stoller with good results. Her vital signs remain stable. She participates in the interview but notes "nothing has changed" and voices continued plans to terminate her life. She asserts suicide as her right. Her physician recommends hospitali-

zation; she wants to go home. He then recommends commitment. Her boyfriend thinks she will hate him forever, but, knowing she needs help, he supports the physician's recommendation. Together they begin to arrange for involuntary hospitalization. Her mother, reached by telephone, concurs in this decision. Miss Stoller only then accepts psychiatric hospital admission.

Once in the hospital, she discovers others with similar problems. She participates in group therapy and individual therapy. Her psychiatrist prescribes an antidepressant. She starts to resolve her loss, recognizes her contributions to the communication problem, and resumes interest in her master's program.

After four weeks in the hospital she returns to her apartment. She arranges for a roommate and continues the medication and individual psychotherapy sessions. When stressed, she again thinks about suicide, but finds talking about it a better alternative. She explores her reactions to her father's suicide and discovers her attempts to recreate his life. She likes herself and finds meaning for her life through her studies and eventually through her career. As she gains confidence academically, she again ventures into the dating world. Later she meets a young man and develops a sharing relationship with him.

Care of suicidal patients after they leave the ED involves hospitalization, day treatment, and individual therapy.

Hospitalization

Hospitalization becomes the treatment of choice for the suicidal patient in a number of situations. For patients who still plan to kill themselves despite all intervention, the physician must arrange inpatient treatment. When the family expresses death wishes for the patient or reacts with indifference to the suicide attempt, the doctor must remove the patient from this fatal environment. Patients who live alone, have made very serious attempts, or have histories of impulsive self-destructive acts must be admitted to a hospital. When delusions of self-annihilation persist, voices continue to command suicide, or delirium produces self-destructive behavior, the physician must secure inpatient treatment.

Hospitalization provides many benefits for the suicidal patient. It offers protection and surveillance 24 hours a day. During the acute phase, patients continue with strong drives to injure themselves. The staff interrupts this self-destructive activity. They take responsibility for the patients. The physician can administer the proper medications in therapeutic dosages to treat the underlying psychiatric condition, for example, thought disorder or depression, and can monitor their effects. The milieu offers support; other patients, help; group therapy, shared experiences; and occupational therapy, successes. Inpatient psychiatry gives the patient help and hope.

Day Treatment

Day treatment offers several advantages to the suicidal patient. It provides a bridge from inpatient treatment to outpatient psychotherapy, and it furnishes the patient daily structure, monitoring, activity, and support. It does require the patient to live in a safe, supportive, and concerned environment. It continues the provision of help and hope but permits the patient greater autonomy than an inpatient unit.

Outpatient Psychotherapy

Successful outpatient psychotherapy revolves about several basic principles. The physician must schedule regular appointments. Patients need to know they will see the doctor at an appointed time each week. The physician must prescribe a limited amount of medication. Patients can have their prescriptions refilled rather than receive a lethal amount of drugs.

The physician must emphasize talking about thoughts and feelings in contrast to taking self-destructive action. The physician must be available to the patient. If the patient becomes suicidal, he or she must have someone to call. The suicidal patient represents an outpatient challenge and an opportunity. The patient, by having the choice to die, decides to live.

REFERENCES

1. Murphy GE: Suicide and alcoholism. *Arch Gen Psychiatry* 36:65-69, 1977.
2. Farberow HL, Shneidman ES: *The Cry for Help.* New York, McGraw-Hill Book Co, 1965.
3. Dubin CI: *Suicide: A Sociological and Statistical Study.* New York, Ronald Press, 1963.
4. Frankl VE: *The Unheard Cry for Meaning.* New York, Simon & Schuster, 1979.
5. Nietzsche FN: *Beyond Good and Evil: Prelude to a Philosophy of the Future.* New York, Random House, 1966, vol 4, p 91.
6. Zung WWK: Suicide prevention by suicide detection. *Psychosomatics* 20:149-159, 1979.
7. Blachly PH, Disher W, Roduner G: Suicide by physicians. *Bulletin of Suicidology,* pp 1-18, 1969.
8. Heiman MT: Suicide among police. *Am J Psychiatry* 134:1286-1290, 1977.
9. Smialek JE, Spitz WU: Death behind bars. *JAMA* 240:2563-2564, 1978.
10. Abram HS, Moore GL, Westervelt FB: Suicidal behavior in chronic dialysis patients. *Am J Psychiatry* 127:1199-1207, 1971.

11. Slater P: *Footholds*. New York, EP Dutton & Co, 1977.
12. Munoz R: Treatment of tricyclic intoxication. *Am J Psychiatry* 133:1085-1087, 1976.
13. Shepherd DM, Barraclough BM: The aftermath of parental suicide for children. *Br J Psychiatry* 129:267-276, 1976.
14. Myers DH, Neal CD: Suicide in psychiatric patients. *Br J Psychiatry* 133:38-44, 1978.
15. Winokov G, Tsuang M: The Iowa 500: Suicide in mania, depression, and schizophrenia. *Am J Psychiatry* 132:650-651, 1975.
16. Avery D, Winokur G: Suicide, attempted suicide, and relapse rates in depression. *Arch Gen Psychiatry* 35:749-753, 1978.
17. Kolb L: *Modern Clinical Psychiatry*, ed 8. Philadelphia, WB Saunders Co, 1973.

11
The Patient With a Thought Disorder

THE PATIENT

Thought disorder means schizophrenia. This disorder is a profound disturbance of thoughts and affects and their integration.

Bill Peterson stares at his dormitory room wall. He faintly acknowledges his roommate's concern, responds only in single words to questions, and does not spontaneously speak. Occasionally he launches into long, illogical discourses about God, pollution, and zoos. His freshman year is due to be completed in one week, and everyone else—friends, faculty, and family—worries about Bill; he does not.

Bill graduated from high school at the top of his class. Although he was a "loner," people had liked him and he had participated in many school and family activities. He had experienced a blue period in his junior year. He rarely had dated.

During his year in college he gradually becomes aloof. Vague, mystical thinking invades his career orientation. He ponders the seven levels of thought and attends a variety of religious functions. Since one week ago he "knows" a particular professor is "out to get him" and control his mind. He spends long time periods alone in his room on weekends and even during vacations. He hears voices arguing in his head and later his thoughts clash there. He is convinced that the school newspaper wrote messages intended for him. His mood swings become extreme and dramatic. Without provocation he quarrels with his roommate. At times he thinks he and his roommate are the same person. He has stopped going to classes.

Bill Peterson manifests profound disturbances in his mood, perceptions, and behavior. Schizophrenia pervades all aspects of the personality.

The Patient's Mood

The patient with a thought disorder displays a number of mood disturbances. Some of these mood problems are present throughout the person's life; others are late manifestations. Schizophrenic patients commonly demonstrate flat affect, inappropriate affect, anhedonia, elements of both depression and anxiety, and aloofness.

A flat affect characterizes the schizophrenic patient. Bleuler (1) considered this one of the four primary symptoms of thought disorder. The patient's discourse portrays the flat affect. These patients talk in a monotone and display poverty of feelings. Their mood is colorless, bland, and emotionally dull (2).

Inappropriateness also describes their affect. A disharmony exists between what patients say (the content) and how they say it (the emotion). Bill Peterson discusses in a monotone the professor's plot to control his mind and then to kill him. He portrays no excitement over this possibility, only a bland, matter-of-fact level of concern. The incongruity between thought and affect is striking.

Anhedonia is the absence of pleasure. The schizophrenic patient lives joylessly. Interpersonal situations bring no happiness (3). The person's developmental history shows no pleasure experiences. Kayton and Koh (4,p413) believe the person with schizophrenia possesses "an intrinsic or acquired pleasure deficit." Bill displays no pleasure, joy, or happiness.

Schizophrenic patients often manifest depression and anxiety. They feel sad over their life's course and the absence of pleasure. They wonder why they are different from others and feel apart from the mainstream of society. They may also show anxiety. This anxiety can take the form of acute panic attack, especially when patients are too pressured, confined, or overwhelmed. Additionally, they experience anxiety over their physical health.

Schizophrenic patients are emotionally aloof. Their interpersonal dullness, monotonous way of relating to others, and anhedonia serve to isolate them. The patients want this retreat. Bill Peterson confined himself to *his* room and *his* wall.

The Patient's Perceptions

A marked perceptional disturbance is the cardinal feature of schizophrenia. Schizophrenic patients develop major distortions in their views of both their internal and external world. As a consequence, their judgment and reason become disturbed. The principle perceptional manifestations of schizophrenia are disordered thoughts, egocentrism, identity confusion, somatic distortions, delusions, hallucinations, and referential thinking.

First and foremost, the patient exhibits a thought disorder. The patient displays this disorder in a number of ways: fragmented thoughts, "predicate thinking," overinclusive logic, overly abstract reasoning, concrete conceptualization, thought blockage, and ambivalence.

The patient's thought processes become fragmented, illogical, and confused. Ideas appear to be totally unrelated, and the person moves from one topic to another with apparent ease and no logical connection. The patient comments, "Horses don't like peanut butter, the sky is blue, and what car do you drive?" This kind of thinking has been described as derailment (5).

The patient uses "predicate thinking." In this type of reasoning, according to Arieti (6), the patient finds people or events identical on the basis of one similarity. For example, the patient is a virgin and so is the Virgin Mary. Then she concludes she is the Virgin Mary.

Schizophrenic patients demonstrate overinclusive thinking and overly abstract reasoning. They draw upon irrelevant data, needless associations, and infinite detail to answer a simple question. Like Bill, they employ overly abstract reasoning. Bill worries about astronautical projects and not about his school work. His view is too global and not pertinent to his life.

Patients may employ concrete thinking and experience blockage of their thoughts. In concrete reasoning, patients focus on the most obvious and physical meaning of an event or statement. They avoid any abstract understanding of it. They take things literally. In thought blockage, patients stop in the middle of a sentence. They have "thought deprivation" (1,p1). The mind goes blank; patients forget what they were saying. In the midst of thinking, the person suddenly has no thought.

Thought disorder is also manifested by another cardinal feature of the disease, ambivalence. Patients experience conflicting thoughts and feelings at the same time. They go back and forth in their emotions, thinking, and behavior. They become paralyzed by indecisiveness.

Schizophrenic patients are preoccupied with themselves and their world. Bleuler (1) termed this autism, and it takes several forms. In one, egocentrism, patients see themselves as the center of the universe. Nothing matters except oneself. In another form of self-absorption, patients live in their own fantasy worlds. An adolescent girl preferred to talk only with her two stuffed animals, which she believed also communicated with her; she avoided her schoolmates and family. In still another type, patients withdraw entirely into themselves. They cease any dialogue with the world. Bill retreats to his room and ultimately just stares at the wall.

Schizophrenic patients experience acute and chronic identity confusion. Their ego boundaries disappear. They become concerned about who they are. Bill on occasion confuses himself with his roommate. One patient expressed the concern, "Am I my inside or outside person?" She did not know how to portray herself in different settings. She had difficulty separating her identity from her mother's, her coworker's, her best friend's, and her roommate's. Patients sometimes lose their sense of sexual identity. Sexual activity then constitutes a threat.

Patients have body image distortions. People with schizophrenia become preoccupied with their physical appearance and imagined changes in it. One patient worried that his lower lip was enlarging. Ultimately, he dwelled on that topic to the exclusion of all other activity. Schizophrenics are concerned about illness. They believe they have "some disease." Or they develop a fascination with their internal organs. They think about them all the time, discuss them, and see them everywhere.

Patients with thought disorder are delusional. The delusions take one of two general forms: persecutory or grandiose. In persecutory delusions, patients believe people, organizations, or interplanetary things are against them. The patients think these forces or people want to hurt or control them. Often the delusion begins with a vague "they" and then evolves into a specific person or organization. This has occurred with Bill. What began as a vague uneasiness untimately emerges as belief that a faculty member desires to control him. In the grandiose type of delusion, patients see themselves as omnipotent. They equate themselves with and occasionally believe they are the President, a great general, or Christ. Recently, one patient came to the ED claiming to be Vice-President of the United States. He wished a speedy evaluation since the helicopter to take him back to Washington was due soon.

Schizophrenic patients hallucinate. Auditory hallucinations constitute the most common type in schizophrenic patients. The patients hear voices of people who are not there — voices expressing conflicts, criticisms, or tasks. These voices occasionally make suggestions that the patients hurt themselves. Patients also hear their own thoughts talking to each other inside their heads (7). Bill hears voices and his own thoughts. Additionally, patients may have tactile, visual, and olfactory hallucinations. One schizophrenic gentlemen felt bugs on his skin all the time.

Patients develop ideas of reference. They find special meaning intended for them alone in newspapers, articles, radio programs, highway signs, or television programs. These ideas of reference serve to reinforce the patient's view that he or she is a special person.

The Patient's Behavior

The major disturbances of mood and perceptions produce profound alterations in the patient's behavior. It is characterized by withdrawal, lability, disorganization, bizarreness, inertia, and violence.

Schizophrenic patients commonly seek withdrawal from the social arena. They desire escape from too much input and too many obligations. Their withdrawal behaviorally symbolizes their aloofness. Bill wants only to be alone in his room.

The schizophrenic patient demonstrates lability of behavior. One moment the patient reads quietly, then for no apparent reason quarrels with a roommate; the next moment the person unexpectedly starts a new project. This erratic behavior mirrors the thought disturbances.

The patients' lives reflect disorganization. People with schizophrenia move frequently from state to state, from job to job, and from person to person.

Patients display bizarreness in language, behavior, and attire. They frequently create their own words, *neologisms,* by mixing up words and ideas. One patient referred to his mother as a "knifebird" because she had a "sharp" tongue. Patients may walk with a peculiar, exaggerated gait. Their clothing may be inappropriate and poorly coordinated. The police brought a woman to the ED after picking her up on the side of the turnpike, where she wore a raccoon coat, wool hat, and gloves in 95-degree weather.

Many patients develop tremendous inertia. They simply do not want to undertake any projects or activities. Moreover, alterations in daily structure are threatening. Patients tolerate change poorly. They seek sameness.

Violence occurs occasionally in schizophrenia. The response to the voices or the delusion can be suicide or homicide. The violence has been generated from within. Bill turns on his roommate for no apparent reason.

THE CAUSES OF THOUGHT DISORDER

Intrapsychic, interpersonal, and biologic factors have been implicated as causative of schizophrenia. Despite over a century of clinical observations and decades of research, the cause remains incompletely understood. Each of these three causes has contributed to the understanding and the treatment of schizophrenia.

Any explanation of schizophrenia must take several basic features of the disease into consideration. The onset generally occurs in late adolescence and young adulthood. Despite its occasionally dramatic occurrence, schizophrenia insidiously develops over one to two years before becoming clinically recognized. Early childhood experiences and personality traits contribute to the syndrome. The prevalence of schizophrenia is 4.78 cases per 1,000 people (8). Schizophrenia is a chronic disease. There is a genetic component to the disease.

Intrapsychic Causes of Thought Disorder

Certain personality traits and individual problems predispose to the development of schizophrenia. These traits include seclusiveness, inability to trust, cognitive deficiency, identity difficulty, and negative attitude.

The potentially schizophrenic patient has often been discussed as a schizoid person. Such a person is shy, withdrawn, isolated, quiet, and introverted. In the resulting seclusion this kind of patient develops his or her own ways of relating and thinking.

Trust is the first and most fundamental step in human development and in the establishment of identity. Trust stands as the cornerstone of interpersonal relationships (9). People lacking trust must resort to a number of maneuvers to protect themselves, including aloofness, talking in monotones to keep people uninterested in them, and avoidance of any dependency.

Often, people who develop schizophrenia are people who have some difficulty obtaining and processing information. They may have difficulty hearing or an internal malfunction of logic and organization. As a consequence they have problems relating to others.

People with identity confusion feel uneasy and disadvantaged in social settings. Often they too readily adopt the characteristics of those about them. They have difficulty distinguishing themselves from others. They struggle to maintain the perimeter of their personality.

Patients commonly have negative attitudes toward themselves and the world. They distort all experiences by focusing on the bad aspects of a situation, and they recall childhood with unhappiness. Schizophrenic people consider themselves worthless.

Interpersonal Causes of Thought Disorder

There has emerged a rich and descriptive literature that ascribes the origin of schizophrenia to interpersonal causes. Lidz and coauthors (10) and Arieti (6) emphasize family conflicts. Bateson et al (11) and Haley (12) stress family communication patterns. Wing (13) advances the social context's role in recurrence of schizophrenia.

Family disturbances result in schizophrenia. The conflicts take many different forms. Lidz et al (10) describe the continual covert and overt warfare between parents. Each rivals the other; neither complements the other. This situation leads to a marital schism with the children in the middle. Arieti (6) explores the intense battle among the hostile, nagging mother, the weak father, and the children. In other families bitter rivalries among siblings are subtly encouraged by a parent to enhance the parent's own position. Protracted, severe family conflict makes it difficult for a child to develop with a positive self-view, basic trust, and a complete identity.

Exposure to bizarre, distorted, and contradictory communication patterns predisposes a person to schizophrenia. Bateson et al (11) presents the double bind theory. Here a significant person, usually a parent, gives two contradictory messages at the same time. A mother gives her son two ties for his birthday. The next day to please her he wears one. She asks why he did not wear the other. The recipient of the messages ultimately feels it is impossible to win. Another form of double bind communication is a split between affect and thought. A father reprimands his son for drinking with a "that's my boy" smile on his face. In some homes the family members talk past one another, not to each other. The patient acquires *their* thought disorder.

An optimal level of social stimulation is required for the schizophrenic patient. A high-intensity, high-pressure environment featuring too many people, too many changes, and too many demands becomes overwhelming and frightening. The patient requires a level of sameness and structure. At the other extreme, an asocial environment devoid of interpersonal stimuli promotes the inertia of the schizophrenic patient.

Biologic Causes of Thought Disorder

There is growing evidence that biologic factors play a significant role in the development of schizophrenia. Genetic, biochemical, and pharmacologic data underscore the biologic contribution.

Schizophrenia occurs in families. It is a genetic disease. A high concordance rate of schizophrenia exists among monozygotic twins, but the rate is much lower in dizygotic twins (14). The incidence of schizophrenia is about 1 percent in the general population; in parents of schizophrenics, it is 5 percent; and in siblings and children of schizophrenics, it is 10 percent (15). Children of schizophrenic parents, after adoption by nonschizophrenic parents, still have a significant incidence of schizophrenia (16).

Numerous biochemical abnormalities have been detected in the schizophrenic population. These range from an immunoglobulin called *taraxein* (17) to abnormal dopamine metabolism. The meaning of these abnormalities remains unclear.

A number of drugs produce a schizophrenialike reaction. Hallucinogenic drugs trigger a schizophrenic psychosis (18). Amphetamines produce a schizophrenic syndrome (19). Phencyclidine has been shown to cause a similar clinical manifestation (20). Dopamine causes schizophrenic behavior (21). These facts suggest that there is a biochemical mechanism to schizophrenia.

THE REACTIONS OF OTHERS

Schizophrenic patients cause great disquiet, conflict, and confusion in those about them. The social milieu mirrors the patient's disorganization. The family members feel concerned, friends are puzzled, and coworkers are unsatisfied after their encounters with the patient. Others' reactions include dissatisfaction, confusion, denial, fear, guilt, avoidance, and a deep sense of dread.

The family and friends feel dissatisfied by their relations with the patient. They perceive the patient's deterioration. Bill is no longer the brilliant student with the great future. He seems to be a shell of his former self. Friends and family no longer experience any rapport with him. Their questions go unanswered and they feel distanced by him. They wonder if they failed in the communication. Should they use another approach? As a result of this dissatisfaction they develop a sense of frustration.

People find themselves confused by these patients. Sometimes the patients behave quite warmly toward others, and then at other times they are hostile. People cannot figure out why. The patients' retreat into fantasy is perplexing, and the belief that others are plotting against them seems "stupid," "illogical," "crazy," and "not real." People cannot follow patients' thoughts, arguments or views. The situation is all very puzzling.

The family often exercises denial of the patient's symptoms. They make excuses for the behavior. "Bill just has a little trouble adjusting to school." They rationalize the problem and focus on the few things going right. They search for a physical cause for the symptoms. One family rushed a daughter to the family physician, believing she "must have a thyroid problem." She was having a schizophrenic episode.

Many people experience fear of the schizophrenic patient. The person's unpredictability, violence, delusions, and hallucinations lend credibility to this concern. Bill has attacked his roommate; he feels a faculty member is "out to get him"; and he stares at the wall. His roommate is afraid of him.

The family members feel guilty (22). They believe they caused the schizophrenia. The family literature reinforces this guilt. Professionals have blamed families for the patients' difficulties.

One result of the dissatisfaction, confusion, denial, fear, and guilt is that the family members avoid the patient. They isolate the person in the house. They also seek to decrease the patient's visibility in the community. This avoidance phenomenon emerges particularly clearly as the disease develops a chronic course.

But most importantly, one other reaction occurs: the family and friends recommend and support the patient's obtaining help. The family and friends sense the seriousness of the problem. They have seen the profound disturbances of affect and thoughts. They know the person has a real problem.

THE INITIATION OF THE EMERGENCY

A wide range of events and circumstances trigger a crisis in schizophrenia (23). There are a number of situations and symptoms which the patient finds intolerable: an acute identity confrontation, stimulus overload, loss of control, a drug-induced panic, concretization of the enemy, and self-destructive impulses. The family and friends ask for help in a number of other circumstances: violence, prolonged inertia, and bizarre behavior.

A threat to the schizophrenic's precariously maintained identity triggers a crisis. The threat may come from many sources. A sexual situation in which the patient is expected to become heterosexually involved may be threatening. So can a dormitory situation where the patient feels too close to someone of the same sex. Identity crisis may develop during pregnancy or in the postpartum period. It happens also at graduations and weddings. It occurs when the patient feels intruded upon. In each case the patient's identity changes or comes into question.

The schizophrenic patient functions optimally within a structured, medium-input environment. If demands and changes exceed the patient's stimulus threshold, stress results. One patient worked as a gas station attendant. He functioned well during regular hours, but when his boss switched him to the busier weekends he experienced a resurgence of his persecutory fears. Too frequent work changes or changes of residence create pressure. Too many social and family demands generate stress. Bill seeks the refuge of his room to avoid overstimulation and the changes that occur at the close of the semester.

When patients perceive that they cannot control their environment, a crisis develops. A 16-year-old girl attempted to control her whole life. She lined up all her shoes in a row. She carefully ordered her room. One day her mother cleaned the room and altered her "arrangement." She was shattered. Her last defense, control over her environment, had been breached. Her thoughts became disorganized and her identity became threatened.

A large number of substances and drugs precipitate a schizophrenic episode in a susceptible individual. These include marijuana, LSD, amphetamines, and PCP (24). One schizophrenic individual reported increased feelings of "paranoia" when she smoked marijuana. Adrenocortical steroids precipitate schizophrenic episodes. Panic characterizes many of these drug reactions.

A major turning point in the patient's course occurs when he or she converts from having vague paranoid fears to identifying a definite enemy. A decisive event in Bill's evolution happens when he focuses on a faculty member. No longer does he suspect "they" are after him. Now he knows, and he knows who. The emergence of a specific enemy accelerates the crisis. A vague, persecutory notion leads to reflection. A concrete enemy promotes action.

Suicide is a significant problem in schizophrenia (25). Thoughts, fears, and acts of self-destruction propel the patient to seek help. Several factors contribute to the schizophrenic patient's becoming suicidal. First, in some cases the "voices" tell patients to hurt themselves. One patient said, "The voices want me to jump off a building." Second, patients may wish to die to avoid the battles in their heads. The thoughts clashing inside the mind become too oppressive. Third, the disease sometimes leads to a protracted series of hospitalizations, unemployment, and medications; patients who have this experience can feel depressed by the disease, hopeless, and suicidal.

Violence is a major reason why family, friends, and coworkers seek immediate assistance for the patient. They feel threats to their safety. Danger galvanizes them into action. Bill has threatened his roommate.

In many situations the family simply loses all patience with the patient's inertia. The "sitting around" has become a burden to the family. A source of income has ceased. Their excuses have run out. They want something done.

Finally, the patient's bizarre behavior necessitates intervention. Public nudity, outrageous dress, uncontrollable giggling, or perpetual rhyming challenges the family's and the community's tolerance.

THE EMTs' RESPONSE TO THE EMERGENCY

Bill's roommate is alarmed. He calls the infirmary. The infirmary in turn summons the municipal rescue service. The unit responds. The EMTs enter the room; Bill continues to stare at the wall. Two members of the team approach him directly. He retreats to the corner of the room and accuses them of working for the evil professor. Then they identify themselves. They state their reason for being there and what they hope to achieve. Bill remains silent. One of the team wants to go home, wondering whether Bill "is for real."

A half hour later the EMTs repeat why they are there. Bill starts to talk with a woman on the team. He outlines the history of Western civilization, in response to her inquiry about his major. He then presents a disjointed defense of his Walden existence in his "walled" room. She reiterates his need for help. He does not agree or disagree but gathers his coat. He leaves with them, returns to his wall, and departs again. He reviews the world's religions in the rescue vehicle with her.

A schizophrenic crisis requires a clear, firm, directed EMT response. The EMTs must address the patient's disorganization with a structured approach. The patient's symptoms and behavior necessitate adherence to intervention protocol, underscore the importance of that sequenced program, and challenge the EMTs' management abilities. The approach involves a prompt response, a clear personnel identification, containment, recognition of EMTs' reactions, an orientation of the patient to the plan of treatment and a periodic reiteration of that goal, a control of violence, an avoidance of excess stimulation, and accompaniment of the patient at all times.

A prompt response serves several purposes. It provides the message that the patient is important and worthy to receive intervention. It helps to check an accelerating disorder of the patient's thoughts or an expanding delusional system.

Personnel identification is critical in these crises. Bill quickly misidentifies the EMTs as agents of the faculty member. EMTs must directly tell the patient who they are, both personally and professionally. They must continually clarify their identity and allow no misinterpretation of their role. At the same time EMTs must remind the patient of his or her own identity.

EMTs must contain the patient, both physically and intellectually. They offer limits by their presence and by their vehicle. By engaging the patient in conversations, they have started to limit the mental disorganization. By identifying themselves and the patient, they help the patient locate identity boundaries.

EMTs must appreciate their own reactions to the patient in order to provide a gently directed, open, and unhurried approach. The schizophrenic patient offers the EMTs a confusing, disorganized constellation of symptoms. Not infrequently, the EMTs find themselves overwhelmed by the extensive reply to a simple question and feel alienated by this person whom they want to help. They become frustrated by the amount of time and apparent lack of success involved. EMTs must appreciate the patient's puzzlement and confusion as part of the disease.

EMTs must control violence. Delusional, hallucinating patients can hurt themselves or others. EMTs must remove any weapons or potential weapons. The patient's unpredictability requires EMTs to be especially vigilant. Restraints may be used in extreme situations.

EMTs must control the amount of stimulation the patient receives. Bill is threatened by the presence of two EMTs but tolerates one well. Limiting the number of people involved helps to contain the amount of sensory input. The removal of provoking family members or neighbors reduces the stimulation.

One EMT must be with the patient at all times. This serves a number of functions. The EMT provides the patient with a personal structure. Their interactions reinforce the patient's identity. The EMT also monitors the patient's behavior, controls the violence potential, and precludes elopement.

THE EMERGENCY DEPARTMENT EVALUATION

The ED staff has the responsibility for making order of the confusing array of symptoms and developing a treatment plan. The ED staff must engage the patient, perform a physical examination, elicit the chief complaint, make a psychiatric evaluation, and assess the patient's mental status.

The Reception

The success of the patient's management in the ED depends on the staff's application of a gently directed approach. To engage the schizophrenic person in the ED evaluation process requires that staff to use their skills, their understanding of patient dynamics, and their utmost tactics. The patients, with their ambivalence, vagueness, and aloofness, challenge the ED routine. Schizophrenic patients require staff time.

> *Bill does go to the ED. He initially refuses to sign in. He stands for fifteen minutes in the ED entrance. A secretary, then a nurse, and finally a physician ask him to come in. An intern suggests they talk in a quiet area after signing in. The patient follows him to the social service office. There he launches into a discourse about the Gulag Archipelago. The intern gently brings him back to the subject and the evaluation. An alert nurse asks the roommate to stay and wait for the physician.*

A number of specific techniques enhance staff effectiveness in the management of the schizophrenic patient in crisis. These begin with clear personnel identification and a stated treatment orientation, and they include maintenance of family involvement, reduction of stimuli, containment, and a comfortably distant and mildly directed interview technique. Additionally, someone must be with the patient at all times.

The ED intervention commences with a clearly stated identification of personnel and their pertinence to treatment. Staff must identify themselves by their formal names and professional roles. A handshake helps to establish contact with the patient. Early and with occasional reminders, the staff must tell the patient their plan for assisting him or her.

The family and friends are critical to the evaluation and treatment. Staff must also engage them in the ED. They supply important information overlooked or avoided by the patient. They possess the advantage of having observed the development of the crisis. They wait with the patient if the ED is busy. They assist in the referral process.

The staff must control the amount of stimulation to which the patient is exposed. An overwhelmed patient needs to avoid an overwhelming environment. Bill feels more comfortable in the office than in the entrance of the ED. The physician interviews the patient alone and in privacy.

Patient control requires containment. The staff establish personal and physical limits for the patient. Through their introduction and interview technique, they begin interpersonally to set up boundaries for the patient. The use of an office for interviewing provides structural limits for the patient.

The physician must employ a comfortably distant interview technique. This includes sitting at a respectful but involved distance from the patient—about 30 inches. Moving too close threatens the patient and his or her identity. Staying too far away reinforces the patient's aloofness. The interviewer must display ease with the situation. The physician acknowledges the difficulty the patient experiences in thinking. He or she listens to the patient's full response to questions but also keeps the patient on the topic.

Patients with thought disorder must not be left alone. Their ambivalence not uncommonly leads to elopement. Their unpredictability results in violence to themselves. Their aloofness expands to full withdrawal.

Physical Examination

The schizophrenic patient requires measurements of temperature, pulse, and blood pressure; and a physical examination. The examination helps the patient be assured about physical well-being and identity.

Chief Complaint

The chief complaint manifests many aspects of the disease and focuses on the crisis. It reflects the patient's ambivalence ("I guess I can't cope"); thought disorder ("I can't control my ideas; they're going too fast"); delusions ("Someone puts a transmitter in my spine"); hallucinations ("The voices are getting louder"); and self-destructive potential ("God wants me to kill myself"). These often illustrate the bizarreness of the patient's thinking and are of diagnostic importance. Bill Peterson's chief complaint is "The professor wins."

Psychiatric Evaluation

The pertinent portion includes history of present illness (HPI); social history; family history; developmental review; educational, vocational, and military history; psychiatric history; history of use of alcohol and abused substances; and medical history.

The HPI reviews the recent events which precipitated the crisis and covers personality changes during the preceding year. The physician must explore stresses and conflicts. It is necessary also to investigate life changes—at school, at work, and at home. The physician pays particular attention to the patient's social involvement and job performance for the last two years. Bill Peterson's HPI reveals a striking diminution of his world in the last year.

The social history provides information concerning the patient's interpersonal environment. It reveals where and with whom the person lives. The physician must appreciate the patient's social milieu. It is that milieu which ultimately either sustains or rejects the patient.

The family history offers diagnostic clues. Schizophrenia occurs in families. A history of schizophrenia in a parent, grandparent, or sibling suggests a predisposition to a thought disorder in the patient. Other important family data include histories of "nervous breakdowns" and psychiatric hospitalizations.

A developmental history furnishes a longitudinal view of the patient. Arieti (26) theorizes that schizophrenia emerges from a lifelong process. The patient as a child did not acquire trust. This lack of trust impends over the child's self-image and social interactions. In later childhood the person becomes hypersensitive and handles this by shyness. By adolescence these young people believe themselves inadequate and further withdraw from other people.

The educational, vocational, and military history contributes several pieces of information to the evaluation. First, the education background, when paired with the vocational level, may indicate a discrepancy. An Ivy League graduate's being employed as a sanitation truck worker suggests a problem. Second, frequent job changes because at each place "people were against me" hint strongly at thought disorder. Third, not infrequently the initial episode of schizophrenia occurs in the service. History of a military mental discharge might reflect such an episode.

The psychiatric history constitutes a major part of the evaluation. This history includes hospitalizations, outpatient involvement, and medications. The patient may have had several psychiatric hospitalizations. Often the schizophrenic patient is attending a clinic, seeing a therapist, and taking medication at the time of the crisis. It is not unusual for an exacerbation of the thought disorder to occur when the patient discontinues taking antipsychotic medication.

Finally, the physician explores the patient's use of alcohol and abused substances. An occasional patient seeks to use alcohol to manage withdrawal from social situations. One 45-year-old man demonstrated his thought disorder only during periods of sobriety. LSD, amphetamines, and PCP precipitate schizophrenic episodes.

A medical history includes recent illnesses and medications. Because it appears during young adulthood, schizophrenia must be differentiated from other diseases occurring then. The physician must consider both multiple sclerosis and systemic lupus erythematosus (27).

Mental Status Examination

The mental status examination yields positive findings in all seven aspects. First, the person's appearance reflects the diagnosis in a number of ways. The patient dresses in a bizarre, uncoordinated, inappropriate fashion. One patient wore a checked shirt, plaid pants, striped tie, and orange socks. Another patient, a 24-year-old, single woman, always dressed like a nineteenth-century widow. Often, chronic schizophrenic patients appear disheveled and unkempt. They look dull and have limited spontaneous movement. Many patients, like Bill Peterson, do not look at the interviewer and prefer to stare at the wall.

The patient displays a flat and inappropriate affect and speaks in monotones while depicting the worst horrors. Bill Peterson describes the professor's plan to kill him in a matter-of-fact, flat tone. The interviewer feels bored, distanced, and confused by the patient.

The thought content demonstrates the schizophrenic process in a number of ways. It reveals itself in the way the patient speaks and what the patient says. It includes faulty thought production, delusions, hallucinations, and irrationality.

The patient's thought production reveals schizophrenia. First, the patient produces thoughts in a disorganized and disconnected manner called *derailment.* If the thoughts become extremely fragmented and run together, the manner of speaking is referred to as *word salad.* Second, the patient becomes loquacious, either using much verbiage to answer the question *(circumstantiality)* or never reaching the goal *(tangentiality).* Third, patients exhibit *blocking;* they simply stop in midsentence or in the midst of an idea. Fourth, patients become *mute;* they do not reply or respond.

The patients with thought disorder have delusions. Bill Peterson fully believes in the professor's plot and remains convinced despite all efforts to change his mind. Delusions range from vague to precise. They can be stationary or expanding.

The schizophrenic patient experiences hallucinations. These are usually auditory, although olfactory and tactile hallucinations do occur. Not infrequently patients not only have auditory hallucinations but also hear their own thoughts talking inside their heads.

Patients also develop ideas of reference. They perceive special personal meanings in many different media events: papers, books, television, radio, and billboards.

The physician must find out about the patient's thoughts and plans of both suicide and homicide. Delusions and hallucinations contribute to the risk that patients will harm themselves or others. Bill Peterson wonders about getting a gun and shooting the professor. The physician must make a precise and extensive examination into this area.

The patient often demonstrates impaired judgment. The physician can assess judgment from the manner in which the patients have managed their lives.

The basic intellectual functions remain intact in schizophrenia. The patient does retain intellectual ability, but other things present distractions that reduce intellectual productivity. Bill Peterson can do college work but his delusion interferes.

Patients' insight into themselves and their disease varies. Mr Peterson has no understanding of his problem. Indeed, he believes it is the professor's problem. Other patients comprehend their disease. They discover the "craziness returns" when they stop taking their medication. They know what stresses tend to overwhelm them.

Assessment of the sensorium shows that schizophrenic patients rarely become disoriented to person, place, and time. However, they respond to abstracts in two extreme ways. On the one hand, a patient may concretely interpret the proverb "a stitch in time saves nine" by saying that a needle and thread are necessary. On the other hand, patients may wax eloquent and be severely vague, abstract, and disjointed. One 19-year-old patient revealed his thought disorder through his interpretations of the proverbs and in no other part of the mental status examination. In response to "a stitch in time," he talked for a half hour about the meaning of achievement in Western civilization.

DIAGNOSIS, TREATMENT PLAN, AND IMMEDIATE EMERGENCY DEPARTMENT THERAPY

The evaluation leads to a diagnosis and a treatment plan. The immediate ED therapy bridges the ED investigation and the implementation of the treatment plan. The schizophrenic patient requires a truly comprehensive treatment plan.

Diagnosis

The intern diagnoses Bill Peterson as having a schizophrenia disorder. He bases his diagnosis upon Mr Peterson's delusions (the professor's control over his mind), auditory hallucinations, and derailment. The physician also notes in reaching this diagnosis that the prodromal phase had featured social withdrawal and flattening of affect and that the patient is overly abstract in his reasoning.

The DSM III (5) lists the criteria for the diagnosis of schizophrenia, emphasizing characteristic symptoms and level of function. The diagnosis requires at least one of the 10 listed characteristics. Seven of these features pertain to delusions. They include: delusions that others are controlling the patient; thought broadcasting, in which the patient believes others hear his or her thoughts; thought insertion, a belief that someone is putting ideas into the patient's head; thought withdrawal, the belief that someone is removing the patient's thoughts; other bizarre delusions; somatic, negative, mystical, or religious delusions; and delusions accompanied by hallucinations. The other three diagnostic characteristics involve hallucinations: auditory hallucinations with voices commenting upon the patient's behavior and ideas, or with two or more voices carrying on a discussion; auditory hallucinations on several occasions, not limited to two words and unrelated to depression or elation; and illogical, incoherent thoughts or impoverished speech paired with a flat affect, hallucinations, or delusions. Finally, these characteristic symptoms must be accompanied by significant impairment of the daily routine.

DSM III sets the criteria for chronicity and the prodromal phase. Chronicity means that one or more of the 10 characteristic symptoms must have been present for six months. The prodromal phase requires deterioration in at least two of the following eight categories: social withdrawal; marked functional impairment; grossly eccentric behavior; decline in personal hygiene; flat or inappropriate affect; tangential, vague, circumstantial speech patterns; bizarre or magical thinking; and unusual perceptual experiences.

The DSM III further notes that the patient with schizophrenia does not demonstrate the full manic or depressive syndrome and that the patient does not have organic mental disorder.

The schizophrenic disorder has five subtypes. Each has met the criteria for schizophrenia and has additional features. The disorganized (hebephrenic) subtype is characterized by marked incoherence; silly, labile affect; fragmented delusions and hallucinations; and gross social impairment. Stupor, rigidity, or excitement highlight catatonic schizophrenia. Organized persecutory or grandiose delusions or hallucinations emerge as the prominent feature of the paranoid subtype. A combination of delusions, hallucinations, and disorganization characterize the undifferentiated subtype. In the residual subtype the patient experiences at least one schizophrenic episode but currently is clinically free of symptoms.

Treatment Plan

To formulate a treatment plan the physician combines information from the patient interview, from significant others, and from EMTs. He or she must take into consideration several important aspects of the disease and its treatment. First, the treatment of choice for schizophrenic patients who are having their first episode of the disorder is hospitalization. Hospitalization permits the maximum diagnostic investigation and therapeutic intervention. Second, antipsychotic medications make significant contributions to patients' improvement (13). Third, psychotherapy can benefit the patient. Fourth, effective treatment of the schizophrenic patient involves a coordinated use of the community therapeutic network—halfway houses, clinics, and aftercare. Fifth, both patients and their families may benefit from time away from one another. A brief hospitalization relieves accumulated domestic stresses. The doctor decides to admit Bill Peterson to the hospital's psychiatric unit.

Immediate Emergency Department Therapy

The immediate ED therapy serves a number of functions. It arranges for and encourages hospitalization. It provides rapid control over mounting disorganization. It offers a medication review and pharmacologic support.

One of the major tasks of the ED is to facilitate psychiatric hospitalization. Schizophrenic patients' aloofness, ambivalence, and suspiciousness make them extremely reluctant to accept hospitalization. Staff can gently persuade them and reinforce the benefits. Through their conduct during the reception and evaluation, staff members begin to establish trust with patients. This trust advances the treatment plan. In extreme cases, when a patient is dangerous but declines help, the staff must arrange for involuntary hospitalization.

The staff can rapidly bring a very disorganized patient under some control by a number of techniques. They contain the patient. They restrain a patient who has become violent. They use antipsychotic medications. Chlorpromazine (Thorazine) 50 to 100 mg PO or haloperidol (Haldol) 5 to 10 mg PO have proven quite effective (28). Haldol 2 to 5 mg as often as every half hour has become the drug of choice for IM use (29). It combines maximum antipsychotic properties with limited hypotensive effects.

ED staff provides immediate help to a chronic schizophrenic patient in ⁻everal ways. First, the physician restarts or alters the antipsychotic medications. Second, the physician checks for extrapyramidal signs and administers antiparkinsonian drugs when indicated. Third, staff members arrange for further community treatment. Finally, they are supportive and reassuring to the patient. That may indeed be the real reason why he or she came.

CARE AFTER THE EMERGENCY

The intern recommends and Mr Peterson reluctantly accepts psychiatric hospitalization. Bill Peterson wonders out loud, "What choice do I have?" Yet, he does sign the admission form. His roommate is greatly relieved and his family, contacted by telephone, encourages him to get help.

Once on the inpatient section, Bill Peterson becomes acutely anxious and says, "Now I have no identity." The treating psychiatrist prescribes Thorazine 100 mg four times a day, and then switches to Stelazine 10 mg four times daily when the patient complains of dizziness. Bill initially feels "borderless" without his wall, but through input from the nurses, psychiatric aides, and other patients he starts to find his identity. His physical investigation includes a complete blood cell count (CBC), urinalysis, EEG, blood chemistries (serum calcium, sodium, potassium, and glucose; and BUN), thyroid function tests (T_3 and T_4), a chest film, and lupus erythematosis cell smears. All test results are within normal limits.

Mr Peterson has regular psychotherapy sessions with a psychiatrist. Bill talks about the stresses of being away from home and trying to be a perfect student. He says everything has become overwhelming. Often he wanders off the subject. The therapist asks, "How does that subject relate to what we were just talking about?" After three weeks in the hospital, Bill comes to understand his attributing his college "failure" to the professor. The medication helps focus his thinking; the occupational therapy program helps him organize his efforts; and group therapy assists him to interact with others.

He returns home after six weeks in the hospital. He continues to take medication and attend weekly psychotherapy sessions. He works as a gardener instead of returning to school. He reports feeling "paranoid" when he misses his medication. In the psychotherapy sessions he sorts out his imagination from real events.

The course of treatment after the ED intervention incorporates two basic factors. The first revolves around the physician's extensive use of major portions of the community's treatment network of hospitalization, day treatment, outpatient psychotherapy, and aftercare services. The second involves the physician's proper application of specific psychotherapeutic concepts and medications to the schizophrenic patient.

Community Options

In a number of situations hospitalization is the treatment of choice for a schizophrenic patient in crisis (30). Indications for admission include a first episode of illness, overwhelming disorganization, dangerousness, lack of social support, and pronounced inertia. In most instances the patients benefit from short-term hospitalizations with an emphasis on rapid symptom resolution and restoration of functioning (31).

The treatment of choice for the first episode of schizophrenia is hospitalization. This principle underscores the seriousness of the disease. Hospitalization affords the most comprehensive investigation and treatment. It permits a complete medical examination and psychological testing. It involves the family in the information-gathering process and in the therapeutic approach.

The totally disorganized patient needs hospitalization. He talks in "word salads"; exhibits erratic and disconnected bits of behavior; shows a labile affect, switching from silliness to crying for no apparent reason; and cannot function in the social or employment arenas.

Dangerousness to self or others constitutes a reason for hospitalization. Schizophrenic patients may act in response to hallucinations and delusions. They may become significantly depressed. Hospitalization protects them and others. Staff have the responsibility to hospitalize patients, involuntarily if necessary, under these circumstances.

The social milieu—family, boardinghouse, and friends—under certain conditions cannot tolerate the patient's symptoms. The hospitalization often provides relief for them and ultimately enables them to sustain the patient in the community.

Finally, pronounced inertia is an indication for hospitalization. Some patients' withdrawal results in their just "sitting there." Hospitalization is the only route to help them engage society.

Day treatment provides a bridge between hospitalization and outpatient psychotherapy. It has the advantage of maintaining the patient's participation in the community and interaction with family members. It continues the structure of the hospital program while permitting the patient more autonomy.

Individual outpatient psychotherapy is a major modality for helping schizophrenic patients in the community. The one to one relationship enables patients to evaluate and modify their perceptions. It allows them to try a safe social interaction. It breaks down their isolation.

Home visits by mental health professionals have particular benefits for schizophrenic patients. Aftercare workers help to break the isolation and withdrawal. They encourage social activity when the patient has retreated too far. They observe the medication effects. They assess and report family conditions and stress. They help the patient to relate to a complex series of social agencies.

Psychotherapeutic Principles

A number of psychotherapeutic principles are particularly appropriate and effective in the treatment of schizophrenic patients (32) regardless of setting. They include maintenance of structure, recognition of affect, linkage of affect to symptoms, appreciation of stresses, and respect for the patient.

The therapist must strive to develop and to maintain a structure for the schizophrenic patient. The patient experiences heightened anxiety and disorganization when life lacks order. The structure takes many forms. In the inpatient unit, the physical limits of the building and the ward routine create structure. In day treatment, a fixed daily schedule provides it. In outpatient treatment, regularly set, consistent appointment times furnish it. The therapist must inform the patient well in advance of schedule changes.

The therapist helps the patient recognize emotions. The flat affect protects schizophrenic patients from feelings of anxiety, rejection, fear, and hostility. Patients struggle to deny and avoid their own emotions. The therapist assists the patient to identify these feelings. Bill Peterson experiences inner anxiety at college, but he hides this by withdrawal and delusions.

As patients become able to recognize their emotions, the therapist encourages them to see the link between emotions and symptoms. One 35-year-old schizophrenic man became "paranoid" on a series of jobs. His psychiatrist helped him to realize that he converted his employment anxiety into feelings of persecution. This linkage of emotions and symptoms serves as a vehicle for patients to understand themselves: otherwise they perceive all symptoms as coming "out of the blue."

In the next step the therapist guides the patient to identify the stress. The stress is a family conflict, a recent life change, a loss, or a job. Knowing the source of pressure, the patient avoids or diminishes it. The stress produces the affect.

Above all, the therapist must demonstrate acceptance of and respect for the patient. Schizophrenic patients suffer from chronic feelings of inadequacy and fear of rejection. They secretly believe people are against them, will make fun of them, and will not like them. The therapist partially counters this by developing a respectful relationship and dialogue with the patient.

Antipsychotic Medications

The advent of antipsychotic medication for the treatment of schizophrenia marks a giant advancement in modern psychiatry. Phenothiazines (eg, Thorazine), butyrophenones (eg, Haldol), thioxanthenes (eg, Navane), dihydroindolones (eg, Moban), and dibenzoxazepines (eg, Loxitane) have proven highly effective in diminishing and relieving the schizophrenic symptoms. If antipsychotic medication is discontinued, 65 percent of schizophrenic patients relapse (33).

The physician has the challenge of selecting the best medication for each patient. To make this determination the physician must align the patient's clinical features with the drug's properties. For patients who manifest significant anxiety, chlorpromazine hydrochloride (Thorazine) 100 mg four times daily, haloperidol (Haldol) 5 mg four times a day, and thioridazine hydrochloride (Mellaril) 100 mg four times daily provide sedation in addition to antipsychotic qualities. For patients who exhibit violence, disorganization, and disruption, haloperidol 2 to 5 mg IM has proven effective. Where the physician is concerned about hypotensive reactions, haloperidol 2 to 5 mg four times daily and trifluoperazine (Stelazine) 2 to 10 mg four times a day are useful. For patient with high levels of paranoia and obsessional thinking but little anxiety, trifluoperazine 2 to 10 mg four times daily or fluphenazine (Prolixin Enanthate and Prolixin Decanoate) 2.5 to 10 mg IM every two weeks has great value.

The best short- and long-term therapy for the schizophrenic patient requires a combined psychotherapeutic and pharmacotherapeutic approach (34).

Finally, despite pessimistic reports (35), the majority of diagnosed schizophrenic patients do well and make good social and work adjustments (36).

REFERENCES

1. Bleuler E: *Dementia Praecox, or the Group of Schizophrenias,* Zinkin S (trans). New York, International Universities Press, 1952.

2. Kraepelin E: *Dementia Praecox,* Barclary RM (trans). Edinburgh, ES Livingstone Ltd, 1919.

3. Harrow M, Grinker RR, Holzman PS, et al: Anhedonia and schizophrenia. *Am J Psychiatry* 134:794–797, 1977.

4. Kayton L, Koh SD: Hypohedonia in schizophrenia. *J Nerv Ment Dis* 161:412–420, 1975.

5. *Diagnostic and Statistical Manual of Mental Disorders,* ed 3. Washington DC, American Psychiatric Association, 1980.

6. Arieti S: *Interpretation of Schizophrenia.* New York, Brunner, 1955.

7. Schneider K: *Clinical Psychopathology,* Hamilton MW (trans). New York, Grune & Stratton, 1959.

8. Talbott JA (ed): *The Chronic Mental Patient.* Washington DC, American Psychiatric Association, 1978.

9. Erikson EH: Growth and crises of the healthy personality. *Psychol Issues* 1(monograph 1):50-100, 1959.

10. Lidz T, Fleck S, Cornelison AR: *Schizophrenia and the Family.* New York, International Universities Press, 1965.

11. Bateson G, Jackson DD, Haley J, et al: Toward a theory of schizophrenia. *Behavioral Science* 1:51-64, 1956.

12. Haley J: Testing parental instructions of schizophrenic and normal children. *J Abnorm Psychol* 73:559-565, 1968.

13. Wing JK: The social context of schizophrenia. *Am J Psychiatry* 135:1333-1339, 1978.

14. Kety SS: Genetic aspects of schizophrenia. *Psychiatric Annals* 6:6-15, 1976.

15. Slater E, Cowie VA: *The Genetics of Mental Disorders.* London, Oxford University Press, 1971.

16. Kety SS, Rosenthal D, Wender PH, et al: Mental illness in the biological and adoptive families of adopted schizophrenics. *Am J Psychiatry* 128:302-305, 1971.

17. Heath RG, Krupp IM: Schizophrenia as a specific biologic disease. *Am J Psychiatry* 124:1483-1490, 1968.

18. Breakey WR, Goodell H, Lorenz PC, et al: Hallucinogenic drugs as precipitants of schizophrenia. *Psychol Med* 4:255-261, 1974.

19. Connell PH: *Amphetamine Psychosis.* London, Chapman & Hall, 1958.

20. Allen RM, Young SJ: Phencyclidine-induced psychosis. *Am J Psychiatry* 135:1081-1084, 1978.

21. Snyder SH: Dopamine and schizophrenia. *Psychiatric Annals* 6:23-32, 1976.

22. Lamb, HR, Oliphant E: Schizophrenia through the eyes of families. *Hosp Community Psychiatry* 29:803-806, 1978.

23. Smith K, Pumphrey MW, Hall JC: The "last straw": The decisive incident resulting in the request for hospitalization in 100 schizophrenic patients. *Am J Psychiatry* 120:228-233, 1964.

24. Slaby AE, Lieb J, Tancredi LR: *Handbook of Psychiatric Emergencies.* Flushing NY, Medical Examination Publishing Co, 1975.

25. Tsuang MT: Suicide in schizophrenics, manics, depressives, and surgical controls. *Arch Gen Psychiatry* 35:153-155, 1978.

26. Arieti S: Schizophrenia: The psychodynamic mechanisms and psychostructural forms, in Arieti S, Brody EB (eds): *American Handbook of Psychiatry,* (ed 2. New York, Basic Books, 1974, vol 3, pp 551-587.

27. Freedman AM, Kaplan HI, Sadock BJ: *Modern Synopsis of Comprehensive Textbook of Psychiatry.* Baltimore, Williams & Wilkins Co, 1972.

28. Shader RI, Jackson AH: Approaches to schizophrenia, in Shader RI (ed): *Manual of Psychiatric Therapeutics.* Boston, Little Brown & Co, 1978, pp 63-100.

29. Donlon PT, Hopkin J, Tupin JP: Overview: Efficacy and safety of the rapid neuroleptization method with injectable haloperidol. *Am J Psychiatry* 136:273-278, 1979.

30. Feigelson EB, Davis EB, MacKinnon R, et al: The decision to hospitalize. *Am J Psychiatry* 135:354-375, 1978.

31. Endicott J, Cohen J, Nee J, et al: Brief vs standard hospitalization. *Arch Gen Psychiatry* 36:706-712, 1979.

32. Fromm-Reichman IF: Psychotherapy of schizophrenia. *Am J Psychiatry* 111:410-419, 1954.

33. Davis JM: Overview: Maintenance therapy in psychiatry: I. Schizophrenia. *Am J Psychiatry* 132:1237-1245, 1975.

34. Grinspoon L, Ewalt JR, Shader R: Psychotherapy and pharmacotherapy in chronic schizophrenia. *Am J Psychiatry* 124:1645-1652, 1968.

35. Harrow M, Grinker RR, Silverstein ML, et al: Is modern-day schizophrenic outcome still negative? *Am J Psychiatry* 135:1156-1162, 1978.

36. Bland RC, Parker JH: Prognosis in schizophrenia. *Arch Gen Psychiatry* 33:949-954, 1976.

12

The Patient Struggling to Control an Impulse

THE PATIENT

Patients struggle with many impulses: to run away, to kill, to drink, to expose themselves, to commit suicide, to eat, to molest children, to steal, to set fires, to take drugs, to have a homosexual relationship, to hit their children, to fight, to mutilate themselves.

Torn between the impulse and the wish to resist it, between the urge and the knowledge that it is wrong, and between the act and the need to talk about it, patients come to the ED. These self-referred patients seek to maintain control and to understand themselves and their behavior.

> Carol Wallace wants to run away from home. At 34 years of age and with two children, ages 5 and 7, she finds herself trapped, angry, isolated, frustrated, and stalled. Her husband, a 36-year-old executive, spends most of his life focused on a career. She loved him, but she now hates him for reasons which she does not understand. She feels boredom and emptiness at home despite the statement by her friends, "You have it made." She wants to run; she has to stay. She does not know; yet she knows too much.
>
> She centers her life on the flight. She schemes, packs, and then unpacks. She gets in the car but stops. She thinks of an affair, of suicide, of homicide, and of alcohol. But she finds each "immoral" and "not her." She dwells on escape, dreams about it, and fantasies about it. She tries to talk to friends, but they have their own problems. She does not want to hurt her aging parents. The minister only preaches to her. She wants to run to somewhere. She feels an explosion building in her head. She runs to the ED for help.

The patient struggling to control an impulse displays a number of emotions, experiences a variety of perceptional changes, and exhibits a series of behaviors.

191

Each represents the conflict; each adds to the torment; and each pushes the patient toward a solution.

The Patient's Mood

The conflict produces a number of intensely contrasting and provocative emotions. These include pleasure, anger, guilt, depression, cravings, wonderment, and anxiety. In the end the patient feels caught in an incredible emotional turmoil.

Pleasure generates the power that keeps the impulse recurring. Fantasies about what the patient wants bring immediate gratification and moments of delight. A 42-year-old, married college professor struggles to avoid an affair with a student. In the thoughts and the preparation, he feels excitement, anticipation, and joy. He balances the consequence of employment termination and divorce against the pleasure. The sober alcoholic struggles against the elation of *just one drink*. The impulse represents a very potent source of intense pleasure to the patient. Carol Wallace would feel great exhilaration if she could just escape.

But the patients also feel anger for a variety of reasons. First, they are frustrated because they simply cannot follow the impulse. Mrs Wallace wonders with annoyance why she cannot just run away. Second, patients are angry that they have these impulses at all. Why do other people seem to have no control problems? The dieting patient is angry because others do not spend their lives fighting the desire to eat every minute. Third, patients express annoyance at the amount of time and energy they expend in controlling the impulses. Mrs Wallace becomes furious at herself for "allowing herself" to be so wrapped up in the dilemma.

Guilt comes to dominate much of the patient's mood. It serves as the counterpoint and counterbalance to the pleasure power of the impulse. Emanating from the clash between the impulse and religious beliefs, professional ethics, community standards, family orientation, and personal convictions, guilt is a powerful emotion. It causes containment of the initial impulse and continues to check the action. Mrs Wallace becomes increasingly guilty as she contemplates running away.

The patient feels depressed for many reasons. Indeed, a sense of depression not infrequently serves as the genesis of the impulse. Mrs Wallace's desire for flight represents her wish to escape her sad, empty home. The unfulfilled impulse becomes a source of depression. Patients long for what they cannot have. The conflict itself produces feelings of melancholy. The patients experience sadness as they find themselves caught up in their own turmoil.

The patient frequently experiences a wave of craving, feeling such an intense desire to act upon the impulse that nothing else in the world matters. The person will sacrifice family, friends, and position to fulfill the desire. A 45-year-old mother of four, wife of a prominent official, wants diet pills. She was addicted for several years. She successfully abstained for one year after inpatient detoxification and treatment. Now she feels "possessed" by an intense craving for "just one pill." At that moment her children and her husband cease to matter. She will do anything to get a pill.

Patients are perplexed by the illogic of their behavior. In moments of insight and objective self-observation, the patient expresses amazement at the entire situation. Mrs Wallace puzzles over her predicament. How could she leave her beautiful children? For what? To go where? She amazes herself.

The impulse, the pleasure, the guilt, and the depression combine to produce the overriding feeling of anxiety. The patient experiences unbearable tension. The conflict causes a continual pressure and pain. The anxiety propels the patient to seek help. Carol Wallace comes to the ED not only as a form of flight but also to escape the tension of her dilemma.

The Patient's Perceptions

The struggle with an impulse affects the patient's perceptions in a number of ways. It produces a pervasive preoccupation, referential thinking, and loss of options and priorities. It causes one to adopt a surreptitious attitude.

The struggle for impulse control becomes a pervasive preoccupation. The patient dwells on the dilemma, spends endless hours pondering the predicament, and interminably wrestles with the conflict. What begins as a concern expands to an obsession. It involves the person's dreams and fantasies. Mrs Wallace has become preoccupied by thoughts of flight. Her fantasied journey dominates her life.

In addition to worrying about the conflict all the time, the patient finds reference to the impulse everywhere. The sober alcoholic discovers hundreds of liquor advertisements in the newspaper and magazines and on television. The patient fighting the urge to molest children sees youngsters everywhere.

Patients confront a paucity of options. By the time the conflict has reached the crisis phase, patients see only two alternatives: either act upon it or not. They become myopic in their outlook. They have trapped themselves.

The conflict has also altered the patients' priorities. They have elevated the impulse so that it is the most important item in life. The role of family and career has degenerated. The impulse has become everything.

Finally, the impulse produces a surreptitious way of thinking. Patients feel so ashamed of the impulse that they keep it to themselves. They do not dare risk telling anyone. They become secretive. Mrs Wallace feels she cannot share her dilemma with anyone—husband, friends, or minister. She keeps the explosion to herself.

The Patient's Behavior

The conflict generates a number of kinds of behavior. These include avoidance patterns of behavior and rehearsal of the impulse. Additionally, the patient exhibits many of the manifestations of anxiety. Yet, most importantly, it is what the patient does *not* do that constitutes the most significant behavior.

Patients attempt to avoid the places where the impulse might be acted upon. They control the impulse by restricting their activities. The sober alcoholic turns down invitations to parties where drinking predominates. The patient struggling with child molesting impulses goes out the the way to avoid playgrounds and parks. Mrs Wallace prefers to stay at home and refuses to drive her car, secretly fearing a trip to the store will lead to flight.

Frequently the patients rehearse the tempting impulse, but each time they stop short of completing the act. They toy with it, play with it, and then at the last moment back off. A 35-year-old, depressed man struggled against the impulse to kill himself. Each night he took out his .38 caliber revolver and held it to his head. He never loaded the gun. He wanted to die; he wanted to live; he wanted help.

These conflicted patients portray all the behavior of the anxious patient (see Chapter 5). They pace, have difficulty eating and sleeping, and appear restless. Their acts reflect anxiety, tension, and agitation.

Yet, it is what the patients do *not* do that contributes the critical part of the behavior. They do *not* run, kill, commit suicide, drink, or expose themselves. Mrs Wallace does not run away from home. The impulse is resisted.

THE CAUSES OF IMPULSIVE BEHAVIOR

Intrapsychic, interpersonal, and biologic factors cause or contribute to the impulse and the struggle to control it. Often the interplay of the three creates the conflict both by prompting the impulse and by providing the barrier against its activation.

Intrapsychic Causes of Impulsive Behavior

Personality attributes and attitudes contribute to the conflict. Some people have characteristics and attitudes that lead to impulsive behavior. On the other hand, other personal features produce impulse restraint. Additionally, the patient with a thought disorder or severe depression is driven by internal commands.

The impulsive personality has difficulty with control. From birth through childhood development, this kind of person exhibits little restraint (1). These patients impulsively pursue their own aims as they mature.

Certain attitudes lead to impulsive behavior. Some people believe they are entitled to all the pleasure they can "get." They see continual enjoyment as a right. A 37-year-old salesman believed he would die by age 38 of a cardiac condition. He based all his life and behavior on that assumption. He drank, used drugs, spent money, and had affairs because "tomorrow will never come!" He discovered, with depression, that he would live beyond the age of 38. He had to reassess painfully his entire life's goal and orientation.

In contrast, other personality attributes and attitudes lead to excessive restraint and restrictions. These generate conflict to any expression of an impulse. This kind of person comes from a repressing family, where even the mention of certain activities was taboo. A 50-year-old, depressed housewife came to the ED because she "thought about suicide." She had never before had the idea; she knew it was a sin; and she felt "bad" because she had experienced even the thought.

Paradoxically, the patient also derives enjoyment from the impulse because of the family's and society's restraint. The concept of "getting away with something" is appealing.

The patient with a thought disorder or someone who is in the midst of severe depression not infrequently responds to voices commanding him or her to do something, for example, to commit suicide or kill someone else. These patients experience auditory hallucinations. The voices order them to perform drastic, repugnant deeds. A 20-year-old man who had been at the state hospital twice for schizophrenic episodes stopped taking his Thorazine. He began to hear voices telling him he was Satan, he must die, and he must jump off the tallest structure in town. With insight based on prior episodes, he came to the ED for help.

Interpersonal Causes of Impulsive Behavior

Interpersonal factors both generate and restrain the impulse. They cause it, and they check its expression. Together they produce the conflict.

Interpersonal factors promote the impulse in two ways: by their endorsement of it and by their causing the situation which prompted it. In the former, family, friends, and employers overtly and covertly support the impulsive behavior. The patient struggling to avoid drugs and alcohol finds his entire social milieu pushing these upon him. A salesman attempting to remain sober finds himself at a business conference where he is "supposed to drink" and discovers his wife still keeps a few beers in the refrigerator. An 18-year-old college student encounters massive pressure from her roommates and her dates to do things she morally objects to.

Interpersonal factors in the social situation sometimes actually cause the impulse. A 14-year-old wants to run away from home because of sexual threats from her brother and protracted battles between her parents. Mrs Wallace desires flight to escape her boredom, her husband, and her house.

On the other hand, the social milieu also serves to check the expression of the impulse. The patient risks suspension from school, expulsion from the family, termination from employment, or divorce by the spouse as a consequence of following the impulse. Mrs Wallace feels constrained from flight by her society, her parents, her family, and her religion.

Biologic Causes of Impulsive Behavior

A number of biologic factors act to heighten the power of an impulse and accelerate the conflict. These include medications, alcohol, abused substances, central nervous system illnesses, and manic episodes.

Certain medications have been known to lead to increased impulsive activity. Goodwin (2) reports that use of L-dihydroxyphenylalanine (L-dopa) heightens sexual drives and activities. Similarly, more aggressive and impulsive behavior has been observed following androgen administration (3). Antidepressants have precipitated impulse control problems in schizophrenic patients and triggered manic episodes in manic-depressive patients.

Alcohol and abused substances create impulse control problems in two ways. First, in the intoxicated phase the patient experiences surges of impulses which remain in check during sobriety. Second, in the withdrawal phase the person develops an intense craving for the drug.

During alcohol and drug intoxication the person experiences strong impulses. Alcohol has been especially implicated. The patients exhibit aggressiveness and heightened sexuality (4). They attempt suicide or homicide. Numerous other abused substances produce increased impulsiveness; these include amphetamines (5), barbiturates (6), cocaine (7), LSD (8), and PCP (9). A 25-year-old man came to the ED in a panic. While mildly intoxicated he had discovered himself getting very close with another man. He was on the verge of "picking him up" when he "realized what I was doing." For the last five years he had been struggling with issues of his own sexuality. While he was under the influence of alcohol the conflict had finally erupted.

Withdrawal from alcohol and abused substances lead to intense craving. Physiologic and psychologic factors combine to make withdrawal from alcohol, amphetamines, cocaine, cigarettes, and opiates extremely difficult. A 28-year-old opiate user comes to the ED for help. He wants to stop his habit but knows without assistance the craving will overwhelm him and he will "get another hit."

Head trauma, intracranial hemorrhages, and seizures produce difficulty with impulse control (10). The patients frequently become boisterous, aggressive, and hypersexual. They exhibit inappropriate, sudden, impulsive behavior. A 24-year-old motorcyclist sustained massive head trauma in an accident. During the acute stage of the recovery and later he displayed "wild," violent behavior in the face of minor stresses.

Additionally, the manic episode of manic-depressive illness leads to increased impulsiveness. Murphy and colleagues (11) note that manic patients experience a pressure and drive resulting in hypersexuality and aggressiveness. Not infrequently these patients seek the ED as they note themselves getting "high."

THE REACTIONS OF OTHERS

Family members, friends, and employers display a wide range of reactions to the impulsive patient. On one extreme they do not even know the problem exists; on the other they encourage the person to obtain assistance. Additional reactions include distance, disbelief, denigration, and avoidance.

Family members and friends frequently do not even know about the problem. The patient has successfully kept a secret of the impulse. Those around the person remain unaware of the conflict. Indeed, her family and friends do not know of Mrs Wallace's struggle.

As a consequence of the secret life, the patient becomes distanced from the social support system. Other people in turn distance the patient but do not realize why. They sense they are not part of the person's life and can never be. Coworkers wonder why the struggling, alcoholic person routinely declines social invitations.

When family and friends do become aware of the impulse, often they simply do not believe it. They do not see the patient as "that type of person" and dismiss the entire notion.

Others react with denigration of the patient and the conflict. They not only refuse to believe the seriousness of the impulse conflict but also ridicule the patient and the problem. They see it as foolish and stupid. "Why can't you drink?"; "What's wrong with eating?"; or "Why are you so hung up about running away?"

Still others avoid the patient when they learn of the impulse. They do not want to be associated with a potential child molester, alcoholic, or drug user. Their action provides evidence for the patient to remain secretive about the conflict.

Some families and friends recognize the patient's torment, anguish, and pain over the conflict and recommend help. They support the person in obtaining therapy. They appreciate the significance of the dilemma.

THE INITIATION OF THE EMERGENCY

Under certain circumstances the patient or the family and friends seek immediate assistance. Although the patient may have tolerated the conflict for decades, it always has the potential to produce a crisis. The situations which create a crisis include overwhelming anxiety, a greatly restricted life, a heightened impulse, the advent of an opportunity to act upon the impulse, and the concern of others.

The conflict generates anxiety. When the anxiety exceeds the patient's tolerance, he or she looks for help. The person discovers the apprehension, tension, and pressure unbearable and seeks relief. Mrs Wallace feels overwhelmed by anxiety. Her dilemma has produced an incredible tension without any release or relief.

Sometimes patients seek help after discovering that the conflict has become their sole preoccupation. They have virtually ceased to function and ignore their jobs and families. The resultant paralysis creates the crisis. A 40-year-old, single woman struggled with an intense desire to eat. Yet she wanted to be thin. Food became her major focus. If she went out she would eat; if she stayed home she would eat. But she wanted to avoid food. She dreamed about food. When her conflict precluded her going to work, she sought help.

Patients request immediate assistance when they perceive a heightened potency to the impulse. They sense an increased drive to harm someone, to hurt themselves, or to drink again. They recognize the growing potential for loss of control. They want immediate help to maintain command over the impulse.

In response to impending opportunity to act upon the impulse, patients seek help. Suddenly they find themselves in a position where they must confront the dreaded, desired object; they cannot avoid it. A 25-year-old man struggled with amorous desires toward children. He managed to keep these impulses in check by avoiding places where he would be alone with youngsters. Then his sister asked him to care for her three children for several days. He panicked; he went to the ED to find out how to get into therapy.

Finally, family and friends, when they become aware of the conflict, often insist that the patient obtain help. Sometimes they seek assistance because of their own apprehension. A mother rushed her 14-year-old son to the ED when he mentioned liking other boys. Other times the social milieu recognizes the toll which the conflict exacts from the patient and urges the person to seek therapy.

THE EMTs' RESPONSE TO THE EMERGENCY

An effective EMT intervention facilitates treatment. The EMTs function in a unique capacity to support and encourage the patient; they help maintian control. Their approach requires a sensitivity to the patient's dilemma, a prompt response, introduction and identification, accompaniment of the patient, a controlled involvement of the family, and—most important—a positive treatment attitude.

A 40-year-old executive, newly separated from his wife and four children, sits in his new apartment and looks at a large bottle of sleeping pills. He wants to kill himself to "show" his wife, but he does not want "to hurt the kids." He calls the suicide hot line; the volunteers there, with his approval, request the rescue unit to pick him up and bring him to the hospital. Speed in response in essential. Proper EMT technique prevents the suicide, supports his control, and facilitates psychiatric treatment.

The entire EMT response and the subsequent ED evaluation must be based on an appreciation of these patients' dynamics and conflict. They feel frightened, ashamed, and embarrassed. They must share the secret, yet this scares them. They tentatively, skeptically, and hesitantly approach help. EMTs' and ED staff members' insensitivity leads patients to withdrawal from the intervention.

A prompt response serves several purposes. First, it provides immediate support and encouragement to patients before they change their minds. Second, it underscores the EMTs' interest in and concern for the patient and their awareness of the seriousness of the crisis. Rapid response tells patients they are important and their problems are significant. Third, by their presence they help the patient to maintain control. The person will not act upon the impulse while they are there.

EMTs must introduce and identify themselves. Doing this establishes a formal and professional approach. It creates a sense of confidence and trust for the patient; it says, "We are trained, interested professionals."

EMTs must accompany the patient throughout the transport. They provide support, preclude withdrawal, and check the impulse. They offer comfort to the anxious patient, encouragement to the frightened patient, and professional concern to the embarrassed patient.

The EMTs must control the family's and friends' involvement. In certain circumstances the family proves detrimental to the intervention. Family members' anxiety or prejudices interfere with treatment and cause the patient to decline help. A mother panics when she discovers her 20-year-old son's child-molesting impulse. Her anger and emotional display cause him even greater apprehension. The EMTs request that she not accompany them to the ED. In other situations family involvement helps and comforts the patient. Family members support and reinforce the seeking of treatment.

The most important function of the EMTs is their presentation of a positive treatment attitude. Covert or overt reactions of "I don't believe that," "You must be sick," "That's a stupid problem," or "Therapy is a waste of time" shatter the frail intervention process. The patient intensely scrutinizes EMTs' words and faces for evidence of scorn and rejection. On the other hand, the EMTs' positive attitude promotes treatment and supports the patient's decision to seek help.

THE EMERGERCY DEPARTMENT EVALUATION

Mrs Wallace goes to an ED. There she shyly, anxiously, and ambivalently signs in. She politely declines to discuss her problem with the triage nurse. Several times while waiting she starts to leave. A nurse persuades her to stay.

The physician interviews her in a quiet room. There for the first time in her long struggle she talks to someone about her impulse to run. The doctor listens; she feels relief. During the interview she discovers the depth of the problem and some of its origins.

She debates and then decides not to involve her husband in the ED evaluation. She welcomes the physician's suggestion of outpatient psychotherapy, and he arranges an appointment with a therapist.

She returns home with "a load off her mind," relieved and helped. She feels good that someone listened without lecturing her and understood her dilemma. She welcomes the opportunity to continue her therapy.

The ED evaluation not only constitutes the turning point in the crisis but also begins the psychotherapeutic process. Through it the staff helps the patient to maintain control, to understand the origin of the impulse, and to become involved in treatment. The evaluation includes the reception, the physical examination, the chief complaint, a psychiatric evaluation, and a mental status examination.

The Reception

The ED reception continues the approach developed by the EMTs, engages the patient, and commences therapy. It facilitates the evaluation and provides treatment. The reception involves promptness; staff identification; the use of a quiet, private room; a positive staff attitude; a judicious involvement of family; constant accompaniment of the patient; and, most important, therapy.

Impulsive patients benefit from prompt reception in the ED. They are ambivalent about having come; delays heighten the urge to leave, and waiting increases apprehension. Mrs Wallace anxiously sits in the ED waiting room. Only because of staff reassurance does she stay.

ED staff must introduce and identify themselves, using both formal names and professional titles. This introduction helps the patient to establish trust and confidence in the ED staff. The staff must also address the patient by formal name. This approach reinforces the patient's adult role. Carol Wallace is addressed as Mrs Wallace, not as Carol, in order to emphasize her responsible, mature role and control.

The physician conducts the interview in a quiet, private room. The office setting promotes a feeling of trust, privileged communication, and security. Mrs Wallace refuses to talk about her problem at the triage desk in the middle of the ED. She feels comfortable in the office.

ED staff promote and make treatment possible by their positive attitude toward the patient. Staff sometimes display many of the reactions cited as occurring within the family and among the friends. They express anger toward the patient struggling with alcohol, drugs, or child-molesting impulses. They see the patient who is fighting for control as immature, irresponsible, or foolish. They underestimate the patient's dilemma and conflict, and they fail to appreciate the gravity of the situation. The patient often perceives these staff attitudes as rejection. More important, a positive attitude makes treatment possible. In the author's experience, the patient asking for help with control represents a very treatable emergency. These patients come to talk about the impulse rather than act upon it. They seek therapy and avoid impulsive behavior.

ED staff must judiciously involve family and friends. In many situations the patient wishes the family not to be notified or otherwise involved. The physician must ask the patient's permission to contact family and friends. A 17-year-old high school senior wanted to run away from home, but at her request a school counselor brought her to the ED. She allowed the physician to call her parents. They came to the ED. There for the first time they realized the depth of the problem. In contrast, Mrs Wallace chooses not to have her husband involved. The physician honors her wishes.

Most patients benefit from having someone stay with them during the evaluation. This reduces anxiety, helps the patients maintain impulse control, and precludes their prematurely leaving the ED. A staff nurse reassures Mrs Wallace during the wait.

Finally, and paramount, the evaluation itself is therapeutic. It provides patients with the unique opportunity to talk about themselves and the conflict. Open disclosure in a private, confidential setting benefits people. They discover they *can* "talk about it."

Physical Examination

The physician must secure a pulse, blood pressure, and temperature. A more extensive examination is undertaken if indicated.

Chief Complaint

The chief complaint encapsulates, highlights, and characterizes the crisis: "Stop me from drinking"; "I have a loaded gun; I'm afraid I might use it"; "Voices are commanding me to jump"; "I want to expose myself"; and Mrs Wallace's "I want to run away from home." These chief complaints also are cries for help and demonstrate insight. "I need help with control"; "I have a fear of touching children"; or "I have to talk about it or I'll do something I'll regret."

Psychiatric Evaluation

The physician focuses on certain key portions of the psychiatric evaluation in the interview of the impulsive patient. Particularly important parts are the history of present illness (HPI), social history, family and developmental history, psychiatric history, and history of use of alcohol, substances, and medications.

The HPI constitutes the cornerstone of the evaluation. In eliciting it the physician must ask specific questions concerning the impulse: How long has the patient struggled with it? When is it worse? When is it better? Has the person ever acted on it? If the patient did act on it, what would happen? When did the impulse first arise? Has it ever occurred before? What effect has the conflict had upon the person's life? Has the patient ever previously discussed it with anyone? How have people reacted to the problem? Does the patient feel in control of himself or herself and the impulse? What can be done to help?

The social history furnishes information concerning where and with whom the patient resides. It offers clues about the social milieu. This knowledge helps the physician to understand the genesis of the impulse and to appreciate the environment to which the patient will ultimately return. The physician discovers Mrs Wallace's social and family life impoverished, empty, and "boring." She seeks flight from her unsatisfying emotional climate. Finding out about the environment to which the patient will return after the emergency is of paramount importance. A 16-year-old boy had urges to set fires. He lived in a wooden tenement district and received no supervision at home. The physician hospitalized him.

The family and developmental history provides further information. The physician inquires whether there are other family members with impulsive conflicts and struggles. Not infrequently a father with problems of impulse control rears a child with similar struggles. The physician also searches the patient's developmental history for impulsive behavior. An impulsive, acting-up youth often grows into an aggressive adult. This history also reveals what impulses the patient *has* acted upon.

The psychiatric history yields important data. Like the patient with a chronic thought disorder, the person with impulse control problems may have a history of hallucinations or commands and may have had psychiatric treatment. The impulse may constitute the first sign of a manic episode. A history of manic-depressive illness provides vital diagnostic information. The patient might have had treatment for a previous episode of erupting impulses. On prior occasions medications may have proved effective in controlling the impulse: if so, the physician needs to find out what they were.

Finally, the physician must make specific inquiry into the patient's use of alcohol, substances, and medications. These not only are responsible for withdrawal craving, but also for the potential increase in the pressure to act upon the impulse. The investigation must be thorough and detailed: What pills? How much alcohol? For how long? When was the last substance taken?

Mental Status Examination

The physician pays particular attention to certain aspects of the mental status examination when assessing patients for impulse control problems. These aspects include affect, thought content, plans for suicide and homicide, judgment, insight, and intellect.

The affect both provides the emotional power to the impulse and reflects the degree of turmoil and conflict. The more potent the affect, for example, craving, the stronger the patient's urge to act upon the impulse. The affect explains the reason why the crisis happened now. Mrs Wallace experiences an intense impulse to run and the bitter turmoil causes her to get help.

In exploring the patient's thought content, the physician examines for hallucinations and obsessions. Auditory hallucinations drive the patient toward impulsive behavior. Obsessions mirror the patient's level of preoccupation.

The physician must assess the potential for suicide and homicide for two reasons. First, the patient may be struggling with an impulse to commit suicide or kill someone else. Second, the patient contemplates suicide as an alternative to either acting upon the impulse or having it publicly exposed. One patient preferred suicide to hitting her child again. A 40-year-old attorney feared professional and public censure for his "secret wish" to dress in women's clothing. He thought of killing himself as an alternative.

The assessment of the patient's judgment reveals how the patient has handled the impulse, the conflict, and the resultant crisis. Has the person maintained control? Has he or she acted responsibly? By coming to the ED instead of acting on the impulse, the patient demonstrates appropriate judgment. Mrs Wallace shows good judgment by "running" to the ED instead of just going away.

The patient's insightfulness indicates both how much has been gained from the interview and how much the person may be expected to benefit from psychotherapy. Very often the patient derives an understanding of the crisis during the intervention. In her interview, Mrs Wallace recognizes the source of her impulse. Insight promotes therapy. The more interest patients have in examining their dynamics, the more inclined they are toward therapy. Mrs Wallace wants to learn more about herself.

The person's intellect offers clues to the best treatment. The more verbal and intelligent the patient, the better the opportunity for psychotherapy.

DIAGNOSIS, TREATMENT PLAN, AND IMMEDIATE EMERGENCY DEPARTMENT THERAPY

As a result of the evaluation and initial intervention, the physician reaches a diagnosis, determines a treatment plan, and undertakes immediate therapy. In this process the physician uses the information and impressions from the patient's evaluation; reports, when appropriate, from significant others; and the observations reported by the EMTs. The physician relies most heavily upon the patient interview.

Diagnosis

The impulse and the struggle to control it can be manifestations of a wide variety of diagnostic categories. These include the psychoses; dependency on alcohol, substances, tobacco, or caffeine; disorders of impulse control; and adjustment reactions.

In both the schizophrenic disorders and the affective disorders, the impulse struggle can be the presenting symptom. Schizophrenic patients, usually of the paranoid or undifferentiated type, complain of voices outside their heads, or thoughts arguing inside their heads, telling them to do something. The patients feel the command is wrong and seek help to oppose it. With affective disorders, impulse issues arise in both the depressed and manic phases. Patients with depressive disorder most often struggle with the impulse to kill themselves. They realize they need help to control their suicidal course. Patients with manic disorder become aware that they are getting "high" and want assistance to check their mood change.

Alcohol, amphetamines, barbiturates, cocaine, opiates, marijuana, tobacco, and caffeine all produce dependency. The diagnosis of dependence includes several criteria. First, the patient develops a strong craving to use the substance on a regular basis. Second, over a period of time the patient uses the substance more frequently and in increasing amounts to obtain the desired effect. Third, the patient discovers upon discontinuance of the substance that he or she feels uncomfortable, anxious, depressed, and driven to resume use of the substance.

The patient may have a disorder of impulse control (12). These disorders include pathological gambling, kleptomania, pyromania, intermittent explosive disorder, and isolated explosive disorder. These diagnoses all feature difficulty in controlling the impulse, tension before the act, and gratification, pleasure, or release at the time of the act. An increasing preoccupation with gambling and a resultant impairment of family and work relations characterize pathological gambling. Kleptomania involves the impulse to steal, followed by pleasure in theft. It is notable that the object stolen is of no direct concern to the patient. The patient with pyromania has the impulse to set fires, feels rising tension before the act, and derives pleasure from the event. The patient has no regard for the consequences of the fire and does not derive financial gain from the blaze. The explosive disorders are characterized by either an isolated episode of violence or intermittent episodes of at least three incidents. In either situation the patient acts out aggression in gross excess of the social standards and then later experiences genuine regret. Between episodes the patient does not manifest aggressiveness.

Finally, the impulse may represent an adjustment disorder. In this diagnosis the patient is reacting to identifiable stresses or situations. The conflict does not represent an exacerbation of a prior mental disorder and will remit once the stress diminishes. The ED physician diagnosed Mrs Wallace as having adjustment disorder with mixed emotional features.

Treatment Plan

The treatment plan focuses on immediate therapy and referral. The referral involves hospitalization, outpatient psychotherapy, or self-help groups. The patient requires a definite referral. The ED intervention has commenced a vital psychotherapeutic program.

Immediate Emergency Department Therapy

The ED intervention must achieve several objectives. These include the patient's recognition and appreciation of the conflict, a positive reception with reinforcement for control, a therapeutic experience, medications if appropriate, and a definite follow-up.

Through the evaluation the patient begins to recognize and understand the conflict. The patient starts to comprehend the depth to which the problem has dominated life. From the history the person realizes the extent, seriousness, and development of the impulse. Mrs Wallace, after the interview, understands the dimensions and the significance of flight.

The ED therapy consists of a positive reception and a reinforcement for the patient's control. The physician must point out to the patient the advantages of having come to the ED rather than acting on the impulse. By the interview, by the attention, and by the follow-up, the staff supports the notion of *talking* about the impulse.

The ED experience must be therapeutic. The patient must have the opportunity to explore an intimate problem openly with a professional. The ED intervention not infrequently represents the first time in the patient's life that he or she has "opened up" to anyone. If the physician performs this exploration with interest, concern, openness, and engagement, the patient feels something has been achieved.

Medications are occasionally of value in the immediate situation. Where anxiety is a serious symptom, a minor tranquilizer for a short time has been useful. Where the patient struggles against violence and wants medicine to keep control, chlorpromazine (Thorazine) 50 to 100 mg PO has been effective. In the vast majority of cases, discussion of the impulse is the most important way to deal with it.

The physician arranges for a definite referral. The control maintained and strengthened in the ED must be continued. Effective ED therapy facilitates the establishment of a treatment program.

CARE AFTER THE EMERGENCY

Mrs Carol Wallace starts outpatient, weekly, individual psychotherapy sessions. She discovers a basic dissatisfaction with her life since her last child commenced school. Her housework and her husband are empty, boring, and uninteresting. Her children seem to need her less than before. From this "hollow" home she seeks to run away.

After recognizing the genesis of her impulse, she begins to explore herself and the solution. She has always used escape to solve problems. She examines alternatives—divorce, career, volunteer activities, more interest in housework, or athletics. She confronts her husband; he responds at first with perplexity and then with support. She returns to school and obtains a part-time position. The impulse dissolves as the underlying problem is resolved.

After the emergency, treatment to help patients continue and enhance their impulse control involves a number of options. These include hospitalization, both individual and group outpatient psychotherapy, medications, and self-help organizations.

Hospitalization

Hospitalization is the treatment of choice for impulse control in many situations. These include situations in which patients ask for further controls, their social environment feels too threatened by them, the patients find the conflict too incapacitating, and the ED physician judges that the patients require continuous support and restraint.

Quite frequently these patients request hospitalization (13). The very insight which brings them to the ED also tells them that the ED intervention is not enough. They feel inadequate to control the impulse. A 44-year-old man came to the ED because he wanted to kill his "adulterous" wife. After the interview he realized he still planned to murder her. He asked to be hospitalized.

In some situations the family is so threatened by the patient that hospitalization is indicated. Struggles to control impulses to kill, to molest, and to set fires disturb, and terrify people in the patient's social environment. Hospital treatment protects the family.

In other situations the conflict dominates patients' lives. They have become so preoccupied by it that they have ceased to function. They have abandoned family and work. In that situation hospitalization provides the necessary controls to permit the person to resolve the conflict.

Finally, in certain situations the physician determines that hospitalization is indicated. On the basis of the examination the physician judges that the patient does not have sufficient control of the impulse. The impulse to kill, commit suicide, abuse a child or spouse, molest, or set fires remains too great to permit discharge to home. The physician either recommends inpatient treatment or arranges for involuntary hospitalization. A 20-year-old woman had the rescue unit bring her to the ED because she felt she was going to strike her daughter. She had struck her 18-month-old child several times for "crying too much." The patient's parents had beaten her during her childhood. She believes she is losing her control. The ED physician insists on her hospitalization. She reluctantly accepts this recommendation.

The principle asset of hospitalization is its ability massively, continuously, and directly to support and reinforce the patient's control. Through its structure and staff the hospital can control the impulse.

Outpatient Treatment

The patient struggling to control an impulse benefits from outpatient treatment, both individual and group. These therapies offer exploration, support, and shared emotional experiences while at the same time permitting the patient maximum autonomy.

Several principles of outpatient psychotherapy apply to the patient conflicted with an impulse. First, the patient requires regularly scheduled sessions. These serve as check points in the struggle to help to establish trust and confidence. Second, treatment focuses on discussion of the impulse. Furthermore, the treatment helps the patient to develop alternatives to the impulse.

Medications

In certain situations, medications help the patient maintain control. For the manic patient lithium carbonate has proved very effective. For the violent patient chlorpromazine (Thorazine) takes the edge off the aggression. For the patient struggling to avoid alcohol, disulfiram (Antabuse) has been of assistance. Methadone helps the patient to control the urge to use opiates. For the schizophrenic patient, phenothiazines such as fluphenazine (Prolixin), butyrophenones such as haloperidol

(Haldol), and thioxanthenes such as thiothixene (Navane) have demonstrated effectiveness in controlling impulse symptoms.

Finally, self-help groups have helped patients with the struggle to control an impulse. Alcoholics Anonymous has been extremely effective. It offers the patient direct, personal, and continuous support. Other groups help parents who want to control their destructive behavior toward their children, people who want to stop smoking, those who wish to curb their excessive eating, or people who are trying to resist drugs.

REFERENCES

1. Reich W: *Character Analysis.* New York, Ferrar Straus & Giroux, 1971.
2. Goodwin KF: Behavioral effect of L-dopa in man, in Shader RI (ed): *Psychiatric Complications of Medical Drugs.* New York, Raven Press, 1972, pp 148–174.
3. Rose RM: The psychological effects of androgens and estrogens–a review, in Shader RI (ed): *Psychiatric Complications of Medical Drugs.* New York, Raven Press, 1972, pp 251–293.
4. Tamerin JS, Mendelson JH: The psychodynamics of chronic inebriation: Observations of alcoholics during the process of drinking in an experimental group setting. *Am J Psychiatry* 125:886–899, 1969.
5. Ellinwood EH Jr: Amphetamine psychosis: I. Description of the individuals and process. *J Nerv Ment Dis* 144:273–283, 1967.
6. Shader RI, Caine ED, Meyer RE: Treatment of dependence on barbiturates and sedatives-hypnotics, in Shader RI (ed): *Manual of Psychiatric Therapeutics.* Boston, Little Brown & Co, 1978, pp 195–202.
7. Post RM: Cocaine psychoses: A continuum model. *Am J Psychiatry* 132:225–231, 1975.
8. Louria DB: Lysergic acid diethylamide. *N Engl J Med* 278:435–438, 1968.
9. Liden CB, Lovejoy FH Jr, Costello CE: Phencyclidine. *JAMA* 234:513–516, 1975.
10. Slaby AE, Lieb J, Tancredi LR: *Handbook of Psychiatric Emergencies.* Flushing NY, Medical Examination Publishing Co, 1975.
11. Murphy DL, Goodwin FK, Bunney WE Jr: The psychobiology of mania, in Arieti S (ed): *American Handbook of Psychiatry,* 2 ed. New York, Basic Books, 1975, vol 6, pp 502–532.
12. *Diagnostic and Statistical Manual of Mental Disorders,* ed 3. Washington DC, American Psychiatric Association, 1980.
13. Lion JR, Bach-y-Rita G, Ervin FR: Violent patients in the emergency room. *Am J Psychiatry* 125:1706–1711, 1969.

13

The Patient Reacting to Alcohol or Abused Substances

Alcohol and abused substances alter patients' minds, change their internal controls, and affect their bodies. The resultant moods and perceptions—and especially the behavior—impact on those about these patients and challenge the skill of the EMTs and the ED staff. A person under the influence of alcohol or abused substances is a person out of control.

This chapter focuses on the effects of alcohol, amphetamines, barbiturates, cocaine, LSD, marijuana, opiates, and phencyclidine (PCP). These are the substances usually involved when EMTs and ED staff encounter patients experiencing drug reactions. The principles apply to other drug reactions as well.

This chapter examines the reactions to alcohol and the abused substances in three phases of their use: intoxication, chronic use, and withdrawal. The intoxication phase covers the effects of ingestion, inhalation, or intravenous administration. The chronic phase deals with the results of a long period of profound substance use. The withdrawal phase involves the impact of the cessation of substance use.

THE PATIENT

Alcohol and abused substances propel patients into an unreal chemical world where the milestones seem confusing and distorted. People who abuse alcohol or other drugs find life bewildering, exciting, and terrifying. Their behavior resembles that of disoriented patients with thought disorders.

Frank Turner, a 35-year-old executive, sees animals on the wall, hears wild screams, feels "things" on his arms, hits the table with his fist, accuses those about him of plotting against him, does not know where

209

he is, speaks incoherently, and experiences waves of terror. He has been drinking and taking drugs with several friends when suddenly he loses control of himself and the situation. His colleagues retreat with fear and summon aid.

Frank Turner has always liked alcohol and, later, drugs. In college and the service he drank a great deal—a six-pack daily on weekends, three whiskeys at the officers' club, and always a "nightcap." He prides himself on his ability to hold his liquor. He took his first drink of wine when he was 12 years old. He uses drugs recreationally: these include marijuana, cocaine, LSD, and PCP. Substance use and abuse has become imbedded into the very fibers of life, although he claims he "can stop anytime."

Frank's father used alcohol to excess. His mother has required a sleeping preparation for the last fifteen years. Frank always feels "a little empty."

The responding rescue unit workers find themselves confronting a "wild man." Frank Turner dramatically changes from crying and dependency to anger and withdrawal within seconds. He welcomes the EMTs and then accuses them of being Communist Party agents. A confounded but persistent EMT team insists he accompany them to the hospital. His terrified friends agree. The EMTs take along several white pills they find in the apartment.

Alcohol and abused substances produce profound alterations in the patient's mood, perceptions, and behavior.

The Patient's Mood

Alcohol and substances affect the mood in two ways. First, they produce a number of intense feelings. These include anxiety, apathy, depression, euphoria, and anger. Second, they also cause an abrupt, dramatic shift from one emotion to another. The resultant lability of affect is a major characteristic of a person reacting to alcohol or abused substances.

Patients who abuse drugs feel depressed. They become sad. Fictional literature all too frequently lionizes the depression which follows a siege of drinking. The chronic alcoholic patient is often a melancholic (1). The amphetamine user experiences an acute, intense depression after discontinuing the drug. Barbiturates produce a depression and are frequently referred to as "downers" or "downs" (2). In small doses they cause sadness and lethargy; in larger doses they lead to drowsiness, ataxia, and coma. Cocaine in moderate amounts causes depression, often of psychotic proportions (3).

Alcohol and the abused substances cause the patient to feel anxiety. This anxiety ranges from mild apprehension to a panic attack. Alcohol use produces mild anxiety (4). Hence the familiar paradox that the substance ingested to relieve tension ultimately results in greater anxiety. Alcohol withdrawal is accompanied by massive apprehension and fear (5). Explosive agitation characterizes the delirium tremens. Amphetamines produce uneasiness, anxiety, and vague fears in the intoxicated phase (6). In the withdrawal period the amphetamine addict develops intense anxiety and craving. Similarly, the opiate addict feels acutely anxious during abstinence (7). Panic reactions have accompanied the use of LSD, marijuana, and PCP (8). Additionally, in withdrawal from barbiturates the patient feels anxious and apprehensive.

Often the patient derives a sense of euphoria from an alcohol or drug experience. This feeling of well-being, confidence, and being "high" is a major reason for the use of the substance. Alcohol makes people feel good. Frank Turner likes to drink. Amphetamines produce a feeling of energy, decisiveness, and greatness. A college student reported that while on amphetamines he "wrote brilliantly all through the night." Cocaine and opiates cause the user to feel good. Similarly, LSD, marijuana, and PCP produce a euphoric experience (9).

Not infrequently, alcohol or these other abused substances cause users to become apathetic. They develop a bland, monotonous feeling. The chronic user seems to have this sense of apathy. The chronic alcoholic displays dejection and resignation.

On the other hand, patients may become angry and hostile. Alcohol converts a quiet person into a belligerent potential combatant. Amphetamines especially have been involved in the generation of patients' hostility during both intoxication and withdrawal. Withdrawal from alcohol and opiates is associated with anger. Cocaine in large amounts, LSD, and PCP have produced anger, rage, and hostility during the intoxication phase (7). Frank Turner clearly demonstrates an alcohol and drug-induced rage.

Patients under the influence of alcohol or drugs display a lability of affect of often dramatic proportions. Like Frank Turner, at one moment they sob penitently and beg for forgiveness, then suddenly turn to attack those about them and accuse the others of working against them. Abruptly they may again lapse into self-pity and resignation.

The Patient's Perceptions

Alcohol, amphetamines, barbiturates, cocaine, LSD, opiates, and PCP produce profound alterations in one's perceptions. They affect all spheres of mental activity. They cause changes in the patient's social orientation, level of awareness, self-image, and body image. They trigger a diverse group of sensations: depersonalization, illusions, hallucinations, and delusions. They affect patients' sense of time, their memory, and their ability to orient themselves to the environment. All these drugs disturb the ability to communicate. What often starts as an experience to enhance one's perceptions results in the loss of control over them.

Alcohol and abused substances affect the patient's sociability. Occasionally people prefer a solitary drug experience. They want to drink in seclusion or smoke marijuana privately. However, most often alcohol or abused substances are used specifically to enhance the social occasion (10). The person obtains increased social ease and heightened affability as the result of a few drinks, some "grass," LSD, or cocaine. Frank Turner originally had discovered alcohol to be a great social facilitator. Later he found drugs achieved the same results.

Alcohol and abused substances alter the patient's level of awareness. Alcohol, barbiturates, and opiates often diminish the patient's alertness and reactions. The user becomes less concerned with the immediate environment and has difficulty with concentration. On the other hand, amphetamines, cocaine, and marijuana heighten the patient's general level of awareness. The amphetamines make people excessively alert and vigilant. Marijuana users report with delight that physical sensations, for example, the sound of music or the taste of food, are enhanced.

Alcohol and abused substances alter people's self-image. In some instances users like themselves less because of the experience. A "bad trip" often produces a negative self-image. More significantly, patients struggling to rid themselves of alcohol or other substances depreciate themselves each time they use the drug. Each drink confirms the inability to stop. But in most situations the experience enhances self-image. As a result of using alcohol, cocaine, marijuana, opiates, or PCP, patients like themselves more and see themselves as having more capabilities and more energy than without the substance.

These substances alter body image. The patient experiences a number of somatic distortions. A marijuana user reported that his arms lengthened and "hung by his side like [those of] a gibbon monkey" (11, p40). A 16-year-old girl on a bad LSD trip screamed that her fingernails were "growing and looking like bayonets." Cocaine and PCP use also lead to body image distortions. The drug user frequently finds a few distortions interesting and amusing, but in excess the changes can be overwhelming and terrifying.

Depersonalization accompanies the use of a number of substances. Patients find either themselves or those about them unreal. They see people as "cardboard," distant, and uninvolved, or they perceive their own bodies as strange and become detached observers of themselves. Not infrequently, depersonalization results from repressed, massive anxiety. Marijuana, LSD, and PCP most commonly produce this reaction. An 18-year-old used LSD with friends. During the trip he felt as if he left his body, watched the proceedings for a while, then rejoined himself.

The patient under the influence of alcohol or abused substances experiences illusions, mistaking one thing in the environment for something else. A 54-year-old man, while intoxicated in the ED, perceived the intravenous line as a snake and became acutely agitated.

Hallucinations frequently accompany and often dominate the drug experience and crisis. They take a number of forms: visual, auditory, olfactory, tactile, and gustatory. Additionally, substances produce pseudohallucinations.

Visual hallucinations are one of the most frequently encountered drug-induced mental experiences. Alcohol withdrawal causes people to experience visual images. In alcohol hallucinosis, patients see people or animals while being fully oriented. They often enjoy this experience. A 48-year-old man stopped drinking two days ago and now comes to the ED complaining of "thousands of naked women" pursuing him. In delirium tremens, the patient sees terrifying figures or animals. Cocaine and LSD produce rich visual imagery and hallucinatory experiences. In large doses both amphetamines and marijuana cause visual hallucinations.

Auditory hallucinations occur with alcohol and substance use. Alcohol, amphetamines, cocaine, LSD, and rarely PCP have been known to produce these auditory events. Patients experience these far less frequently than the visual type. The auditory hallucinations take many forms, including voices both accusing and praising, ranging from whispers to screams; music; and strange sounds.

Abused substances also lead to olfactory, tactile, and gustatory hallucinations. Cocaine produces olfactory and tactile hallucinations. In the olfactory type, the patient smells gasoline, natural gas, garbage, or feces. In the tactile type, the patient complains of things or "bugs" crawling on or under the skin. The tactile hallucination follows a number of days of intense cocaine use. LSD has been known to cause a metallic taste in the mouth.

Certain substances produce pseudohallucinations (7). The patient sees a visual image, most frequently a geometric design, but also knows the figure is not real. LSD and cocaine are the chief causes of such experiences.

Use of alcohol and abused substances leads to two types of delusions, grandiose and persecutory. In the first, which is encountered less frequently, the feeling of well-being generates delusions of world leadership, of personal messiahship, and of grand schemes. In the second, suspicion and fear predominate. Patients feel their spouses have been unfaithful or imagine people are plotting against them. Alcohol has been especially implicated in the delusion of infidelity. In alcoholic hallucinosis and alcoholic paranoia, the delusion often centers on the spouse's extramarital activities. Amphetamines produce paranoid delusions during both intoxication and withdrawal. A 45-year-old housewife had used "diet pills" for years. Two weeks after her physician refused to fill another prescription she became acutely paranoid. She obtained a gun and barricaded herself at home. She claimed a motorcycle gang was after her. Cocaine, LSD, marijuana, and PCP sometimes generate persecutory delusions during the intoxication phase. Opiate users become very suspicious during withdrawal.

Alcohol and abused substances alter one's sense of time. Certain substances such as marijuana make the user perceive time as passing slower than it actually does. Other drugs, especially amphetamines, produce a perception of speed. Time is hurrying; everything happens quickly.

Alcohol and the abused substances disturb the user's memory. They interfere with recent recall in particular, although chronic alcohol ingestion leads to a Korsakoff's psychosis, in which both recent and distant memory become profoundly disrupted. Many times patients who abuse alcohol cannot recall events that occurred during a bout of drinking (12). They experience *blackouts,* which are amnesic episodes and which constitute a cardinal manifestation of alcohol addiction. Similarly, according to Jellinek (13), the patient intoxicated from barbiturates subsequently has difficulty in recalling earlier activities. Frank Turner has no recollection of events in his home the night of the emergency.

Disorientation is one of the most significant effects of alcohol and abused substance use. The patients have difficulty knowing where they are and what time it is. All the abused substances under discussion here have the ability to alter the patient's orientation during high-dosage intoxication. Additionally, chronic use and withdrawal affects the patient's sense of place and time. Disorientation ranks as the critical ingredient in the diagnosis of delirium tremens. During the crisis Frank Turner did not really know where he was and what time or even what day it was.

Patients may lose the ability to communicate with others. Some users become so preoccupied with their internal world and themselves that they prefer to avoid contact with anyone else. But in most crisis situations the patients cannot communicate because they have become incoherent. They leap from one subject to another; they develop their ideas illogically, circumstantially, and tangentially. They have lost control of their thoughts.

The Patient's Behavior

Marked behavioral disturbances reflect the profound changes in these patients' mood and perceptions. Patients exhibit alterations in activity level, sexuality, appetite, sleep, and coordination. They may have seizures. Additionally, they may become either suicidal or homicidal.

Alcohol and abused substances alter the user's activity level in one of three ways: (1) increase it, (2) decrease it, or (3) produce an oscillation between the first two. A number of drugs cause users to become very active. These patients meet people, work long hours, exhibit restlessness, and appear always on the go. Amphetamines especially have this capability. Opiate withdrawal often propels the user into hyperactivity to obtain more drugs. Other drugs tend to promote less activity. The person displays lethargy and apathy. He or she has less energy, undertakes few projects, and avoids people. Chronic use of alcohol, barbiturates, marijuana, and opiates tends to promote hypoactivity. However, not infrequently the patient dramatically fluctuates between hyperactivity and hypoactivity, manifesting labile affect and perceptual alternation.

Alcohol and abused substances affect the patient's sexuality. Certain drugs, such as marijuana, enhance sexual activity. These drugs intensify the sensations involved. Alcohol by legend increases the desire but decreases the performer's ability. Chronic use of alcohol, barbiturates, or opiates tends to lead to less interest in sexual activity.

Alcohol and abused substances affect the user's appetite. Some substances, especially marijuana, enhance appetite and thirst. Many substances, including amphetamines, alcohol (when used habitually), barbiturates, cocaine, and opiates produce a decreased appetite, weight loss, and malnutrition. Indeed, historically, physicians prescribed amphetamines for appetite appeasement.

The patient's sleep pattern reflects the use of alcohol and abused substances. Alcohol intoxication, both intoxication and chronic use of barbiturates, and use of opiates lead to increased sleep. On the other hand, amphetamine intoxication, cocaine use, and alcohol and barbiturate withdrawal produce insomnia. The drug and the stage of its use directly affect the patient's sleep pattern.

The patient's coordination mirrors the drug use. Certain drugs, notably amphetamines, improve coordination. Alcohol and barbiturate intoxication lead to incoordination. Alcohol withdrawal causes tremors.

Seizures constitute a dramatic behavioral consequence of alcohol and substance use. They occur during alcohol or barbiturate withdrawal. The alcoholic patient experiences seizures during the first 12 to 48 hours of abstinence, as "rum fits," or after three to five days of sobriety, as delirium tremens. Abrupt cessation of barbiturate use leads to status epilepticus. Cocaine and PCP intoxication can result in seizures.

Alcohol and certain substances have been associated with suicidal and homicidal behavior. The implicated substances include amphetamines, cocaine, LSD, and PCP. Alcohol appears to diminish conscious prohibitions and controls. The depressed patient attempts suicide while intoxicated; the angry patient strikes out while under the influence. Both later express remorse. The patient can get hurt or can injure others in the turmoil of a "bad trip," delusions of persecution, or the disorientation produced by amphetamines, LSD, or PCP. Frank Turner threatens to kill his friends.

THE CAUSES OF ALCOHOL AND SUBSTANCE ABUSE

Intrapsychic, interpersonal, and biologic factors govern the use of drugs and each person's experiences with them.

Intrapsychic Causes of Alcohol and Substance Abuse

Intrapsychic dynamics play a significant role in drug use. Intrapsychic factors provide the impetus to begin using alcohol or substances. Important motivations include the wish to escape from emptiness and the quest for answers, recreation, calmness, or euphoria. Intrapsychic influences cause continuation of drug use and also lead to its termination.

Inner feelings of emptiness and anhedonia (inability to experience joy) lead some people to try alcohol or drugs. These people experience deep loneliness, unhappiness, and nothingness. Often they are schizophrenic or depressed. They believe drugs will fill their emptiness. Frequently they experiment with a series of drugs. Frank Turner has tried alcohol, marijuana, LSD, amphetamines, and cocaine.

Patients may seek drug experiences to solve religious, philosophical, or psychotherapeutic problems (14). People most frequently use hallucinogens, especially LSD, in these quests. They look to the drug to provide insights, offer visions, and give answers.

Many people use alcohol or drugs recreationally. Alcohol, marijuana, cocaine, LSD, opiates, and PCP are used to reward work and to provide enjoyment. In college, and then in the Army, Frank Turner had looked forward to drinking. Alcohol had provided his predominant recreational activity.

Others turn to alcohol or drugs as self-medication for anxiety. They feel tense, fearful, and apprehensive. Alcohol, barbiturates, and opiates provide relief.

In some instances people find euphoria through drugs. These people go beyond filling the emptiness and obtaining calmness and reach the level of ecstasy. Drugs bring them exhilaration and elation. They use amphetamines, opiates, and cocaine to achieve this "high." Life offers these users no comparable experience.

Those who continue to derive a sense of fullness, insight through imagery, pleasure, calmness, or euphoria from the substances persist in using them. Frank Turner enjoys his drinks and he continues to drink.

On the other hand, intrapsychic factors also influence people to stop substance use. A "bad trip" on marijuana or LSD, or a painful flashback, causes some people to cease their use of the substance. The drug itself causes anxiety. Instead of promoting calmness, it induces apprehension. So the user decides to quit. The experiences with alcohol and abused substances produce guilt. Some people become disturbed by allowing chemicals to control their lives. They then stop using the substances.

Interpersonal Causes of Alcohol and Substance Abuse

The social milieu contributes to drug use in many ways. In certain situations the family and friends promote and support substance use; in others they "drive" the person to want to escape through drugs. But frequently it is the family or friends who demand the termination of the person's drug involvement.

Many social settings promote alcohol and drug use. Frank Turner had encountered pressure to drink, both at college and in the Army. His friends had urged him to be "one of the boys." Certain avant garde groups foster drug use (15). Some families support, encourage, and reinforce alcohol use (16). In certain socioeconomic settings heroin use is the group norm (17). The environment initiates, reinforces, and sustains drug use.

Because of family conflicts, work stresses, or neighborhood pressures, people may seek a chemical escape. They feel victimized at the office and at home or depressed by their environment. Substances seem to offer a way out of the trap.

But the social milieu can also demand termination of drug use. Interpersonal dynamics frequently play a major role in the decision to quit. Powerful motivations for cessation include threats of divorce, challenges from the children, and confrontation by the boss. A 55-year-old gas company executive had been progressively increasing his alcohol use and decreasing his job performance. He "knew" he had a drinking problem but procrastinated about getting help. Only after his employer demanded he stop drinking and obtain assistance did he cease his alcohol use.

Biologic Causes of Alcohol and Substance Abuse

Biologic considerations enter into all phases of the patient's drug involvement. Alcohol and the abused substances directly affect the central nervous system (CNS) and the rest of the body. The user develops tolerance to certain substances. A variety of physiologic reactions accompany substance withdrawal.

Alcohol and the abused substances directly affect the CNS and the rest of the body. Alcohol and barbiturates act as CNS depressants. In the intoxicated person they produce ataxia, vertigo, tremors, and vomiting. In large amounts they cause coma. Amphetamines cause a catecholaminergic response producing tremors, increased reflexes, hypertension, pupillary dilation, tachycardia, and dry mouth. Cocaine also acts through the catecholaminergic mechanism to cause dilated pupils, tachycardia, hypertension, sweating, and tremors. Additionally, cocaine precipitates seizures. LSD increases the manufacture of serotonin and decreases norepinephrine production in the CNS (18), resulting in dilated pupils, sweating, and tachycardia. Marijuana acts on the CNS like LSD and leads to profuse sweating, injected conjunctiva, nystagmus, ataxia, urinary frequency, dry mouth, and tachycardia. Opiates function as CNS depressants and cause constricted (pinpoint) pupils, decreased blood pressure, slow pulse, flushing, and a lowered body temperature. PCP has sympathomimetic properties and acts as both a CNS stimulant and depressant. It causes nystagmus, blurred vision, ataxia, and opisthotonos; PCP also interferes with proprioception and decreases pain sensitivity and temperature appreciation (19).

Tolerance develops as a result of prolonged substance use. Through increased enzymatic activity, the drug is metabolized more rapidly as usage continues, with the result that the patient requires more of the substance to achieve the initial good feeling. Tolerance occurs especially with alcohol, amphetamines, barbiturates, and opiates.

During the withdrawal phase, the patient experiences many physiologic reactions. Withdrawal from alcohol or barbiturates involves tremors, diaphoresis, tachycardia, dilated pupils, ataxia, and seizures. After prolonged alcohol use, the withdrawing patient exhibits Wernicke's encephalopathy with ophthalmoplegia, nystagmus, ptosis, polyneuritis, papilledema, convulsions, and hypotension. Amphetamine cessation manifests itself through hypersomniance. Opiate withdrawal is accompanied by sweating, yawning, rhinorrhea, tremors, lacrimation, piloerection (erection of the body hair) and dilated pupils.

THE REACTIONS OF OTHERS

Family, friends, and employers display a number of reactions to patients who abuse alcohol or other drugs. Some support, encourage, and extol their social participation; some do not care; some sermonize. Others reject and avoid the patients. Still others express concern and suggest getting help.

In a wide variety of social settings, the significant people in the patient's life support and positively reinforce drug-taking behavior. College fraternities, many clubs, and gatherings after athletic competitions boast of their alcohol consumption. Some fathers proudly enjoy "belting" one down with their sons. In certain social situations hosts encourage the recreational use of drugs such as cocaine, LSD, and marijuana. Friends share their "coke" or "trip" together. Frank Turner's friends endorse and promote his drug use. They enjoy experimenting with new "stuff."

Many people ignore the patient's alcohol or drug use. They see it as the person's private business and choose not to interfere. They observe, but at a distance.

Some family members, friends, and employers preach at the patient. They equate any alcohol use or drug participation as evidence of moral and spiritual decay. Alcohol and drugs represent sin.

Other people reject and avoid the patient. A spouse divorces the partner because of the alcohol or drug excesses. Parents eject children, and children leave home because of their own or parents' alcohol or drug use. The employer terminates a worker for drinking or taking drugs on the job. A 60-year-old man drank to excess over many years. When intoxicated he railed against his family. Ultimately his wife divorced him and his children refused even to visit him. As an intoxicated Mr Flood laments in a poem by Edwin Arlington Robinson (20,p739):

And there was nothing in the town below—
Where strangers would have shut the many doors
That many friends had opened long ago.

Often family members, friends, and employers recognize patients' excesses and recommend help. The people in the social environment objectively observe the use and monitor its effects. Their concern and interest encourage users to seek assistance.

THE INITIATION OF THE EMERGENCY

Alcohol or substance use initiates a psychiatric emergency in a number of ways. "Bad trips," panic attacks, and acute disorganization constitute drug-induced crises. Other emergencies involve withdrawal symptoms, seizures, self-destructive behavior, and violence. A request for help with control by either the patient or family also initiates the emergency.

A "bad trip" propels a person to the ED. Cocaine, LSD, and PCP especially produce violent, terrifying, and overwhelming images in the user. The new drug participant is at particular risk for this reaction. A 16-year-old girl attended a high school party where "sugar cubes" were passed around. She took one. Suddenly she saw everyone with knives and spears, heard wild animal sounds, felt her body getting smaller, and focused on her heart beat. Her frightened friends immediately brought her to the ED. Tripping also can lead to the flashback phenomenon. Flashbacks are vivid, horrifying recollections of a nightmarish drug experience (11).

Amphetamines, cocaine, LSD, marijuana, and PCP precipitate panic attacks. The panic involves overwhelming fear, loss of control, massive anxiety, expectations of impending doom, and a total sense of urgency. The patient becomes completely dominated by the experience and believes death is imminent.

Use of alcohol or abused substances leads to the patient's complete disorganization and disorientation. The profound alterations include anxiety, loose associations, paranoia, hallucinations, delusions, distortions of body image, and disorientation. The patient is psychotic. Alcohol intoxication, pathologic intoxication, amphetamine intoxication and withdrawal, cocaine intoxication, LSD intoxication, and PCP intoxication can all produce symptoms of psychosis.

Withdrawal reactions constitute serious medical and psychiatric emergencies. The patient experiences a diminution or cessation of the supply of the substance and plunges into a state of withdrawal. In alcoholic hallucinosis, alcohol withdrawal symptoms begin in the first two days with auditory and visual hallucinations in a clear sensorium. Seizures which occur in the first 12 to 48 hours are known as "rum fits." After three to five days delirium tremens sets in with tremors, visual hallucinations, disorientation, and seizures. The amphetamine user during withdrawal demonstrates an intense craving for the drug. The barbiturate user during withdrawal, which commences within 72 hours after the last sedative ingestion, exhibits anxiety, restlessness, insomnia, anorexia, nausea, vomiting, and convulsions. The opiate patient within 8 to 12 hours after the last dose develops drug craving, sweating, lacrimation, yawning, rhinorrhea, tremors, and piloerection (21).

Seizures create an emergency situation. In the intoxication phase cocaine and PCP cause convulsions. Alcohol withdrawal in the first 12 to 48 hours and then after 3 to 5 days leads to convulsions. Barbiturate withdrawal causes convulsions between the third and seventh day and can result in status epilepticus.

Substance use promotes self-destructive behavior in two ways. First, alcohol and barbiturates potentiate underlying depressions and activate latent suicidal desires. Second, substances provide an avenue for either purposeful or accidental suicide. Too many barbiturates or heroin of unexpectedly high quality have resulted in death.

A number of drugs promote violence. Alcohol, amphetamines, cocaine, LSD, and PCP have been particularly associated with assaultive behavior. The patient who is intoxicated or withdrawing from alcohol becomes combative. Amphetamine use leads to violence. PCP has been implicated in acts of homicide.

Patients or their families turn to the EMTs and the ED for help in controlling the alcohol or substance use. They want detoxification and assistance in terminating drug use. A 24-year-old housewife drank too much. She became progressively more irritable and began to strike out at her infant daughter. One day she realized she needed help. She went to the ED. The staff took her request seriously and set her up with an alcoholism counselor. After being sober for five months she remarked, "I felt I had just one moment when I was open for help. I'm glad someone listened."

THE EMTs' RESPONSE TO THE EMERGENCY

The EMTs' response to the patient reacting to alcohol or other substances must include structure and direction. The response involves promptness, early and repeated identification, securing the substance, stating and restating the intervention plan, awareness of the EMTs' attitudes, containment, continued involvement of the family and friends, and constant patient supervision. The EMTs help the patient to reestablish control.

EMTs must respond promptly to a patient in an alcohol or drug crisis. The patient's lability of affect, alterations of consciousness, and rapid changes in behavior dictate early intervention. Frank Turner's condition dramatically fluctuates from violence to withdrawal.

EMTs must clearly identify themselves at the commencement of the intervention and periodically repeat that introduction. They must use both their names and their titles. This initial identification helps the patient to distinguish the EMTs from imagined enemies. The EMTs' professional titles and uniforms assist the patient in this recognition process. The periodic reidentification serves the important function of reassuring and reorienting the patient.

The EMTs must secure the alcohol or the substances. There are a number of reasons for this step. First, it removes from the patient a source of intoxication. Second, the pills, especially, represent a convenient source for an overdose. The patient who is depressed or under the influence of substances can take an overdose during the intervention process. Third, the EMTs must bring the substances with them to the ED. This helps the ED staff to identify the pills and render proper and specific treatment.

EMTs must state and periodically restate the intervention plan. Doing this provides the patient with a sequence structure and also supplies the family and friends with information about the intervention. In view of the patient's fluctuating mental status, the EMTs must periodically remind him or her of the plan.

EMTs must be aware of their own feelings toward the patient. Not infrequently they feel angry and inclined to reject the patient. They express many of society's prejudices. They want to lecture and scold. The patient requires professional intervention.

The patient also requires containment. The intervention plan, the EMTs' presence, and the transport vehicle provide a structure and containment. Disorganized, disoriented, and wandering behavior must be limited.

The family and friends provide valuable help in the intervention. They furnish information as to what the patient has consumed. They can be with the patient. They can help decrease and diffuse the person's anger.

Someone must be with the patient at all times. This person monitors the patient's condition, prevents elopement, and intervenes if the patient becomes self-destructive. The accompanying person also furnishes reassurance and companionship to the patient in crisis. A 20-year-old girl experienced a "bad trip" on LSD. Her friend stayed with her all the way to the hospital. The friend continually helped to orient, reassure, and comfort her.

THE EMERGENCY DEPARTMENT EVALUATION

The ED evaluation marks the turning point in the patient's alcohol or drug crisis. The ED staff through the evaluation process must establish patient control and derive the information upon which to reach a diagnosis and base immediate and referral treatment. The evaluation involves the ED reception of the patient, the physical examination, the chief complaint, the psychiatric evaluation, and the mental status examination.

> Frank Turner reaches the ED in the rescue vehicle with the supervision of the EMTs and the support of his friends. He demonstrates significant reluctance to enter the ED, declaring he is in control now. With staff support he does agree to talk to someone and to have a physical examination. At least one staff member of the ED recommends he not be seen or "logged" in, believing "he is just another junkie."
>
> The physician remains uncertain as to what, if anything, Mr Turner has ingested. His friends mention recent experimentation with PCP. The EMTs bring a sample of some white powder with them. The physician examines Mr Turner in a quiet room; When Frank Turner had been on a stretcher in the middle of the ED, he had incorporated much of the noise into his delusions and had become demonstratively more agitated. The examination reveals nystagmus and unusual neurological findings.
>
> During the evaluation Frank Turner's mood changes dramatically; he continues to hallucinate and periodically attempts to wander about the ED.

The Reception

The reception is the key step for the entire evaluation process. The reception continues, advances, and refines the approach developed by the EMTs. It includes a prompt intervention, early and repeated staff identification, establishment of control of the situation, recognition of personnel attitudes toward the patient, involvement of the family and friends, and having someone with the patient at all times.

The patient reacting to alcohol or drugs requires prompt ED intervention (22). Promptness achieves several things. First, it ensures the patient's admission to the ED. Many patients remain extremely ambivalent about receiving help. They proclaim, "I can do it myself." Without a prompt response they often simply walk out. Second, in view of the patient's labile affect, unstable consciousness, and fluctuating behavior, early, swift reception precludes an escalation of symptoms. Third, and most important, promptness provides the message that the ED has something to offer this patient.

Staff must identify themselves to the patient and repeat this process periodically. The introduction promotes a positive patient response to being in the ED. It serves to help the patient distinguish between medical personnel and imagined enemies. The reminder of staff identification continues to orient the patient throughout the evaluation process.

Staff must establish control of the situation. Taking control commences with their introduction. It involves the use of a quiet, isolated treatment room. The patient must be contained, both emotionally and physically. Staff members must confront and control the violence. They must use security personnel, restraints, and medications as necessary. Keeping in verbal contact with the patient is another way ED personnel secure patient control. The physical examination, psychiatric evaluation, and mental status examination all promote the patient's involvement with reality.

Staff attitudes often hinder intervention. "Repeaters," "not motivated," "manipulators," "sinful," "irresponsible," and "a waste of time" represent many of the staff views toward the patient. At least one staff member rejects Mr Turner's right even to be in the ED.

The family and friends make valuable contributions to the evaluation. They supply information about the crisis and the patient's history. They offer companionship and orientation to the patient. They help determine and provide for the referral.

Someone must be with the patient at all times. This provides essential support. This person monitors the patient's emotional and physical condition and precludes elopement.

Physical Examination

The physician must perform a physical examination on the patient reacting to alcohol or other substances. The vital signs, the patient's appearance, and the cardiopulmonary, abdominal, and neurologic parts of the examination require particular attention. A number of laboratory studies may be indicated.

The patient's temperature, pulse, and blood pressure provide the physician with vital information. An elevated temperature is one of the cardinal features of delirium tremens. It also occurs in cocaine and LSD intoxication and during barbiturate and opiate withdrawal. Opiate intoxication and alcoholic coma cause a decreased temperature. Patients exhibit tachycardia during the following conditions: alcoholic hallucinosis, delirium tremens, amphetamine intoxication, cocaine intoxication, LSD intoxication, marijuana intoxication, and PCP intoxication. A slow pulse occurs during opiate intoxication. Hypertension occurs in a variety of alcohol- and drug-related situations: amphetamine intoxication, cocaine intoxication, LSD intoxication, and PCP intoxication. Hypotension occurs in Wernicke's encephalopathy, barbiturate withdrawal, and opiate withdrawal (7).

The patient's physical appearance often reveals the medical status. The chronic alcoholic patient shows spider angiomas over the upper trunk and extremities. The patient with amphetamine intoxication not infrequently looks malnour-ished and has tremors and needle marks. The person with cocaine intoxication is pale. The marijuana user exhibits injected conjunctivae. Patients with opiate intox-ication demonstrate flushing; during opiate withdrawal they have pilomotor erec-tion, "goose flesh."

The physician must pay particular attention to the cardiopulmonary and abdominal examinations. Alcohol use causes hepatitis, cirrhosis, gastritis, pancrea-titis, and myocarditis. Chronic alcoholics frequently have pneumonia. Intravenous amphetamine or opiate use leads to hepatitis and subacute endocarditis.

The physician must undertake a thorough neurologic examination. Use of alco-hol or abused substances leads to a variety of neurologic changes. Alcohol intox-ication produces ataxia, vertigo, tremors, and slurred speech. Alcohol withdrawal leads to a number of changes: alcohol hallucinosis is accompanied by nystagmus and a fine tremor; delirium tremens produces ataxia, dilated pupils, and a coarse tremor; Wernicke's encephalopathy causes ataxia, nystagmus, opthalmoplegia, palsy of the lateral rectus muscles of the eyes, ptosis, polyneuritis, and papille-dema. Amphetamine intoxication causes dilated pupils, tremors, and hyperactive reflexes. Barbiturate withdrawal leads to muscle weakness, tremors, and hyper-active reflexes. Cocaine intoxication produces dilated pupils and tremors. LSD intoxication also leads to dilated pupils. Marijuana intoxication results in ataxia, nystagmus, and tremors. Opiate intoxication causes constricted pupils. PCP intox-ication produces ataxia, miotic pupils, nystagmus, blurred vision, clonus, hyper-active reflexes, slurred speech, opisthotonos, and tremors.

The physician must consider a number of laboratory studies. A blood alcohol study helps to determine the patient's level of intoxication. Similarly, a barbiturate level establishes the amount of the drug the patient has consumed. Measurements of hematocrit and hemoglobin prove useful since excessive alcohol use leads to anemia. Liver function studies and measurement of serum amylase are also val-uable.

Chief Complaint

The patient's chief complaint reveals a great deal of information about his or her involvement with alcohol or abused substances and the role drugs have played in the crisis. Patients often focus on the loss of control: "I took some LSD and now I think I'm losing my mind"; "Everything is going too fast"; "I'm dying"; "My world is ending." Some patients express concern about perceptual alterations: "I feel remote from everyone"; "My hands are changing shape"; "I see coffins everywhere"; "I keep hearing this angry voice"; "I smell urine all the time." Other chief complaints concentrate on the delusional aspects of the patient's experience: "I am God and want to save you," or "They are all coming after me." The chief complaint may reflect the family dynamics: "My wife said I need help." Patients occasionally just request more drugs: "I'm withdrawing, I need a prescription." Some patients ask for assistance in regaining control: "I want to drink again, but I don't want to; please help me."

Psychiatric Evaluation

The physician must focus upon certain aspects of the psychiatric examination. These include history of the present illness (HPI), social history, family history, history of alcohol and drug use, psychiatric history, and medical history. The physician must employ information derived not only from the patient interview but also from family, friends, other doctors, therapists, and the EMTs.

The HPI must answer a number of key questions; they include "Why is the crisis occurring now?" The interview for patients who have been drinking must include the following areas: How much do they drink? When did they stop? What caused them to stop? What has been their experience when they have stopped before? Where durgs are involved the physician looks into the following areas: What did the person take? When? Has the patient ever used it before and with what effects? Under what circumstances was the drug taken? Who was there? The HPI must provide specific information concerning the patient, the substance, and the dynamics of its use.

The social history furnishes important data concerning the patient's living situation. The social milieu and the physical environment play roles in alcohol or drug use. A person living alone has many hurdles to overcome in the struggle with drinking. No one checks the patient's urges. Conversely, some home environments promote alcohol or drug use. Knowing where patients have come from and where they will return to helps the physician to understand the dynamics of the substance-related behavior and assists in making the most appropriate referral.

The family history emphasizing alcohol and drug use provides the physician with further useful information. Alcohol use and drinking problems run in families (23).

The physician must concentrate on the patient's alcohol and drug history. The patient's experiences with substances must be pursued in detail, as emphasized in the preceding discussion of the HPI. What has the person used? When, where, and with what results? Finding out the quantity of alcohol, amphetamines, barbiturates, or opiates consumed daily provides data upon which to predict withdrawal patterns. Interestingly, the patient with an alcohol problem often can recall vividly his or her first drinking experience (24). The physician must inquire into the patient's alcohol or drug career. This history must include the patient's experiences in treatment for alcohol or drug abuse.

The physician must inquire about the patient's psychiatric history and use of psychotropic medications. Not infrequently, psychiatric patients seek alcohol or drug experiences. Further, these patients often are taking prescribed psychotropic medications.

The physician must emphasize the medical history. Addiction to alcohol or other drugs produces a wide variety of illnesses (25,26). These range broadly and include, for example, anemia, gastritis, myocarditis, hepatitis, local infections, and septicemia. Additionally, the patient may have begun using drugs because of a painful disease.

Mental Status Examination

The physician must perform a careful and thorough mental status examination. This procedure as it particularly pertains to patients who abuse alcohol or other drugs is described in the paragraphs that follow. In addition to examining the patient's mental status, the physician must record and document the results in the patient's record. These notes provide an important means of assessing changes that may occur later.

Appearance.   Patients reveal a great deal about themselves through their appearance. Chronic alcoholic patients are often disheveled, with uncoordinated clothes, cigarette holes in their clothing, and blank stares. Amphetamine users appear restless and anxious; they often wear sunglasses, and they avoid eye contact. Barbiturate users, when intoxicated, exhibit lethargy and indifference. Opiate users have needle tracks.

Affect.   The patient displays a wide range of intense affects. These include depression, anxiety, panic, euphoria, apathy, and anger. More important, the patient reacting to alcohol or drugs frequently displays a pronounced lability of affect. Frank Turner demonstrates a remarkable range of emotions during the evaluation. He laughs, cries, shows anger, and feels joy, all within the space of several minutes.

Thought Content.   The physician must explore the patient's thought content. The thought content encompasses body image distortions, feelings of depersonalization, illusions, hallucinations, delusions, and ability to communicate. The patient can exhibit a variety of hallucinatory experiences: visual, auditory, olfactory, tactile, and gustatory. The patient may talk illogically, disconnectedly, and incoherently. The physician must listen particularly to the thought content and its expression.

Suicide and Homicide.   The physician must assess the patient's potential for attempting suicide or homicide. Patients must be asked specifically whether they have any thoughts or plans about hurting themselves or someone else. The HPI furnishes information concerning recent suicidal and homicidal behavior.

Judgement.   The physician must assess the patient's judgement. How has the person handled his or her life, especially the crisis? The HPI provides the most important clues in this determination.

Insight.   The physician must also assess the patient's level of insight. Occasionally a patient demonstrates remarkably clear comprehension of the problem. Some alcoholics, for example, know they *cannot* drink. One drink destroys years of sobriety. But in most situations the alcohol or drugs act as great deluders, depriving the users of the ability to see themselves as they really are.

Sensorium.   The physician must make a critical evaluation of the patient's sensorium. The assessment of sensorium includes testing the patient's orientation (to person, place, and time), ability to do calculations (subtraction by serial 7's), recall (immediate, recent, and distant), and ability to interpret proverbs. The hallmarks of the patient reacting to alcohol or drugs are disturbance in the sensorium and fluctuation in level of consciousness. The sensorium examination helps to establish the difference between alcohol hallucinosis and delirium tremens. In the former, the patient has a clear sensorium; in the latter, the patient displays disorientation and loss of immediate and recent memory. A patient with a chronic alcohol problem often interprets proverbs concretely.

DIAGNOSIS, TREATMENT PLAN, AND IMMEDIATE EMERGENCY DEPARTMENT THERAPY

The ED evaluation culminates in a diagnosis and treatment plan and leads to immediate ED therapy. The physician makes a diagnosis and treatment plan from information derived from the physical examination; chief complaint; psychiatric evaluation and mental status examination; the history obtained from family, friends, and often physicians and therapists; and the observations made by the EMTs and ED staff. The diagnosis is the basis for the immediate therapy.

Diagnosis

A number of psychiatric diagnoses apply to patients reacting to alcohol or drugs (27). The following discussion deals with the most frequently encountered ED diagnoses.

Alcohol induces a number of organic mental disorders in the three phases of its use. Intoxication produces both alcohol intoxication and alcohol idiosyncratic intoxication. Chronic excessive use causes dementia. Withdrawal leads to alcohol tremulousness, "rum fits," alcohol hallucinosis, delirium tremens, and alcohol amnestic syndrome (28).

Alcohol intoxication results from the patient's consumption of alcohol. Depending upon the person, a blood alcohol level between 30 and 150 mg/100 ml produces the typical inebriated condition. The drinker demonstrates stupor at 200 mg/100 ml and can lose consciousness above 300 mg/100 ml.

The diagnosis of alcohol idiosyncratic intoxication (pathological intoxication) is made when a person consumes a small amount of alcohol, becomes aggressive, and then has amnesia for the episode. Dementia associated with alcoholism, another diagnosis, is a significant organic impairment which persists at least three weeks after the patient ceases to drink. Alcohol tremulousness, "the shakes," peaks 24 hours after the patient stops drinking. The person with alcohol tremulousness exhibits irritability, insomnia, and tremulousness without hallucinations or disorientation. This is a self-limited, benign condition.

Alcohol hallucinosis is the diagnosis for patients who, while maintaining a clear sensorium, experience auditory or visual hallucinations or both in the first two weeks of abstinence. This condition often precedes delirium tremens. "Rum fits" are grand mal seizures occurring only between 12 and 48 hours after the patient stops drinking. Alcohol amnestic syndrome (Korsakoff's syndrome) occurs in some patients with histories of heavy alcohol consumption. These patients demonstrate recent memory deficiency, but their immediate recall is intact. Alcohol withdrawal delirium (delirium tremens) develops within the week, usually three to five days after a person who is habituated to alcohol terminates or drastically diminishes alcohol intake. It manifests itself in autonomic hyperactivity, elevated temperature, attention disruptions, memory and orientation impairment, seizures, and rapidly fluctuating clinical condition.

Amphetamine use leads to four diagnostic categories: intoxication, delirium, delirium delusional syndrome, and withdrawal. Amphetamines are discussed here as representative of many sympathomimetic drugs.

Amphetamine intoxication occurs within one hour after amphetamine use. The mental manifestations are elation, grandiosity, hypervigilance, and insusceptibility to fatigue. Physical signs and symptoms are hypertension, sweating, nausea, vomiting, anorexia, and insomnia. Behavioral results include poor judgement and impaired functioning. Amphetamine delirium is delirium developing within 24 hours of amphetamine use. Amphetamine delusional syndrome is characterized by a paranoid delusional system marked by referential thinking, aggressiveness, anxiety, and hyperactivity; the syndrome develops in chronic users and is precipitated by a recent use of amphetamine. Amphetamine withdrawal occurs in the abstinent heavy user. These patients have fatigue, sleep disturbances, and increased dreaming.

Barbiturate use causes crises in all three phases: acute ingestion produces barbiturate intoxication; chronic use leads to barbiturate amnestic syndrome; and withdrawal produces delirium.

Barbiturate intoxication manifests itself through mood disturbances or impulsiveness, incoordination, slurred speech, ataxia, difficulty with attention, and impaired judgement. Barbiturate amnestic syndrome (short-term recall deficiency but intactness of immediate and long-term memory) occurs in people with long histories of heavy use. Barbiturate withdrawal delirium is delirium occurring within the week after barbiturate cessation. The patient displays impaired attention, disorientation, memory deficiency, insomnia, illusions, hallucinations, and a rapidly fluctuating clinical course.

Cocaine intoxication occurs within the first hour of cocaine use. Mental manifestations include grandiosity, increased vigilance, insusceptibility to fatigue, excitement, elation, and excessive talking. Physical signs and symptoms include tachycardia, increased blood pressure, dilated pupils, sweating, nausea, vomiting, insomnia, and anorexia. Behavioral concomitants of cocaine intoxication include impairment of judgement and functioning.

LSD, discussed here as a representative hallucinogen, leads to hallucinosis, delusional syndrome, and affective syndrome.

Hallucinogen hallucinosis occurs after LSD ingestion and is characterized by perceptual alterations including illusions, hallucinations, depersonalization, and intensified sensations. The patient exhibits tachycardia, tremors, incoordination, and dilated pupils. Hallucinogen delusional syndrome is the persistence of a delusional system induced by LSD use. Hallucinogen affective syndrome occurs when use of LSD precipitates a persistent affective episode characterized by either anxiety or depression.

Marijuana produces intoxication and a delusional syndrome. Cannabis intoxication results from marijuana use. The patient develops euphoria, enhanced sensations, a feeling that time is progressing very slowly, and indifference. Tachycardia, injected conjunctivae, and increased appetite accompany cannabis intoxication. Cannabis delusional syndrome refers to a delusion, usually paranoid, which occurs within two hours after marijuana use and does not persist more than six hours after use has been discontinued.

Opioid use results in diagnoses of intoxication and withdrawal. Opioid intoxication is characterized by constricted pupils, either euphoria or dysphoria, drowsiness, slurred speech, and impaired attention. Opioid withdrawal occurs several days after heavy drug use and manifests itself in tachycardia, elevated temperature, mild hypertension, rhinorrhea, lacrimation, dilated pupils, yawning, diarrhea, piloerection, and insomnia.

PCP results in intoxication. PCP intoxication manifests itself in flushing, gross incoordination, excitement, nystagmus, unresponsiveness to pinprick, rigidity, distorted body image, estrangement, hostility, and apathy (29).

The physician diagnoses Frank Turner as having substance induced delirium. The drug cannot be identified, but the physician suspects PCP. The friends think it is either LSD or PCP.

Treatment Plan

The treatment plan must encompass immediate control, inpatient detoxification, and long-term therapy. These steps represent the integrated, integral sequence the patient must follow for effective treatment. The immediate control will be discussed below in the section on immediate emergency department therapy.

Inpatient detoxification constitutes the most critical and crucial step in the treatment sequence. No treatment can be undertaken while the patient is under the influence of alcohol or other drugs. From a practical standpoint, it is impossible to detoxify a patient outside a structured, substance-free environment. The patient's craving becomes a driving force. People who are withdrawing require massive support, frequently including medication. A secure, structured milieu provides such support.

Addiction requires long-term therapy. The desire to use alcohol or drugs again does not disappear with detoxification. In many cases the patient experiences a life-long struggle with alcohol or drugs. A 50-year-old executive, a member of Alcoholics Anonymous, notes he has been sober 10 years, 9 months, and 4 days. He knows that with just one drink he returns to his addiction.

Immediate Emergency Department Therapy

The patient reacting to alcohol or drugs requires immediate therapy. This intervention aims to help the patient reestablish control. The therapy involves containment, a treatment orientation, medication, and a referral.

Containment means control. The major initial function of the ED staff must be to establish patient control. They employ a prompt reception, an identification of themselves, a quiet room, security personnel, and restraints if necessary. Having one person continually converse with the patient on an LSD trip helps to establish contact and control. A quiet, low-stimulus environment benefits the patient on PCP.

Staff must present a treatment orientation to the patient. They must appreciate that they have something to offer the patient.

A number of medications have been effective in the immediate intervention into an alcohol or drug crisis. Each abused substance requires specific medication.

The selection of medications for patients reacting to alcohol depends on the symptoms and the stage of use. The intoxicated patient needs only tincture of time. The patient with pathological intoxication benefits from chlordiazepoxide hydrochloride (Librium) or haloperidol (Haldol), either PO or IM. For alcohol tremulousness, chlordiazepoxide hydrochloride provides mild sedation. "Rum fits" are treated with IV diazepam (Valium) to stop the convulsions and 100 to 300 mg of phenobarbital PO daily during the withdrawal period. Alcohol hallucinosis is treated with chlordiazepoxide hydrochloride. Delirium tremens necessitates either paraldehyde 8 to 12 ml every 4 hours or chlordiazepoxide hydrochloride (30).

Pharmacologic treatment of Amphetamine users depends on the situation. Intoxication is treated with haloperidol PO or IM. If anticholinergic drugs have been taken in addition to amphetamines, then the use of diazepam PO or IM is indicated. For withdrawal, haloperidol PO or IM is effective.

Barbiturate use also involves two situations. Intoxication requires no medications. An overdose calls for general supportive measures. Withdrawal necessitates hospitalization. If status epilepticus develops, IV diazepam is effective.

Cocaine intoxication responds to haloperidol (Haldol) PO or IM. A cocaine overdose necessitates general supportive measures.

LSD intoxication in mild forms is treated with diazepam 5 to 20 mg PO or 5 to 15 mg IM; or chlordiazepoxide hydrochloride 25 to 100 mg PO or IM. For more severe forms of LSD intoxication the treatment is haloperidol PO or IM.

Marijuana intoxication in mild form responds to diazepam or chlordiazepoxide hydrochloride PO or IM; in severe form, haloperidol or chlorpromazine hydrochloride (Thorazine) PO or IM is indicated.

Opiate use manifests itself in two ways, intoxication and withdrawal. Intoxication in overdose requires naloxone (Narcan) 0.4 mg IV. Acute withdrawal responds to chlorpromazine hydrochloride 25 to 100 mg PO or chloral hydrate 500 to 1,000 mg PO. Methadone treatment necessitates inpatient detoxification.

PCP intoxication is treated with haloperidol PO or IM.

Finally, as part of the immediate therapy, the physician must initiate and implement the referral.

CARE AFTER THE EMERGENCY

Frank Turner, at the insistence of the physician and his friends, is admitted to the psychiatric unit of the hospital. There he continues to exhibit the symptoms which precipitated his admission. His psychiatrist does a complete physical examination, obtains a psychiatric history, documents the mental status examination, and prescribes haloperidol 2 mg every four hours. He also orders a barbiturate level and a urine amphetamine determination (both prove negative).

During the first several days on the unit, the staff members spend a great deal of time and effort orienting Frank Turner and structuring his days. Too many visitors make him more disorganized. Gradually he emerges from the chaos and feels very distant from the crisis. He voices shame for his behavior and starts to talk to a therapist about his drug problem.

During his hospitalization and then in his outpatient psychotherapy sessions, Frank Turner explores his loneliness, emptiness, and purposelessness. He discovers the void the drugs have filled.

His therapist establishes regularly scheduled sessions. Mr Turner recognizes the depression and business stresses that promoted his drug use. He discusses his new fear of drugs—a dread of "going crazy" again. Several years later, he looks back with wonder at his "drug days."

The comprehensive approach to the patient reacting to alcohol or substances demands a definite referral. The course of therapy after the emergency involves inpatient treatment, halfway houses, medication maintenance, group therapy, individual therapy, and self-help organizations.

Inpatient Treatment

The significant issues of inpatient treatment are (1) admission criteria, (2) specific drug detoxification programs, (3) provision of a structured, supportive approach, and (4) establishment of proper outpatient therapy.

The indications for inpatient admission include the need for detoxification, disorientation, disorganization, family disruption, barbiturate withdrawal, medical emergency, suicidal behavior, and threats of homicide.

Detoxification is the cardinal indication for admission. Effective treatment of the patient reacting to alcohol or substances requires a drug-free environment.

Disorientation and disorganization are also major indications for inpatient treatment. Delirium requires control. Frank Turner's severe disorientation and disorganization marked by lability of affect, hallucinations, delusions, and fluctuating behavior necessitate his admission.

Family disruptions often lead to an admission. The patient's abuse and behavior become intolerable for the family and friends. They feel threatened, angry, and frightened. They need a short rest from the patient.

Barbiturate withdrawal carries with it the potential for the patient to develop status epilepticus. Barbiturate withdrawal must be done only in a hospital setting.

Alcohol or drug use leads to a number of medical conditions which necessitate hospital treatment. These include pancreatitis, delirium tremens, seizures, septicemia, urinary retention, hepatitis, gastritis, endocarditis, malnutrition, and profound anemia.

Alcohol or drug use promotes suicidal and homicidal threats and behavior. These become absolute indicators for inpatient treatment. The hospital provides security, structure, control, and containment.

Alcohol and certain drugs require specific detoxification programs. For alcohol withdrawal, chlordiazepoxide hydrochloride (Librium) has proven the drug of choice. For barbiturate withdrawal, the physician substitutes, then decreases, pentobarbital. To establish the initial dose, the physician gives the patient 200 mg of pentobarbital and then observes the patient's reactions after one hour. A patient who uses up to 500 mg of barbiturates daily develops somnolence, nystagmus, and ataxia after the test dose. If the customary daily intake is 500 to 600 mg, mild ataxia and nystagmus result. Those who use 700 to 800 mg develop only nystagmus; and patients whose daily intake is greater than 900 mg show no evidence of intoxication. After the pentobarbital tolerance level has been established, pentobarbital at the tolerance dosage is given in divided doses every 4 to 6 hours. Then the pentobarbital is decreased at a rate of 100 mg daily until it is discontinued (2).

For opiate withdrawal, methadone therapy is effective. The patient receives methadone 10 to 20 mg PO initially and then an additional 5 to 15 mg PO within the next 24 hours until withdrawal signs cease. Once stabilization has been established, the methadone dosage is decreased as much as 20 percent daily over a maximum of 21 days.

The inpatient treatment features structure and support. The disoriented and disorganized patient needs containment, schedules, and control. Withdrawal causes the patient stress, fear, pain, anxiety, and dread. The unit offers the patient 24-hour-a-day support and encouragement.

Finally, the inpatient experience must prepare the patient to continue the treatment beyond the period of hospitalization. It must establish the patient in a definite outpatient treatment program. The treatment linkages must be forged before discharge and positively endorsed by the unit and the community referral agency (31). One particularly useful technique involves having the outpatient therapist visit the patient in the hospital.

Halfway houses provide a strong, significant, and useful treatment bridge between the inpatient unit and the home. Halfway houses feature structure, support, and therapy; at the same time they permit the patient to resume employment. A number of these houses have been successfully established for patients with alcohol or drug problems.

Two maintenance medications help patients control alcohol or drug use: disulfiram (Antabuse) and methadone. Disulfiram interferes with alcohol metabolism. If a person taking disulfiram consumes alcohol, within 15 minutes the patient experiences flushing, sensations of heat, headache, nausea, vomiting, hyperventilation, dyspnea, and feelings of impending death. The dosage of disulfiram is 500 mg PO daily. Methadone works to curb the craving and to decrease the pleasurable sensation from any opiates that may be taken. Methadone is given orally in doses of 40 to 120 mg daily.

Group and individual therapy have been beneficial to detoxificated and abstaining patients. The therapy must be scheduled, supportive, confronting, and not rejecting (32). Patients require regular sessions. They benefit from realistic encouragement and frank appraisal of their progress. For many patients the crisis commences a life-long struggle to curb craving. With the help of therapy the patient must develop a new life with different priorities and a different orientation.

Self-help groups make a very valuable contribution to the patient's successful control of alcohol or drug use. Alcoholics Anonymous has an outstanding record of achievement, effectiveness, and support. Self-help promotes self-control.

REFERENCES

1. Pottenger M, McKernon J, Patrie LE, et al: The frequency and persistence of depressive symptoms in the alcohol user. *J Nerv Ment Dis* 166: 562–570, 1978.
2. Shader RI, Caine ED, Meyer RE: Treatment of dependence on barbiturates and sedative-hyp-

notics, in Shader RI (ed). *Manual of Psychiatric Therapeutics.* Boston, Little Brown & Co, 1978, pp 195-202.

3. Post RM: Cocaine psychoses: A continuum model. *Am J Psychiatry* 132:225-231, 1975.

4. Loque PE, Gentry WD, Linnoila M, et al: Effect of alcohol consumption on state anxiety changes in male and female nonalcoholics. *Am J Psychiatry* 135:1079-1081, 1978.

5. Greenblatt DJ, Shader RI: Treatment of the alcohol withdrawal syndrome, in Shader RI (ed): *Manual of Psychiatric Therapeutics.* Boston, Little Brown & Co., 1978, pp 211-235.

6. Angrist BM: Toxic manifestations of amphetamines. *Psychiatric Annals* 8:443-446, 1978.

7. Slaby AE, Lieb I, Tancredi LR: *Handbook of Psychiatric Emergencies.* Flushing NY, Medical Examination Publishing Co, 1975.

8. Tong TG, Benowitz NC, Becker CE, et al: Phencyclidine poisoning. *JAMA* 234:512-516, 1975.

9. Weil AT, Zinberg HE, Nelsen JM: Clinical and psychological effects of marihuana in man. *Science* 162:1234-1242, 1968.

10. Petersen RC, Stillman RC (eds): *Cocaine 1977: National Institute on Drug Research Monograph #13.* Rockville, US Department of Health Education & Welfare, 1977.

11. Siegel RK: Hallucinogens and perceptual changes. *Drug Therapy,* 1:34-44, 1971.

12. Fine EW, Steer RA: Short-term spatial memory deficits in men arrested for drinking while intoxicated. *Am J Psychiatry* 136:594-597, 1979.

13. Jellinek EM: Phases of alcohol addiction. *Quart J Stud Alcohol* 13:673-684, 1962.

14. Louria DB: Lysergic acid diethylamide. *N Engl J Med* 278:435-438, 1968.

15. Wolfe T: *The Electric Kool-Aid Acid Test.* New York, Bantam, 1969.

16. Wolin SJ, Bennett LA, Noonan DL: Family rituals and the recurrence of alcoholism over generations. *Am J Psychiatry* 136:589-593, 1979.

17. Scher J: Patterns and profiles of addiction and drug abuse. *Arch Gen Psychiatry* 15:539-551, 1966.

18. Valzelli L: *Psychopharmacology.* Flushing NY, Spectrum Publishers, 1973.

19. Liden CB, Lovejoy FH, Costello CE: Phencyclidine, nine cases of poisoning. *JAMA* 234:513-516, 1975.

20. Robinson EA: Mr Flood's party, in Ciardi J: *How Does a Poem Mean?* Boston, Houghton Mifflin Co, 1959, pp 738-739.

21. Green AI, Meyer RE, Shader RI: Heroin and methadone abuse: Acute and chronic management, in Shader RI (ed): *Manual of Psychiatric Therapeutics.* Boston, Little Brown & Co, 1978, pp 203-210.

22. Dilts SL, Berns BR, Casper E: The alcohol emergency room in a general hospital: A model for crisis intervention. *Hosp Community Psychiatry* 29:795-796, 1978.

23. Winokur G, Reich T, Rimmer J, et al: Alcoholism III: Diagnosis and familial psychiatric illness in 259 alcoholics. *Arch Gen Psychiatry* 23:104-111, 1970.

24. Ullman AD: The first drinking experience of addictive and of "normal" drinkers. *Quart J Stud Alcohol* 14:181-191, 1953.

25. Mendelson JH: Biologic concomitants of alcoholism: Part I. *N Engl J Med* 283:24-32, 1970.

26. Mendelson JH: Biologic concomitants of alcoholism: Part II. *N Engl J Med* 283:71-81, 1970.

27. *Diagnostic and Statistical Manual of Mental Disorders,* 3rd ed Washington DC, American Psychiatric Association, 1980.

28. Victor M: The alcohol withdrawal syndrome. *Postgrad Med* 47:68-72, 1970.

29. Aronow R, Dore AK: Phencyclidine overdose: An emerging concept of management. *JACEP* 7:56–59, 1978.

30. Kaim SC, Kleff CJ, Rothfeld B: Treatment of the acute alcohol withdrawal state: A comparison of four drugs. *Am J Psychiatry* 125:1640–1646, 1969.

31. Klerman GI: Dealing with alcohol and drug abuse and mental illness. *Public Health Rep* 93:622–626, 1978.

32. DiCicco L, Unterberger H, Mack JE: Confronting denial: An alcoholism intervention strategy. *Psychiatric Annals* 8.596–606, 1978.

14
The Victim of a Traumatic, Brutal Experience

The catastrophes of life bring the survivors and the victims to the EMTs' attention and to the ED. Death, rape, suicide, incest, and trauma produce a group of people sharing a private and public hell. The victim of a traumatic event or the survivor of a brutal experience is a person in emotional crisis who requires emergency intervention.

THE SURVIVOR AND THE VICTIM

A bus strikes 10-year-old Peggy Somers as she walks to her violin lesson. Despite heroic efforts by the EMTs and the ED staff, the physician pronounces her dead an hour after arrival at the ED. Personnel feel both frustrated and sad. The physician meets the parents and tells them of the death. They emotionally disintegrate and recoil with pain, overwhelming grief, and guilt. They insist on seeing their daughter.

A businessman watches from the alley as 35-year-old Miss Sally Randall prepares for bed. He moves in through the window, holds a knife at her throat, and forces her to have intercourse with him. He leaves; she is devastated, ashamed, afraid, and terrified. She calls the police; they take her to the ED. There she feels angry and bewildered. She believes everyone knows and people do not care. The event haunts her.

As 27-year-old William Pattern drives his motorcycle north on Route 1, a vehicle heading south comes toward him out of control. The accident causes extreme damage to his left leg. Despite swift EMT and ED intervention, the orthopedic surgeon has to remove the leg. William Pattern

*is in pain; he blames himself; he blames the other driver; he feels alone
and helpless. He wants to cry.*

Despite the apparent differences, Peggy Somers's parents, Sally Randall, and
William Pattern share a common cluster of moods, perceptions, and behaviors as
each struggles to confront the devastation. The survivors of a completed suicide,
patients with a wide variety of medical and surgical emergencies, and the victims
of incest share these reactions (1–3).

The Mood

The survivor or the victim grapples with a series of intense, unanticipated emotions. As Stevenson (4) describes, the very nature of the traumatic event — a death
or a life-threatening experience — generates a feeling of incredible depth and pain
that is unequaled in any other aspect of life. The unexpected quality of the catastrophe further intensifies the reaction (5). The survivor or victim feels depressed,
numb, bewildered, exhausted, anxious, frightened, angry, and helpless.

A deep, intense depression emerges as the central emotional experience. The
survivor or victim has sustained a devastating loss. The person grieves and feels
profoundly sorrowful. Mr Somers experiences an "incalculable emptiness" as he
reacts to the doctor's report. He feels the dread of death and struggles with its
sudden finality.

Survivors and victims react with a feeling of numbness and enter into a period
of emotional shock. A mother rushed her unresponsive 6-month-old son to the ED.
He died there from sudden infant death syndrome. She withdrew into herself and
felt "numb." This numbness lasted for the next month.

Survivors and victims also feel bewildered by the entire series of events. They
struggle with a host of conflicting and profound emotions. Sally Randall felt glad
to be alive, yet ashamed of her silence during the attack. She cried one moment,
then laughed. She is perplexed by the episode.

Survivors feel exhausted by the entire experience (6). They feel drained,
washed out, incredibly tired, and worn out. Mrs Somers feels so exhausted she
has difficulty getting to her feet. She wants to "just sit here awhile and get my
strength."

People confronted with traumatic situations often feel anxious. They must cope
with a reality they had not prepared for nor anticipated. It is with great apprehension that William Pattern faces his decision about amputation.

Frequently people react with fear. They have been frightened by the experience. Perhaps they could have been killed. "He threatened to kill me" dominates
Sally Randall's feeling. She is more frightened that the man had held a knife to
her throat than she is by the sexual assault.

The survivor or victim feels anger. The trauma has shattered the person's life.

Sally Randall expresses rage, indignation, and hostility. Women who have been raped feel angry not only toward their assailants but also toward the men staffing the ED (7). The family of a person who has committed suicide not only grieves the loss but expresses anger (8).

The survivor or victim emerges from the traumatic experience with a deep sense of helplessness (9). Each person is impotent in the face of death. Each has events happen to him or her; none feels in command of the immediate situation. William Pattern loses control of the motorcycle. Sally Randall finds herself powerless against her assailant (9).

The Perceptions

The traumatic event creates a large number of perceptual experiences for the survivor or victim. The catastrophe produces preoccupation with the loss or event, guilt, shame, identification with the deceased, dreams and nightmares, distrust, recollection of earlier times, disbelief, and a search for an explanation.

The loss and the event become a major preoccupation for the survivor or victim. The Somers's see their daughter's image everywhere. As Lindemann (6) notes, the mental picture of the deceased dominates the survivor's thoughts. The images help the survivor keep the dead alive. The victim of brutality continually reviews the event. Sally Randall cannot get the rapist's face out of her mind. William Pattern keeps recalling the accident. He searches his memory for details of the event. Then he pictures his leg.

Guilt is a universal reaction to the loss or trauma. The family and friends instantly believe they caused the death. One woman worried for decades about the altercation she had with her father the night he died. The survivor of a suicide struggles with the concept of having caused it. The suicide note often reinforces such guilt. Victims believe they are culpable. Sally Randall wonders whether she had left the window unlocked. William Pattern dwells on his contribution to the accident—had he been speeding?

Shame often accompanies victims' guilt. They feel humiliated by the event. Sally Randall views herself with disgust and shame for having been raped. Victims suffer at the hands of the attacker and then, mentally, at their own.

The survivor identifies with the deceased. He or she adopts attitudes and behavior of the person who died. Mrs Somers finds herself wondering about Peggy's dolls. Her daughter loved dolls.

The survivor's or victim's dreams and nightmares reflect the loss or event. Mr Somers has a recurrent dream that his daughter comes home from a trip. Sally Randall, when she can sleep, frequently awakes in terror from a nightmare of being chased. William Pattern keeps dreaming of himself engaged in a wide variety of athletic events; in his dreams he has both legs.

Often people emerge from traumatic experiences with distrust. The event has shattered their confidence in themselves and in others. They wonder why the tragedy could not have been averted, why medical intervention failed when on television the EMTs and the ED always triumph. Or they feel betrayed. Sally Randall not only does not trust her assailant but also now wonders whether she can trust any man. The survivor of a loved one who has committed suicide believes the dead person, in taking his or her life, betrayed a trust and relationship.

The survivor or victim mentally reverts to earlier times. Malinak and colleagues (10) note that all the members of the family vividly recall when they last saw the deceased. Survivors reflect on happy occasions, on better times. The victim recalls other circumstances, when things used to be good.

The devastation leaves in its wake a tremendous sense of disbelief. People often state, "I don't believe this is happening to me!" The entire experience seems unreal. People feel like spectators at their own crises.

Each searches for an explanation for the catastrophe. Each looks for a cause. Why? becomes the person's basic thought, either stated or implied. The swiftness of the event intensifies the quest.

The Behavior

The devastation impacts upon the survivor's or victim's behavior in many ways. It alters appetite and activities. Each person reacts in his or her own individual way and has individualized needs for solitude or companionship. Somatic complaints and sleep disturbances are common. Survivors usually wish to see the body. They become either hyperalert or numb.

Many people report loss of appetite following a traumatic event. Food has no flavor, and the distressed person just does not want to eat. Food seems very unimportant.

Daily activities become totally disrupted. Even after the funeral the Somerses find it impossible to resume their lives. Sally Randall is unable to return to work the day after the rape. Her fears, distrust, and shame keep her a prisoner at home.

People vary in the degree of interpersonal interaction they seek after the tragedy. Some handle the crisis by withdrawing into themselves. They want to be alone. Upon learning of the sudden death of his best friend, a man felt the strong urge to be alone in the woods. There he privately cried. Others desire to be surrounded by people. They fear being alone; they reach out, demanding closeness; they want to be held. Whether people want solitude or closeness, they all want to be away from the rest of the patients and families in the ED.

Survivors and victims frequently develop a number of physical ailments. They complain of headaches, colds, chest pain, and just exhaustion. Frequently they describe somatic symptoms not unlike the physical problems of the deceased. A young man developed wheezing shortly after learning of the death of his father, who had succumbed to the effects of chronic obstructive pulmonary disease.

Survivors and victims often experience insomnia. Sleep eludes them as they lie in bed reviewing in infinite detail the traumatic experience. The survivor keeps seeing the dear one.

Family members frequently wish to see the body of the deceased. They have last seen the loved one earlier in the day when everything was fine. Now, suddenly, a doctor says the person is dead. The Somerses want to view their daughter. They cannot believe what has happened. Seeing her confronts them with devastating reality.

The survivor or victim may react with hyperalertness. The person listens intently to everything the staff says, scans the EMTs' and the ED personnel's faces for clues and cues, and hears every hallway conversation. Sally Randall looks about carefully for any sign of disapproval from police or ED staff. William Pattern watches with jealousy everyone walking with two legs.

Other survivors and victims recoil into numbness. They go into shock. Only hours, days, or weeks later do they emerge and attempt to deal with the devastation. Then and only then will all the remarks made by the EMTs and the ED staff come back to these people. They *have* heard everything that has been said.

THE DETERMINANTS OF RESPONSES TO TRAUMATIC EVENTS

The therapeutic approach to survivors or victims must be based on two considerations: (1) intrapsychic, interpersonal, and biologic factors contribute to each person's response to the crisis, and (2) EMTs and ED staff must move beyond the cause of death, the dynamics of the assailant, and the reason for the injury, and must focus on helping the survivor or victim. All too often the actual cause of the tragedy eludes discovery: the mechanism of sudden infant death syndrome remains unclear, the attacker escapes, and the reason for an accident frequently is unknown. Often, as Frankl (11) observes, fate and chance seem to play roles in these events. But the survivor or victim is a clear and immediate reality and must become the focus of intervention.

Intrapsychic Factors

A number of intrapsychic factors influence how survivors or victims handle the event. These include their fundamental orientation to life, their concept of death, their self-concept, and their body image.

One's basic orientation toward life influences how one deals with the event. The person with a pessimistic view finds the death or trauma further confirmation of that pessimism. People who ordinarily use a great deal of denial attempt to isolate, segregate, and distance themselves from the experience. The person with a religious orientation can put the event into a greater perspective. And the person with an optimistic outlook places the event into a framework of hopefulness.

Survivors' feelings about death play a significant role in how they consider the *end* (12,13). People who believe in an afterlife and who have strong religious convictions discover hope in the tragedy and find meaning in the event. Some people in other circumstances find only utter devastation. Survivors' views about suicide influence their reactions to suicidal death. Occasionally a survivor views suicide as a sin and the committer as ineligible for Heaven (14).

The event challenges the survivor's or victim's self-concept. The wife of a 58-year-old man died suddenly of a myocardial infarction. They had been married for 40 years, during which she had made all the family decisions. He then found himself incapable of making any decisions. He had never viewed himself as autonomous. The person with self-disdain finds rape or incest a justification of this low self-esteem.

Physical injury confronts and challenges the victim's self-image (body image). Each person carries a conscious and unconscious view of himself or herself as a complete person. William Pattern cannot conceive of himself without a leg. A 48-year-old woman became involved in an automobile accident and sustained a facial laceration. She had prided herself on her beauty. She felt so devastated by the accident that she considered suicide.

Interpersonal Factors

The relationship the survivor has had with the deceased, the victim's relationship with the attacker, and the relationships between the injured person and a significant other all influence reactions.

The feelings of the survivor toward the deceased contributes to the survivor's reaction to the death. Survivors who had related to the dead person with marked ambivalence experience difficulty in the mourning process (15). Their hostility, often unexpressed, exaggerates guilt feelings. A 70-year-old wife cared diligently and selflessly for decades for her bedridden husband without ever feeling frustration. Upon his death she became psychotically depressed as she struggled to suppress all hostile feelings toward him.

Sudden death deprives the survivor of any opportunity to say good-bye and achieve a sense of closure. As a result, the last interaction becomes very significant to the survivor and sets the tone for the person's feelings about the death.

The victim's relationship to the offender influences responses. In cases where the rape victim knew the assailant, the sense of betrayal is great. In cases of incest, the victim is caught in a very difficult situation. A middle-aged executive made advances to his 14-year-old daughter. She felt paralyzed by fear, love, and hate. She loved her father, yet she knew what he was doing was wrong. She felt guilty about telling her mother.

The relationship of the injured with significant others affects reaction to the trauma. Injured people who believe their personal relationships are governed by their physical appearance and ability become even further devastated by the loss. William Pattern believes his girl friend will leave him as a result of the accident.

Biologic Factors

Two biologic factors contribute to survivors' and victims' reactions to the traumatic event: alcohol and pain. Alcohol distorts people's views and colors their interpretations and understanding. Not infrequently the patient needs to sober up before being able to appreciate the extent of the injury. Pain heightens all reactions. All injuries appear worse when the patient is experiencing great pain. William Pattern can think only about the pain.

THE REACTIONS OF OTHERS

The family and friends display a wide variety of reactions toward the survivor or victim. Their responses play a major part in the survivor's or victim's acceptance of the event. Their reactions range from accusations to support and include avoidance, apathy, and empathy.

Some family members, friends, and acquaintances blame the survivor or the victim for the event. They accuse the person of negligence, malice, irresponsibility, impulsiveness, immaturity, provocativeness, impudence, carelessness, recklessness, or rashness (16). They invoke a vindictive, wrathful condemnation of the survivor or the victim. A young mother lost her firstborn to sudden infant death syndrome. Her mother-in-law, who had vehemently objected to the wedding for religious reasons, believed the death proved the union and seed were "bad." She informed the grief-stricken mother of her view. As Sally Randall recoils from the rape, a coworker implies she has invited the assailant by her "loose clothing and life style." William Pattern's father remarks upon hearing of the accident, "I told him not to buy the stupid motorcycle."

Others react by avoiding the survivor or the victim. A friend of the Somerses noted he experienced too great a pain when he saw them. A girl friend of Sally Randall confesses she "does not know what to say," so she does not want to call

Sally "right away." William Pattern's girl friend has difficulty coming to see him the first time and procrastinates for a week.

Still others respond with apathy. They isolate themselves from the event, the survivor, and the victim. They employ rationalizations, use denial, and react with blandness. The survivor or victim feels no support, interest, or concern. These people display a matter-of-fact, business-as-usual attitude.

In most cases the family and friends provide meaningful, empathic support. They respond with concern, love, and warmth. They come to the survivor's side and share the grief, sorrow, and pain. They stand by the victim and offer continued acceptance. Through their care they help to sustain the survivor or victim through the crisis.

THE INITIATION OF THE EMERGENCY

The death, the assault, the accident, or the molestation precipitates the crisis. It comes abruptly and unexpectedly.

THE EMTs' RESPONSE TO THE EMERGENCY

This section emphasizes the EMTs' response to the survivor and concern for emotional reactions of the victim. By training, orientation, and the medical emergency confronting them, the EMTs focus upon the patient's physical requirements. The comprehensive approach calls for them to expand their intervention. It demands an increased level of awareness and sensitivity. It means that even if the patient dies they can still help the family and the friends.

The EMTs' response involves a number of factors. First, EMTs must monitor their communications throughout the intervention. Second, they must keep the family informed of the activities during the intervention. Third, they must appreciate and check their own reactions toward the survivor or victim. Fourth, they must listen to the survivor or victim. Fifth, they must recognize their own responses to the event.

EMTs must monitor their own dialogue throughout the entire intervention. The family and friends listen intensively and recall for decades what the EMTs say. They hear, amplify, and occasionally distort the EMTs' remarks. For the family already struggling with guilt, a "smart" comment by a callous EMT confirms their blame. Trauma victims carefully listen to everything said about their condition. *Everyone* hears the EMTs' radio-transmitted reports to the hospital. A mother discovered that her baby was not breathing and called for help. The responding EMT inquired how long she had left the infant unattended. She perceived this question as an attack on her mothering.

The EMTs must inform the patient and the family of their activities throughout the intervention. They employ an increasingly elaborate variety of techniques and equipment in their treatment, ranging from intravenous medications to defibrillators. Although routine to the EMTs, these terrify many people. Additionally EMTs fairly frequently treat a patient in one room with the family anxiously waiting in another; whenever this is the case, one of the EMTs must periodically tell the family what is happening.

The EMTs must appreciate their own reactions to the survivor or victim. They may indeed judge as irresponsible the mother whose child got into the medicine cabinet and took brightly colored pills. They may think rape victims invite the attack or motorcycle operators flirt with danger. These attitudes interfere with intervention.

Whenever possible the EMTs must allot time just to listen to the survivor or victim. The person is struggling with a devastating event and benefits from talking about it. William Pattern begs for someone to talk with him as the ambulance speeds him to the hospital.

Finally, the EMTs must recognize their own reactions to the trauma to which they are exposed. They witness many brutal scenes and catastrophes. These affect them — they feel sad, angry, and bewildered. They worry about whether they did enough or the right thing. They experience difficulty sleeping and have nightmares. A new volunteer rescue worker helped transport a 43-year-old man with chest pain to the ED. The patient had a cardiac arrest and died en route. The EMT became so overwhelmed with a sense of failure that he dropped out of the local unit. EMTs need to talk and listen to each other, especially after a difficult case.

THE EMERGENCY DEPARTMENT EVALUATION

The ED staff advances and amplifies the EMTs' response to the survivor and the concern for the victim's emotional reactions. The ED, too, must expand its focus and has a responsibility beyond the immediate medical evaluation and treatment.

The Reception

The reception involves proper telephone techniques, use of a private room, management of communications between the staff and the family or patient as well as of comments among the ED personnel, appreciation of the staff's own reactions, and accompaniment of the patient throughout the treatment.

Telephone communication technique is extremely important. Not infrequently, the patient is brought to the ED and then the ED staff has the responsibility of contacting the family. When the staff initiates the telephone call, the ED staff member must first identify himself or herself to the family. In cases where the patient has died, it is preferable to have the family come to the ED rather than inform them over the telephone of the death. An effective technique is to tell the family that the loved one has sustained a serious injury and to ask them to come to the ED. Staff may also recommend that the family have a close friend drive them there. The staff person tells Peggy Somers's parents only that she is in the ED. Then, when they arrive, the physician informs them personally and privately of the death.

The family requires a private, quiet, dignified room to wait in; the room should have a telephone. There they can meet with the doctors, cry without being observed, and be away from the confusion and activity of the ED. The telephone is very important, for there are many calls to be made. One chaplain insists that the family call the funeral home *before* they leave the ED.

Communications between staff and family stand as the key part of the comprehensive approach. Interaction commences when the family arrives. Whenever possible, the physician and the staff must introduce themselves to the family. Then throughout the intervention the family members must be kept informed of the treatment that is taking place. One useful method of doing this is to have a member of the treatment team visit the family at five-minute intervals throughout the therapy. If the patient dies, the physician must be the one to tell the family. This information must be disclosed in the privacy of the room. At the point of death, the family wants to know that "everything that was possible was done." Then the physician must spend a few minutes with the family, answering their questions and just listening.

The physician must communicate with the injured patient. The physician introduces himself or herself, keeps the patient informed as the treatment evolves, and listens to the patient's reactions. William Pattern bitterly complains that he does not even know his physician's name and no one has told him what is happening.

Staff must monitor their comments during treatment. The family members and the patient scan the milieu for implications as well as factual information. They listen for accusations. A 22-year-old man died of a self-inflicted gunshot wound. In the suicide note he had displayed anger toward his family. When the ED physician joked about the letter to a colleague, the patient's sister overheard the conversation and believed the doctor blamed her. Patients surviving cardiac arrest report staff behavior and comments during the resuscitation.

The ED staff must appreciate their own feelings toward the survivor or the victim and then act professionally. They may feel that the parents' negligence caused the accident or that the patient should have worn a seat belt and should not have been drinking. Such attitudes can interfere with the ED treatment.

In some cases a staff member feels too close emotionally to the survivor. One nurse could not attend to the Somers family; she had lost a child several years ago in a boating accident, and Peggy's death brought back too many memories. Conversely, an ED secretary who had experienced the loss of a younger sister was able to provide comfort and support to the Somerses. The secretary attributes her effectiveness to "having been there."

The ED staff find themselves deeply affected by the traumas and tragedies they encounter in their work. Their patients die. They see families devastated. They experience grief, insomnia, nightmares, and frustration. They, too, benefit by recognizing these feelings and talking about them.

Patients are helped by having someone with them at all times. They feel anxious, angry, and scared. Being alone heightens their anguish. As Sally Randall waits in the examining room, her apprehension increases. When a nurse joins her, she feels relief.

Physical Examination

The rape victim requires a proper gynecological examination with a female nurse present.

Chief Complaint

The chief complaint offers insights into the reactions and struggles of the survivor or victim. Survivors often wonder, "Why me?" They may blame themselves: "I caused her to die." They sometimes accuse the doctor: "They killed her." Many feel very sad: "It hit me like a ton of bricks!" Victims also search for meaning: "Why?" They also castigate themselves—"I was such a fool"—or display hopelessness: "What can I ever do?"

History

The physician must take the approach of listening to survivors and victims rather than asking the customary information-gathering questions. The physician provides treatment to the survivor or victim by permitting the person to talk about the event. In that context the major part of the interview revolves about the history of present illness (HPI). Other areas of importance include history of previous trauma, social history, and religious background.

The history of present illness focuses on the event. Survivors and victims often present a detailed review of the event. They begin the process of resolving the loss by reflecting upon that day's activities. The Somerses talk for hours about what their daughter has recently been doing.

The ways families and individuals can be expected to handle stress can partially be predicted by the ways they have previously dealt with difficult situations. Some families come together in the wake of a traumatic event; others fragment and quarrel. A family history provides clues.

A knowledge of the social situation provides the physician with information about the environment to which the survivor or victim will return. Sally Randall lives alone. The ED physician recommends that she stay with a friend for the next several days.

Religion offers the survivor or victim sustenance, meaning, support, and structure. Knowing the family's religious affiliations and views helps the physician organize assistance. Clergy provide relief to the survivor. Clergy can start to address questions of Why? and can give specific answers to questions about funeral arrangements.

Mental Status Examination

In certain situations the physician must undertake a mental status examination of the survivor or the victim. A woman who had been raped wanted to kill herself because of the assault, believing the experience had ruined her life. However, in the overwhelming majority of cases such an inquiry is totally inappropriate.

One indication of stress is that the family denies the death or the patient denies the injury. Another instance of inadequate coping is seen when a survivor wants to kill the person responsible for the death. Still a third involves a victim who prefers suicide to the consequences of the traumatic event.

The physician must assess the survivor's or victim's understanding of the event. From the interview the physician usually can assess the person's understanding of what has happened. A victim who does not comprehend the extent of the injury frequently refuses treatment and seeks prematurely to leave the ED. A 68-year-old man had a myocardial infarction. He interpreted the pain as indigestion and wanted to go home. Careful attention from his doctor persuaded him to stay for tests.

A distraught family member rarely seeks revenge, but in a few cases the physician must assess the survivor's homicidal potential. As the result of a head-on collision, a 14-year-old girl lay in critical condition in a trauma room. The driver of the other vehicle, who had superficial injuries, sat in a treatment cubicle. The girl's father announced that if his daughter died he would kill the driver.

Similarly, in a few cases the victim reacts to the traumatic event by wanting to die. As a result of the injury or the emotional trauma, the patient feels there is no future. The physician must inquire into the patient's thoughts and plans about suicide.

DIAGNOSIS, TREATMENT PLAN, AND IMMEDIATE EMERGENCY DEPARTMENT THERAPY

The core of the comprehensive approach revolves upon the ED staff members' recognition of and response to the emotional needs of the survivor or victim. Occasionally a diagnosis is called for.

Diagnosis

The diagnosis most commonly applied to survivors and victims is transient situational disorder, either adjustment disorder or post-traumatic disorder (17). The adjustment disorder diagnosis emphasizes the short-term, transitional nature of the disturbance. Making the diagnosis of post-traumatic disorder involves several criteria. They are: (1) a recognizable stressor which all agree would cause significant distress; (2) a reexperiencing of the event by either repeated recollections of it, recurrent dreams, or a sudden repetition of the event triggered by an environmental or ideational stimulus; (3) a numbness marked by either diminished interest in activities, estrangement from others, or affective constriction; and (4) at least two of the following: hyperalertness, sleep disturbance, guilt about surviving, memory difficulty, avoidance of activities which precipitate memories of the event, and heightened symptoms upon exposure to events which resemble the event.

Treatment Plan

The treatment plan consists of the immediate intervention and the treatment that will be provided after the ED visit. The former remains the important focus for the ED staff. The latter involves the family's support, the community's helping network, and the services of religious institutions and specialized groups such as rape counseling centers.

Immediate Emergency Department Therapy

The immediate therapy consists of the care and concern of the ED staff, the assistance clergy, the viewing of the body, and the assistance of specialized groups.

The ED staff members provide vital help through their personal response to the survivor or victim. The steps outlined in the section on ED reception address the emotional needs of the survivor or victim.

Clergy play a significant role in helping the survivors. They can stay with the family. They can start to answer questions of *why*. They can help the family with the funeral arrangements. By training and experience they are particularly able to help the family grieve. The family usually appreciates and is helped by having someone present from the clergy whether or not they are all of the same faith or denomination. A 24-hour ED call schedule for chaplains and other clergy proves quite valuable. The hospital chaplain joins the Somers family in the ED and spends four hours with them. He listens; he guides them; and he helps. They leave very appreciative of his comfort.

Not infrequently, the family wants to view the body in the ED. The unexpected suddenness of the event never permitted them an opportunity to say good-bye. Often the staff has more fears about the family's seeing the body than are justified by the survivors' reactions to the experience. When the deceased person is not completely disfigured and the family requests to view the body, they should be allowed to do so. This event helps them to integrate the loss and challenges their disbelief. The Somerses insist upon seeing their daughter. The ED physician accompanies them but stays in the background.

Some groups have particular skill and experience in dealing with certain types of victims. Rape counselors have demonstrated their effectiveness in working with the assault victim (18).

CARE AFTER THE EMERGENCY

The Somerses spend several minutes with Peggy in the trauma room and say good-bye. After four hours in the ED with the hospital chaplain they make the long, sad journey home. Their families and friends, as well as their minister, provide massive support. Two painful days later they hold a small funeral. During the subsequent year the family experiences particularly difficult times at the winter holidays and on what would have been her eleventh birthday. A year later to the day, the Somerses join the chaplain in the ED and talk about the loss. They thank him for all his help.

Sally Randall stays with a girl friend. She cannot work for the next several days. When she does manage to sleep, she awakes in terror. Scenes of the rape dominate her days; she becomes preoccupied by a sense of guilt for her participation in the event. Although initially interested in pressing charges against a person the police apprehended, she ultimately drops the case after being vigorously questioned by the suspect's attorney.

She obtains help from a rape center counselor whom she has met in the ED. Therapy proves difficult. She stops dating for the next six months. Slowly, her life returns to normal. She moves from the city.

William Pattern undergoes surgery. During his hospitalization he bitterly complains of leg pain in the amputated extremity. He develops a severe depression, for which his physician prescribes imipramine (Tofranil) 50 mg three times daily. The support he receives from his family, girl friend, and hospital staff encourage him. But only when he acquires an artificial limb and starts to use it does he begin to recover substantially from the depression.

In subsequent days the survivors or victims have a variety of experiences during the struggle to integrate the event and to resume life. Most find support in family and friends. For most the feelings which commenced in the ED persist. For some a sense of disbelief continues for years. Some will seek psychotherapy. Many will experience anniversary reactions.

The support of family, friends, and clergy plays a critical role in the adjustment. They demonstrate acceptance of the survivor or victim. They help mourn and share the burden. The neighbors, friends, families, and classmates come together to support the Somerses. Their community and their religion sustain them. William Pattern derives a great deal of encouragement from his family and, especially, his girl friend.

The depression, anguish, guilt, and terror originally felt by the survivor or victim persist and slowly diminish as time passes. Survivors and victims experience waves of these feelings periodically. These reactions are especially intense in the first few weeks and interfere with work, sleep, and appetite. The mourning period normally involves six months to one year. Each person finds an emptiness in life.

In certain situations the survivor continues not to believe the reality of the event. He or she denies the death or the circumstances of the death. A young man lost his father in a fiery airplane crash. The body could never be definitely identified. The man persists in the belief that his father lives. He claims his father never got on the airplane. He keeps waiting for his return. A young woman took a fatal overdose of sleeping pills. She had been seriously depressed before the suicide but had masked this from her parents. Her parents refused to accept the suicide. They went to many physicians to prove she died of "natural causes."

Occasionally survivors or victims benefit from psychotherapy. They wish to remove the trauma of the event so they can continue with their lives. Sally Randall talks with her counselor about her fear of being killed, her guilt for participation in the act, her shame, her recurrent images of the assault, and her terror of being alone. In this fashion she eventually comes to terms with the event.

Not infrequently the survivor or victim remembers the traumatic event with great intensity on the anniversary of its occurrence. It recurs in a dream or is consciously recalled. The anniversary of the event will stand always as a special day. Many religions observe memorial activities on the anniversary of a loved one's death. The Somerses visit the ED one year later.

REFERENCES

1. Glover E: Notes on the psychological effects of war conditions on the civilian population: I. The Munich crisis. *Int J Psychoanal* 22:132–146, 1941.

2. Glover E: Notes on the psychological effects of war conditions on the civilian population: III. The blitz. *Int J Psychoanal* 23:17–37, 1942.

3. Rado S: Pathodynamics and treatment of traumatic war neurosis. *Psychosom Med* 4:362–369, 1942.

4. Stevenson RL: *Virgin: Bus Puerisque and Other Essays in Belles Lettres.* London, William Heinemann Ltd, 1924.

5. Soreff S: Sudden death in the emergency department. *Crit Care Med* 7:321–323, 1979.

6. Lindemann E: Symptomatology and management of acute grief. *Am J Psychiatry* 101:141–148, 1944.

7. Groth AN, Burgess W, Holmstrom LL: Rape: Power, anger, and sexuality. *Am J Psychiatry* 134:1239–1243, 1977.

8. Shneidman ES: Prevention, intervention, and postvention. Ann Intern Med 75:453–458, 1971.

9. McCombie SL, Bassuk E, Savitz R, et al: Development of a medical center rape crisis intervention program. *Am J Psychiatry* 133:418–421, 1976.

10. Malinak DP, Hoyt MF, Patterson V: Adults' reactions to the death of a parent: A preliminary study. *Am J Psychiatry* 136:1152–1156, 1979.

11. Frankl VE: *Man's Search for Meaning: An Introduction to Logotherapy.* Boston, Beacon Press, 1979.

12. Kübler-Ross E: *On Death and Dying.* New York, MacMillan Co, 1970.

13. Becker E: *The Denial of Death.* New York, MacMillan Co, 1973.

14. Shneidman ES: Suicide as a taboo topic, in Shneidman ES, Farberow NL, Litman RE (eds): *The Psychology of Suicide.* New York, Science House, 1970.

15. Freud S: Mourning and melancholia, in Jones E (ed): *Collected papers of Sigmund Freud.* London, Hogarth Press, 1925 vol 4, pp 288–317.

16. Brownmiller S: *Against our will.* New York, Bantam Books Inc, 1976.

17. *Diagnostic and Statistical Manual of Mental Disorders,* 3rd ed. Washington DC, American Psychiatric Association, 1980.

18. Hilberman E: *The Rape Victim.* New York, Basic Books Inc. 1976.

15

The Patient With No Place to Go

To the ED come those who are world-weary, tired, unemployed, outcast, or homeless. As Knowles (1) observed, people now seek the ED who in prior eras would have sought the cathedral for asylum. They ask not only medical and psychiatric help but also food and shelter.

THE PATIENT

Mr Joseph Hart asks a reluctant rescue unit to bring him to the ED. At 50 years of age Mr Hart has no friends, no money, no job, no food, and no place to stay. Although he lives in a "room" occasionally, he frequently hitchhikes or "rides the rails."

He was married and divorced twice many years ago. He has a 25-year-old son "somewhere in California" whom he last saw 10 years ago. He has held a wide variety of jobs for short times, including positions as carpenter, factory worker, grounds keeper, and night watchman. He has been treated at a number of state hospitals over the years but does not take any medications. He has been in jail. He drinks to excess when he can get the "booze." He received a dishonorable discharge from the military.

He comes hopeless, pennyless, familyless, and friendless to the ED. His parents have died; his brothers and sisters have long since ceased to care about him, and he about them. He comes because there is nowhere else to go.

Homeless patients display a wide variety of emotions, perceptual changes, and behaviors.

The Patient's Mood

These patients exhibit a number of emotions. These include depression, apprehension, apathy, bitterness, and helplessness. Their moods frequently appear blunted, beaten, and bland.

The patients feel depressed. They display all the accompaniments of despair: hopelessness, melancholia, sadness, loneliness, purposelessness, and feelings of uselessness. They know they do not fit in. They feel defeated and rejected. Joseph Hart experiences a protracted feeling of emptiness.

The patients do struggle with a sense of apprehension, the apprehension born of necessity. They face the very basic issues of survival—food and shelter. They realize their request for help is of the most fundamental level.

Despite the apprehension they are also apathetic. Paradoxically, their moods reflect indifference and silent resignation. They have been in this predicament before.

The patients' moods portray a tinge of bitterness. They regret a series of lost opportunities; they feel betrayed by a host of relatives, teachers, and employers; and they sense rejection by family and friends.

Above all they feel genuinely helpless. They cannot find their own solutions. They see themselves as powerless, resourceless, and useless.

The Patient's Perceptions

Homeless people typically demonstrate a number of perceptual changes. These, too, are muted by years of fruitless struggle. They include a negative attitude, a rejecting view of life, hallucinations, and mild disorientation.

The patients have developed a negative attitude toward life, activities, the future, and themselves. Why try? is their attitude about everything. They will get fired, so why should they seek work? Their families do not care, so why ask them for help?

Rejection permeates and dominates these patients' thinking. They anticipate rejection. All they have known has been exclusion by family and friends. They even reject themselves. They decline any more than the basic help. They only want food and shelter, not a job, training, or counseling.

Often the patient has hallucinations. The long-term schizophrenic patient reports having had auditory hallucinations for years. The chronic alcoholic patient experiences visual hallucinations during periods of withdrawal.

The patients not infrequently demonstrate evidence of mild disorientation. They have difficulty thinking of the date and recalling recent events. Chronic alcohol use or malnutrition has caused some degree of organic mental disorder. Also, because of their life style, marked by monotonous days and little stimulation, they may simply not know the date.

The Patient's Behavior

Homeless people's behavior reflects their moods and perceptions. They wander; they have few friends; and they seek help only in an emergency.

The patients often are wanderers, drifters. An earlier generation would have called them hoboes. They search the nation for something. Each patient's history reveals many addresses, many jobs, and many places, but no *home*.

They have few if any friends. They have no involved family. They are alone.

They seek help only in the crisis. When they have enough money to survive, they spend it. Only after the government check has been used do they come to the ED. Joseph Hart comes only when he has to.

THE CAUSES OF HOMELESSNESS

Intrapsychic, interpersonal, and biologic factors contribute to the homeless patient's situation. The person's plight often results from a long series of interactions among these three factors.

Intrapsychic Causes of Homelessness

The intrapsychic factors involve the patient's attitudes, views, and ideas. These include distancing, the anticipation of failure, an institutional orientation, the loss of initiative, and idiosyncratic, egocentric, and eccentric reasoning.

Often the patient has developed a pattern of distancing other people. The patient avoids close, intimate, and involved relationships, preferring instead brief, intense encounters terminated by an abrupt withdrawal. In some cases this behavior reflects early losses. Joseph Hart does not desire any close relationships. He wants to be helped and then left alone.

Not uncommonly these patients have anticipated failure all their lives. They believe all their efforts are preordained not to succeed. This self-defeating attitude leads to a chronic lack of participation in the environment. Parents, teachers, or other significant figures throughout the patients' lives have labeled them "no good." They themselves have incorporated this judgement.

All too frequently the patients have been institutionalized (2). They have been in state facilities, hospitals, prisons, or retardation centers for many years. They are unprepared for survival in society. They have derived the basics of life and security "within the walls."

Homeless patients display lack of initiative. They seem incapable of helping themselves. They feel overwhelmed. Joseph Hart has lost heart and any sense of initiative.

Additionally, some of these patients portray an idiosyncratic, egocentric, and eccentric orientation toward life. In the extreme form they suffer from chronic schizophrenia (3). They respond to internal ideas, thoughts, and priorities. They are guided by their delusions and hallucinations. One 36-year-old man came to the ED looking for a place to stay because he had lost his job and had no money. He had left 12 jobs in the last year and a half, each time after discovering his coworkers were spying on him "for the Undersea League of Justice and Revenge."

Interpersonal Causes of Homelessness

Interpersonal factors contribute to the situation in a number of ways. First, these patients do not have the support of family and friends. Second, they have been rejected by employers, landlords, and agencies. Third, they lack the basic skills to succeed in the job market.

They do not have the support of any family members or friends. Usually, family and friends have long since abandoned these patients, either by outright rejection or simply by losing contact. In other cases parents have died and siblings live a great distance away. Joseph Hart has no family, no friends, and no one to turn to.

The patients have confronted a series of rejections by employers, landlords, and agencies. For a variety of reasons, including mental illness, history of state hospital treatment, time spent in jail, substance abuse, lack of skills, and distancing, the patients have found many doors closed in their faces.

Finally, the patients not infrequently lack the interpersonal and employment skills to succeed. They do not possess the trade capability, the needed education, the intellectual grasp, or the interpersonal facility to obtain and sustain jobs.

Biologic Causes of Homelessness

These patients have several physical problems which both cause their condition and result from it. These include alcohol use, chronic illness, and malnutrition.

Frequently the patient has been involved in alcohol abuse. This has produced a deterioration of physical and mental health and has precluded a number of employment opportunities. The alcohol abuse causes dementia. The resultant organicity makes employment even less possible. In addition, the alcohol permits the person to withdraw.

Chronic debilitating illnesses such as chronic obstructive pulmonary disease (COPD), produce a person who is unemployed, depressed, and isolated. The disease precludes employment and distances the patient.

Chronic isolation, homelessness, undereating, and depression cause the patient to become malnourished. The physical effects of malnutrition and vitamin deficiency include weight loss, fatigue, unsteady gait, tremors, hypotension, anemia, disorientation, and apathy.

THE REACTIONS OF OTHERS

Family and friends react in a number of ways to the patient. Some show anger, ridicule, and annoyance. Others either avoid or ignore the person. Some do demonstrate concern but often lack the resources to assist.

The family and previous friends not infrequently display anger, frustration, and annoyance toward these patients. They ridicule, reject, and abandon them. They punitively blame and depreciate them. "It's his own damn fault." "Who needs him, anyway?" "I hate him." They show scorn.

The anger of friends and family often converts to avoidance behavior. They want nothing to do with the patient. When the person comes to visit, the porch light is off and the door is locked. These patients are treated like outcasts or lepers.

As a further step, relatives and former friends become totally indifferent to the patient. They go beyond active avoidance to complete ignoring. They cease to mention the person or include the person in any way in their lives. In their minds, the patient is dead.

Some family and friends do demonstrate care and concern but lack any resources to help. They live too far away or have no room in their homes. They do want the person to get assistance but they do not have sufficient funds.

THE INITIATION OF THE EMERGENCY

Under a number of circumstances the patient seeks the ED. Indeed, the patient may have tolerated a meager existence for years. Yet certain stressors precipitate the crisis: loss of residence, loss of financial support, suicidal behavior, an inability to cope, or deteriorating physical health.

The usual reason for the crisis is loss of shelter. A variety of conditions produce this homeless state: eviction, expulsion, abandonment, discharge, wandering, or the destruction of the house. One patient resided in a boxcar. Whenever the railroad officials searched the yard he would come to the ED for temporary refuge. Joseph Hart has recently wandered into town and has no place to stay.

Being without financial resources produces a crisis also. Without an income or monetary support the patient cannot obtain food and shelter. Losing employment or using up one's government check accounts for this situation.

Occasionally patients react to their homeless, jobless, rootless, and friendless condition with suicide. As they confront their emptiness, suicide becomes an alternative. The police brought a 50-year-old man to the ED after he attempted suicide by walking down the middle of a busy highway. The patient said that with no place to live, no money, no food, and no friends, he had no reason for living.

Frequently patients seek the ED because they are overwhelmed. Some have spent most of their lives in a state hospital and cannot cope with the community stresses. They want to return to the hospital.

Finally, the patients come to the ED because of physical debility and illness. Malnutrition, anemia, tuberculosis, COPD, pneumonia, or neurologic disease make the patient's marginal existence impossible. The sickness makes the homeless condition intolerable.

THE EMTs' RESPONSE TO THE EMERGENCY

The EMTs entire response must be based on the premise that the patient with no place to go represents a psychiatric emergency. This kind of patient does indeed justify and require the EMTs' intervention and an ED evaluation.

The EMTs' response involves a concern and respect for the patient. It includes a response; an introduction and identification; the recognition of their own attitudes, followed by a professional approach; and the accompaniment of the patient.

The most important feature of the EMTs' approach must be that they do respond. They do not ignore, avoid, or reject the patient.

The response involves the EMTs' introducing and identifying themselves. They must use their names and titles. Further, and very critical, they must address patients by their formal names—not "Joey," "Old Man," or "Pops," but Mr Joseph Hart.

EMTs must appreciate their own reactions to these patients and then respond professionally. Not infrequently EMTs share the rejecting, negative attitudes previously described. The EMTs transport Mr Hart only reluctantly and wonder why he does not work, why he "just cannot take control of his life," and why their time and taxes are used in this way.

Someone must accompany the patient during transport. The patient is anxious, frightened, and isolated. EMTs can help by their responses, by not rejecting the person, and by their presence.

THE EMERGENCY DEPARTMENT EVALUATION

For the patient with no place to go, the ED serves as a point of evaluation and of direction. It must confront the challenge and develop alternatives for the patient. The ED evaluation encompasses five aspects: the reception, the physical examination, the chief complaint, the psychiatric evaluation, and the mental status examination.

The Reception

The ED staff must receive the patient. The reception involves an introduction and identification; a quiet, private room; a recognition of staff attitudes; and a complete history and physical examination. The ED staff must continue to advance the concern and respect developed by the EMTs.

The ED staff must introduce and identify themselves. Additionally, they must address the patient by the patient's formal name.

The patient requires a quiet, private place in the ED for the evaluation. It is humiliating and degrading to tell one's story in the middle of the waiting room, in the corridor, or in the midst of the trauma rooms. The office permits a sense of dignity and importance.

Staff must be aware of their attitudes toward this patient and then conduct themselves professionally. ED staff not infrequently evidence annoyance, frustration, anger, and antagonism toward the patient. They express bitterness that these patients come there, that they take up valuable time and space, and that they do not help themselves. Staff may feel that this kind of patient is not their problem. Staff must display responsible and responsive attitudes.

Finally, the patient requires a complete history and physical examination. All too often the ED physician conducts an abbreviated interview and performs a cursory physical examination. Such a hasty procedure misses valuable information and further undercuts the patient. A 50-year-old man came to the ED because he had no place to stay. He had no job, money, friends, or home. He also complained of a productive cough and "not feeling good." After a quick examination he was sent to a local shelter; that night he returned with fever, dyspnea, and delirium. The ED physician hospitalized him with pneumonia complicated by pleural effusion.

Physical Examination

The patient requires a physical examination. Certainly the staff must obtain this patient's pulse, blood pressure, and temperature. All too frequently the person's life situation has produced a number of distressing physical problems. The examination includes blood studies and a chest roentgenogram when they are indicated.

Chief Complaint

The chief complaint highlights, dramatizes, and encapsulates the crisis. The patient states it directly: "I have no place to stay"; "I need help—I have no place to go"; or "I'm hungry and homeless." Some patients describe their emotional need: "I want to go back to the state hospital"; or "I can't cope." Family members or others may describe the crisis: "We found him in the street—do something"; or "We can't help him anymore."

Psychiatric Evaluation

The patient with no place to go requires a thorough psychiatric evaluation. This includes a history of present illness (HPI); social history; family history; psychiatric history; educational, military, and vocational history; criminal history; history of alcohol and substance use; and medical history.

The HPI furnishes details about the recent and immediate events which have precipitated the crisis. The HPI explains why the emergency occurred when it did. This part of the interview reveals where the patient has been staying and with whom, what sources of income the patient has, where the person has been lately, and what caused the emergency. It also suggests what the patient expects from the ED intervention. Mr Hart has just arrived in the community and knows none of the resources. He wants direction.

The social history provides information about the patient's social milieu and support system. The physician inquires about friends, acquaintances, contacts, and personal resources.

The family history explores a once-significant part of the person's life and searches for potential contacts. This history suggests causes of the social isolation: divorces, deaths, abandonments, and rejections. It also points the physician toward possible contacts that can be used in arranging for help.

The psychiatric history offers information in a number of areas. The physician must inquire into the patient's current psychiatric treatment. Not infrequently, the patient is already involved in an outpatient program, such as a clinic or aftercare program, and takes psychotropic medication. Occasionally it is discovered that the patient is actually on a pass from a hospital! The doctor must investigate the person's inpatient experiences. These often indicate significant events and periods of the patient's life. Joseph Hart has been treated at several state hospitals, currently takes no medication, and has no interest in returning to "that institution."

The physician's exploration of the educational, military, and vocational history yields valuable information. It provides a vital description of the patient's background and points to future opportunities. It suggests areas of strengths and resources. The physician finds Mr Hart has some extremely valuable carpentry skills and other work experiences.

The physician also must investigate the patient's alcohol and substance use. Alcohol often has been involved in the patient's life and problem. This part of the history also suggests possible avenues for referral and treatment.

Finally, the physician must obtain a medical history. The patient may have been treated for a variety of physical problems and may have taken a number of medications.

Mental Status Examination

In the complete mental status examination, the physician must pay particular attention to a number of aspects. These include appearance, affect, thought content, plans for suicide and homicide, judgment, and sensorium.

The patient's appearance reveals a great deal of information. The person's dress, cleanliness, kinesis, eye contact, and coordination suggest both the dynamics and the dilemma. Joseph Hart wears an old suit and ill-fitting shoes, and he looks at the physician's face during the interview.

The physician must examine the patient's affect. How does the patient feel? Sad? Bitter? Indifferent? The patient's effect on the interviewer provides clues to the patient's mood.

The doctor must review the patient's thought content. How logical and organized is this person? Does the patient hallucinate or have delusions?

The patient's thoughts about and plans for suicide and homicide must be explored. As patients contemplate their homelessness and joblessness, they also consider suicide as an alternative. As they review the rejection they encounter, they also ponder retaliation, revenge, and homicide. The physician must assess both risks.

The patient's judgment is evaluated. How has the patient handled life in general and the crisis in particular? This information gives the doctor clues that help with referral.

Finally, the physician must assess the patient's sensorium — orientation, recall, and mental ability. The patient's crisis and condition may be the product of organic mental disorder. The person may be disoriented and may have marked memory deficits. Such a finding influences the physician in planning the referral.

DIAGNOSIS, TREATMENT PLAN AND IMMEDIATE EMERGENCY DEPARTMENT THERAPY

The physician must reach a diagnosis, formulate a treatment plan, and undertake immediate therapy.

Diagnosis

The physician bases the diagnosis on the information derived during the patient evaluation, the observations and experiences of the EMTs, and the history obtained from family and friends.

A number of diagnoses apply to the patient with no place to go. These range from psychosis to personality disorder and from psychiatric illness to physical disease. Diagnoses include dementia associated with alcoholism, residual schizophrenia, introverted personality disorder, schizotypal personality disorder, adjustment disorder, and physical illness (4). Not infrequently two diagnoses apply.

Dementia associated with alcoholism involves the protracted heavy consumption of alcohol and the signs of dementia persisting at least three days after the patient has stopped drinking. The dementia criteria include intellectual deterioration, memory impairment with disruption of abstract reasoning, poor judgment, or personality change. Indeed, the crisis may arise as a result of alcohol use in any of its three phases—intoxication, chronic use, and withdrawal.

The patient may fit the diagnosis of residual schizophrenia. In this category, the patient at one time has exhibited a full schizophrenic episode with delusions, hallucinations, and bizarre behavior but now does not have clear and obvious symptoms of psychosis. However, blunted affect, eccentric behavior, social withdrawal, and thought disorder are present. Frequently the history shows that the person has been treated on a psychiatric unit at least once.

The physician diagnoses Mr Hart as a patient with residual schizophrenia. This diagnosis is based on his history of hospitalizations, his blunted, inappropriate affect, his eccentric reasoning processes, and his social withdrawal and isolation.

Other patients fit the description of the introverted personality disorder. In this category the patient portrays a life-long difficulty with interpersonal relationships. The person has few if any close relationships; has marked difficulty in forming interpersonal relationships; shows significant introversion with withdrawal; prefers solitary activities or detachment; and manifests a decidedly bland affect but does not evidence bizarre, eccentric thought processes and communication patterns.

In contrast, the person with schizotypal personality disorder demonstrates many of the characteristics of the introvert but also exhibits thought disorder *almost* as a schizophrenic patient does. These patients have never had a schizophrenic episode. Their moods, perceptions, and behavior do show magical thinking, ideas of reference, illusions, social isolation, bizarre communication, difficulty in interpersonal situations, inappropriate affect, suspiciousness, and social apprehension. Both the introverted and schizotypal personality patterns often lead patients to live a marginal social existence that occasionally results in their having no place to go.

Homeless patients often have adjustment disorders. They exhibit anxiety, depression, and apprehension in response to the direct stress of becoming homeless, jobless, and friendless. They are reacting to identifiable stressors and not just experiencing exacerbations of underlying mental disorders.

Finally, the patient may be diagnosed as suffering from a wide variety of medical diseases. Or, as frequently occurs, the patient has both a mental disorder and a concomitant serious physical illness.

Treatment Plan

The referral constitutes the heart of the treatment plan. The referral involves several aspects. The hospital's department of social services provides remedies and preeminent assistance here. First, the physician must help to solve the crisis of *no place to stay*. One most useful approach is for the ED to maintain a list of available resources and locations. When the patient requires hospitalization, the physician arranges it. Second, the physician can offer the patient direction and guidance as to where to obtain welfare and other financial support. Third, he or she can involve the patient in aftercare programs.

Immediate Emergency Department Therapy

The evaluation provides significant immediate therapy. By treating the patient with dignity and respect, by conducting a thorough physical examination, by participating in a complete psychiatric interview, and by demonstrating concern, the physician helps the person substantially. Patients feel they have been heard and someone has paid attention. Someone shows an interest in helping them to regain control over their lives.

CARE AFTER THE EMERGENCY

Joseph Hart tells the ED doctor about his life, his children, his many jobs, his travels, and himself. Tears come to his eyes as he discusses his family, but he quickly changes the subject. As the physician reviews treatment options, Mr Hart insists he only wants a place to stay and a meal. The physician finds him to be in good physical condition despite his wanderings.

The physician also involves a social worker in the case. The social worker discovers Mr Hart receives a regular government check. He arranges an appointment for Mr Hart with the local agency to continue his financial support. He also directs Mr Hart to the city welfare office, the state employment office, and the aftercare unit.

The physician and the social worker consult the ED list of resources and then secure a bed for Mr Hart at a shelter.

A number of community options aid the patient with no place to go. The physician must know the community resources, as well as the patient's needs. The important resources include hospitals, nursing homes, halfway houses, shelters, aftercare programs, and local, county, and state programs.

Hospitalization

The patient requires hospitalization under a number of circumstances. These situations reflect the patient's unique vulnerability and lack of social support. They include severe disorganization, danger of suicide, detoxification, and medical illnesses.

Hospitalization is indicated for patients who exhibit severe disorganization. The patient shows hallucinations, incoherence, delusions, and thought disorder. This situation occurs in schizophrenic patients. The hospital provides structure, treatment, and order, as well as a place to stay.

Suicide risk constitutes a major reason for hospitalization. The physician must secure inpatient treatment if the danger of suicide is significant. The police brought a 45-year-old man to the ED. His girl friend had just kicked him out; he had no job; he had no friends; and he had walked in front of the police car "hoping it would hit me." The physician arranged for his hospital treatment.

The need for detoxification is another indication for inpatient treatment. Alcohol or substance intoxication or chronic use complicates the clinical condition of the homeless patient and often necessitates hospitalization.

Medical illnesses necessitate hospitalization in two ways. First, many of these patients have medical conditions severe enough to warrant hospital treatment. The patient with pneumonia, congestive heart failure, or gastrointestinal bleeding requires hospitalization. Second, because the patients are homeless and friendless, they often cannot be treated for even relatively simple illnesses as outpatients. A 40-year-old man who lived in boxcars came to the ED with an infected left arm. The physician determined that the man had cellulitis. The doctor hospitalized him when he realized the patient could not purchase the necessary antibiotics, had no place to elevate the arm, and had no one to monitor his condition.

Nursing Home Placement

The nursing home represents the community resource of choice for the homeless patient with physical illness and dementia. It provides structure, treatment, and support. It supplies a place for the patient to stay when the family cannot manage at home. The ED must play an important role in helping families obtain nursing home placement.

Halfway Houses

A variety of halfway houses provide a place to stay and a place for the patient to become reinvolved in the community. Halfway houses offer a less restrictive milieu than the hospital, but they provide major support to the patient.

Shelters

The community offers a variety of shelters and kitchens. The Salvation Army provides this facility in many communities.

Aftercare

Aftercare programs provide support when the hospitalized patient returns to the community. They also help the person find a place to live and transportation to outpatient appointments, and they monitor progress.

Other Agencies

Additionally, a wide variety of local, county, state, and federal agencies assist the patient. The ED must maintain a list of appropriate agencies and make referrals to them when indicated. The social worker refers Mr Hart to the city welfare office and the state employment office.

REFERENCES

1. Knowles, JH: The hospital. *Sci Am* 229:128–137, 1973.
2. *The Chronic Mental Patient in the Community.* New York, Group for the Advancement of Psychiatry, 1978, vol 10, No. 102.
3. Kolb LC: *Modern Clinical Psychiatry,* ed 8. Philadelphia, WB Saunders Co, 1973.
4. *Diagnostic and Statistical Manual of Mental Disorders,* 3rd ed. Washington DC American Psychiatric Association, 1980.

16
Crisis Mission: Treatment and Referral

EMTs and ED staff members have twin missions in emergency psychiatry: treatment and referral. These two functions constitute their basic responsibility and the goal of their intervention.

TREATMENT

This section reviews the extensive treatment modalities which EMTs and especially the ED staff have available. First it examines the principles underlying all psychiatric intervention; then it explores the various treatments.

The Principles

The underlying principle of emergency psychiatric care is that each crisis represents a therapeutic opportunity. In the process of an emergency, patients learn about themselves, their conflicts, their background, their supports, and their potential. The emergency brings to the surface hidden dynamics and feelings; it makes available information and material previously avoided. It provides not only a chance for the patient to regain equilibrium but also an opportunity to gain better self-understanding and to advance.

The other principles involve the staff's prompt, respectful attention, staff identification, patient accompaniment, involvement of significant others, thorough psychiatric and medical evaluation and examination, diagnostic formulation, and listening to the patient. The application of these principles is elaborated in the preceding chapters.

Types of Therapy

The ED physician employs a wide variety of therapies to resolve the crisis. These include a psychotherapeutic session, conjunct therapy, family therapy, network therapy, commitment, medications, rechecks, and referral. The physician may combine several of these as indicated.

Psychotherapy Session. First and foremost, the physician provides the patient with a psychotherapeutic experience. The evaluation interview itself begins the treatment process and provides therapy (1). Furthermore, the physician engages the patient in a psychotherapy session (2). The physician permits the patient to express feelings, discuss the "unmentionables," and review the roots of the dilemma. Patients have a genuine chance to talk about themselves; they have a unique opportunity to examine themselves, explore their emotions and ideas, venture into new concepts, and understand themselves (3). The physician creates this therapeutic session through interest in the patient, by appropriate questions, and by just listening.

Conjunct Therapy. If the patient's major difficulty is with another person, the physician undertakes conjunct therapy—joint treatment of both. This technique proves valuable in crises between spouses, lovers, or roommates. The physician listens, mediates, and confronts their dispute. One particularly productive intervention technique involves the following: The physician interviews the patient alone; then, with the patient's permission, the spouse is interviewed; and finally the physician brings them both together and helps them to address, confront, compromise about, and resolve the problem.

A 20-year-old woman comes to the ED, depressed over the alleged infidelity of her lover, who is also her roommate. She believes he has been meeting another woman. The physician interviews the boyfriend and discovers he has been tutoring a woman student but without any overt sexual behavior. The physician brings the woman and her boyfriend together. The three of them examine the misunderstanding and make plans to avoid such situations.

Family Therapy. Crisis often involves the entire family, and the physician engages the whole family in therapy. Typical situations include conflicts over a truant child, chronic illness of a parent or child, divorce disrupting the entire family, one parent's alcoholism that is devastating the family, or disharmony among three generations living in cramped quarters. The physician brings together the entire family to resolve the problem.

Network Therapy. In certain situations the crisis involves not only the patient, spouse, and family but also many other people. For example, a 35-year-old man with a history of schizophrenia developed conflicts with his wife, his two children, his in-laws, and his landlord. The physician brought together the entire network. Together they recognized the patient's problems, the financial stresses upon his family, and the difficulty with neighborhood teenagers. Together they devised a strategy to handle these problems and averted the patient's psychiatric hospitalization. The physician brings together the patient's entire social network — spouse, children, extended family, landlord, employer, police, aftercare worker, and therapist — to resolve the crisis (4).

Commitment.   The ED physician has available a most powerful treatment — restraint — in the form of commitment (5). Commitment can stop the self-destructive or homicidal behavior. In ordering involuntary commitment, the physician mandates treatment to save lives.

Medications.   The physician employs medication as part of ED therapy. One particularly useful technique involves giving the appropriate medication and monitoring the patient's response for several hours. This is especially helpful when the patient is struggling with anxiety and disorganization.

Rechecks.   Another highly effective treatment technique involves the physician's having the patient back to the ED the next day for a scheduled recheck. This plan provides the patient with a definite, immediate appointment. The doctor then observes the medication's effects and monitors the patient's progress. Often the physician has the patient back several days in a row.

Referral.   Finally, the physician completes the other key aspect of the crisis mission, a definite referral. In most psychiatric emergencies the patient requires treatment after the ED intervention. By establishing a referral, the physician underscores the patient's future, worth, and treatability.

THE REFERRAL

The referral constitutes the other major crisis mission of the ED, and it involves three key aspects (6). First, the ED staff must appreciate its vital function as the center of the community's treatment network. Second, the staff must recognize the referral sources from which patients come to the ED. Third, staff must establish an appropriate referral for each patient in crisis.

Overview of the Referral Process

The ED is the focal point of the community's treatment network. It receives patients from a vast variety of sources including physicians, factories, schools, other hospitals, and jails. A number of sources of transportation bring patients to the ED — EMTs, police, families, or patients themselves. In turn the ED physician refers ED patients to an equally extensive variety of places, for example, physicians, clinics, and hospitals. This receiving of referrals and making of referrals is one of the major functions of the ED.

Staff members' recognition of their vital referral function brings two important consequences. First, from awareness of the importance of referrals, staff personnel derive pride, satisfaction, and an overall comprehension of their work. They see their role in the entire network and their overall participation in the community's treatment programs. Second, to fulfill their referral role responsibility, staff must know the extent of the network. They must have knowledge of where patients come from and where and to whom they are being referred. The ED often refers patients to places that have referred patients to it. This entire referral process represents and requires collaborative participation. The community's mental health referral and treatment network is reviewed at the end of this chapter.

Referrals to the ED

The ED staff has a number of significant interactions with the referral source that go beyond simply receiving the patient. These involve obtaining information prior to the patient's arrival, securing material that has been sent with the patient, and checking with the referral source as part of the complete evaluation. The ED staff must involve themselves with the referral source.

In the first of these three phases of interaction, the referral source calls ahead with information concerning the patient. Staff receiving such information must do several things. They must identify themselves and note the identity of the caller. They must write down the information. They must obtain the caller's telephone number and an estimate of the patient's arrival time. Then, the staff member with the information must communicate it to all the other members of the ED staff. All too frequently information secured by one staff member is lost and no one knows about the patient when he or she appears (7).

Not uncommonly, the patient arrives with pertinent material from the referral source. This material includes records from the physician's office or from another hospital, the jail, or a nursing home. The EMTs may transport with the patient a suicide note or pill bottles. All these materials furnish valuable and useful information to the ED staff.

Finally, and most important, the ED staff must contact the referral source directly as part of the complete evaluation. The physician must call the referring physician, school, hospital, or police. Such contacts produce extremely valuable, often critical, information necessary to complete the evaluation.

Referrals From the ED

The ED physician must establish a referral for the patient having a psychiatric emergency. Rarely does one admission to the ED resolve the serious emotional disruption a psychiatric crisis represents. The physician has the responsibility to arrange for proper treatment (8).

In establishing the referral, the physician must be guided by several principles (9). First, the physician must make a *definite* referral. The patient requiring outpatient treatment needs a scheduled appointment with an identified therapist. The patient requiring inpatient treatment needs a secured bed before being sent to the psychiatric hospital or inpatient unit. Second, with the patient's permission, the ED physician must provide the receiving therapist with the ED record. Third, when the patient requires inpatient treatment at another hospital, the physician must secure safe transportation. The proper referral completes the ED crisis mission.

THE REFERRAL NETWORK

The following compendium is a list of the people and organizations that most commonly refer emergency psychiatric patients to the ED and to which the ED most frequently refers patients (10-20). The list functions as a resource and emphasizes the role of the ED as a focus and as a part of the entire community's mental health treatment network.

I. Inpatient facilities
   A. Medical-surgical hospitals
      1. General hospitals
      2. Veterans Administration hospitals
      3. Military hospitals
   B. Psychiatric hospitals
      1. Psychiatric units within general hospitals
      2. Private psychiatric hospitals
      3. State psychiatric hospitals
      4. Veterans Administration psychiatric hospitals
      5. Military psychiatric facilities
   C. Detoxification centers
      1. General hospitals
      2. Specialized facilities
   D. Nursing homes
II. Alternative living situations
   A. Abstinence settings—residential facilities emphasizing abstinence, drug-free environment, therapy, and rehabilitation
      1. For alcoholics
      2. For drug abusers

270 MANAGEMENT OF THE PSYCHIATRIC EMERGENCY

B. Halfway houses—residential facilities offering a structured, semicontrolled living situation with emphasis on autonomy, employment, and community functioning
   1. For the mentally ill
   2. For ex-prisoners
C. Boardinghouses—residential facilities that provide independent living with opportunities for socialization and therapeutic interaction
D. Runaway centers—facilities that offer temporary shelter and therapy for runaways
E. Shelters—community agencies, for example, the Salvation Army, that offer meals and a place to stay
F. Foster homes—private homes in which a family provides a temporary or long-term home for a small group of people
   1. For children
   2. For patients discharged from psychiatric facilities
   3. For patients with mental retardation
G. Dormitories
   1. School residence halls for matriculated students
      a. High school or preparatory school
      b. College or university
   2. Residence halls associated with community programs
      a. Goodwill Industries
      b. Mental retardation facilities
      c. Training programs
   3. Military barracks
   4. Residence facilities associated with employment, for example, at a resort
   5. YMCA, YWCA, YMHA
H. Refuges for battered wives or children
III. Criminal justice system
A. Police organizations
   1. City police
   2. Sheriff
   3. State police
   4. Federal marshall
B. Probation officers
C. Courts and judges

D. Incarceration facilities
1. City lockup
2. County jail
3. State prison
4. Federal penitentiary
E. Attorneys
1. Legal aid organizations
2. Private attorneys

IV. Home treatment programs—programs promoting and providing treatment in the patient's home; personnel usually include physicians, nurses, mental health workers, physical therapists, and homemakers
A. For the mentally ill
1. Acute intervention
2. Supportive follow-up for patients discharged from psychiatric hospitals (aftercare)
B. For the medically ill
C. For the aged
D. For new mothers

V. Day treatment programs—programs that offer all the advantages of hospital treatment (structure, group and individual therapy, occupational therapy, supervision, and participation) but from which the patient goes home at night

VI. Community resources
A. Individual providers
1. Physicians
2. Psychiatrists
3. Psychologists
4. Social workers
5. Nurses
6. Clergy
B. Organizations for treatment
1. Community mental health centers
2. Hospital clinics
3. Counseling centers
4. Programs affiliated with religious organizations
5. Rape counseling centers
C. Specialized counseling and support groups

1. For alcohol and drug problems
   a. Alcoholics Anonymous
   b. Al-Anon
   c. Alateen
2. Rape counseling centers
3. Child-abusing parent groups
4. Support groups for people who have encountered specific medical problems
   a. Groups for parents who experience sudden infant death syndrome
   b. Ostomy clubs
   c. Lost Cord Club (for people with laryngectomy)
   d. Wheelchair competitions
5. Senior citizen centers
6. Special groups
   a. Big brother and big sister organizations
   b. Single parent groups; divorce workshops
7. Travelers' Aid

D. Treatment within an organization
   1. Schools
      a. Junior high school and high school counselors
      b. College and university mental health programs
   2. Business and industry programs
      a. Mental health programs
      b. Personnel officers
   3. State programs
      a. Welfare social workers
      b. Vocational rehabilitation counselors
      c. Child and adult protective services workers

VII. Telephone-centered programs—programs that deal with patients exclusively by telephone
   A. Information services
      1. Poison control centers
      2. 911 switchboards
   B. Intervention services
      1. Suicide prevention and crisis hot lines
      2. Alcohol and drug hot lines
   C. Referral services

REFERENCES

1. Sullivan HS: *The Psychiatric Interview.* New York, WW Norton & Co, 1954.

2. Marmor J: Short-term dynamic psychotherapy. *Am J Psychiatry* 136:149-155, 1979.

3. Dressler DM, Donovan JM, Geller RA: Life stress and emotional crisis: The idiosyncratic interpretation of the events. *Compr Psychiatry* 17:549-558, 1976.

4. Speck RV, Attneave CL: *Family Networks.* NY, Pantheon Books, 1973.

5. Roth LH: A commitment law for patients, doctors, and lawyers, *Am J Psychiatry* 136:1121-1126, 1979.

6. Gibson G: The social system of emergency medical care, in Noble JH, Wechsler H, LaMontagne ME, et al (eds): *Emergency Medical Services: Behavioral and Planning Perspectives.* New York, Behavioral Publications, 1973, pp 85-125.

7. Soreff SM: Psychiatric consultation in the emergency department. *Psychiatric Annals* 8:189-194, 1978.

8. Redlich F, Kellert SR: Trends in american mental health. *Am J Psychiatry* 135:22-28, 1978.

9. Jellinek M: Referrals from a psychiatric emergency room: Relationship of compliance to demographic and interview variables. *Am J Psychiatry* 135:209-213, 1978.

10. Aldrich CK, Nighswonger C: *A Pastoral Counseling Casebook.* Philadelphia, The Westminster Press, 1968.

11. Donovan JM, Bennett MJ, McElroy CM: The crisis-An outcome study. *Am J Psychiatry* 136:906-910, 1979.

12. Glick ID, Hargreaves WA: *Psychiatric Hospital Treatment for the Nineteen Eighties.* Lexington MA, Lexington Books, 1979.

13. Gordon JS: The runaway center as community mental health center. *Am J Psychiatry* 135:932-935, 1978.

14. Gove WR, Fain T: A comparison of voluntary and committed psychiatric patients. *Arch Gen Psychiatry* 34:669-676, 1977.

15. Grunebaum H, Kates W: Whom to refer for group psychotherapy. *Am J Psychiatry* 134:130-133, 1977.

16. Herz MI, Endicott J, Gibbon M: Brief hospitalization. *Arch Gen Psychiatry* 36:701-712, 1979.

17. Herz MI, Endicott J, Spitzer RI: Brief versus standard hospitalization: The families. *Am J Psychiatry* 133:795-801, 1979.

18. Langsley DG, Kaplan DM: *The Treatment of families in crisis.* New York, Grune & Stratton, 1968.

19. Miller SI, Browning CH, Tyson RI: A study of psychiatric emergencies: Part III. Findings on follow-up. *Psychiatry in Med* 2:133-137, 1971.

20. Rachlin S, Grossman S, Frankel J: Patients without communities: Whose responsibility? *Hosp Community Psychiatry* 30:37-39, 1979.

17

Responsibilities and Restraints: The Legal Dimensions of Treatment

The law constitutes one of the major dimensions of emergency psychiatric intervention. It presents the EMTs, the ED staff, and the psychiatrist with a number of responsibilities and restraints. There are six key issues. First, staff must have a basic appreciation of the nature of law and its application to their work. Second, because of the legal aspects, emergency personnel often view the psychiatric patient as the "unwanted patient." Third, the law gives the emergency staff important responsibilities and mandates, for example, the authority to institute involuntary commitment. Fourth, the law also limits what the ED staff can actually do with and for the patient. Fifth, staff must always remain oriented toward patient care and must exercise sound clinical judgment throughout the intervention. Sixth, emergency personnel must follow basic medicolegal principles that ensure both good patient care and effective staff protection.

THE LAW

The EMTs and ED staff must have an appreciation of the law and its application to their work. The fundamental concepts to be understood involve the basic orientation of the legal system, the variations in laws from state to state and from time to time, and the pioneer status of emergency litigation.

The legal system is oriented around procedure; it follows an internal logic and asserts its own values. The law pays a great deal of attention to order (1). It demands adherence to a particular sequence and stresses proper procedure regardless of the actual events (2). The legal system has its internal logic and order. The legal system also differs in emphasis and orientation from the medical system. The law places a premium on liberty; medicine holds life as the most precious (3).

The law varies from state to state. Each state has its own set of statutes governing psychiatric intervention and commitment. This means emergency personnel must know the legal requirements and procedures for *their* state. This chapter presents general principles.

The law also changes with time. Federal and state laws change. New statutes are added; previous pieces of legislation are revised; and old laws are dropped. As a result the EMTs and ED staff not only must know their state's statutes but also must keep their knowledge current. The author has seen dramatic alterations and limitations in the last decade concerning commitment laws in his state, Maine. The law has changed, the commitment form has been redrafted several times, and the procedure has been varied in a number of ways.

Finally, the EMTs and the ED staff find themselves on a legal frontier when dealing with psychiatric emergency patients. The EMTs' intervention is new; it places emergency personnel in areas only now being legally defined.

PERSONNEL REACTIONS

Not surprisingly, personnel often express concern about the legal implications of emergency psychiatry. Their reactions stem from several sources: lack of knowledge, uneasiness about the malpractice issue, and dissatisfaction with the additional work required by legal stipulations. Together these reasons contribute to the viewpoint that the psychiatric patient in crisis is an unwanted patient.

First, EMTs and ED staff often lack knowledge of the law as it pertains to the care of psychiatric patients. As a result they feel discomfort with psychiatric patients and the related management issues.

Second, many emergency personnel may view the psychiatric patient as a potential plaintiff and themselves as defendants. They wonder whether the family will sue them if they release a patient who subsequently commits suicide or some other act of violence. If they institute commitment, they wonder whether the patient can sue. The malpractice factor provokes great concern and anxiety.

Third, the legal aspects of emergency psychiatry consume time. Staff must follow a number of procedures to commit a patient. Their involvement with the psychiatric patient may lead to a court appearance.

The remainder of this chapter provides EMTs and ED staff with the legal principles concerning psychiatric patients and reviews medicolegal procedures to protect the patient and themselves.

THE RESPONSIBILITIES

The law provides EMTs, ED personnel, and psychiatrists with extraordinary responsibilities to protect patients and other people. It gives them the power and obligation to intervene. Indeed, it demands that they take action. The EMTs and the ED staff have responsibilities in four areas: intervening in the case of suicidal or homicidal patients, committing suicidal or homicidal patients, warning intended homicide victims, and reporting child abuse.

In the first instance, the EMTs must intervene with, contain, and transport the suicidal or homicidal patient. When they respond to a call, they must assess the situation. A patient who is trying to commit suicide must be stopped. EMTs must remove implements of destruction—knives, razors, pills, or ropes. If the patient has a gun, they must summon police. They must act to prevent the suicide and to save the life, regardless of the patient's stated wishes to be left alone and to die. Similarly, they must intervene with the homicidal patient. They must check the person's violence and remove potential victims. In either case they must act decisively to save lives. They must use their best judgment, based on the patient interview and the information from family and friends.

Commitment signifies a more formal, legal intervention. It moves beyond a momentary blockage of destructive behavior and imposes hospitalization. Although involuntary hospitalization has been attacked by some critics (4,5), it does save lives. The suicidal or homicidal patient must be stopped; recovery should be expected. Frequently the patient's suicidal impulses pass within several days and the patient wishes to continue on with life (6).

There are two basic criteria for commitment: mental illness and dangerousness. Each state has its own particular emphasis, wordings, and procedures, but these two aspects are found in most states' laws. First, the patient must have a diagnosable mental illness. Second, the dangerousness must be in the form of a clear and present risk of suicide or homicide. The threat to life must be real, for example, a verbal threat, a suicide note, an overdose, or an announced plan for self-destruction or injury to someone else. The emphasis must be on immediate danger of suicide or homicide (7).

The ED physician's decision to commit a patient must be clearly based on the physician's evaluation of the patient. The evaluation consists of the patient's interview and the information derived from family, friends, EMTs, and significant others. The physician must also clearly record his or her observations and the necessity for involuntary hospitalization.

The ED physician has the responsibility to warn the intended homicide victim in those situations in which a patient with known homicidal intentions remains in the community (8). Recent litigation has emphasized the physician's duty to warn the victim (9).

In many states the EMTs, the ED staff, and the psychiatrists have the responsibility to report cases of suspected or confirmed child abuse to state authorities (10). Health care personnel often are in a position to observe or be aware of the abuse. Statutes require them to act upon this information (11).

STAFF RESTRAINT

EMTs and ED staff must exercise a strong degree of restraint in two areas. The first area pertains to the patient who requires treatment but refuses it. The second area deals with confidentiality. Both aspects demand discipline and ethical adherence.

The psychiatric patient has the right to decline treatment (12). No longer does mental illness alone necessitate commitment. Commitment requires *both* mental illness and immediate danger of suicide or homicide. Staff may recommend treatment and hospitalization, but the patient can refuse. Recent court decisions have said patients have the right to be ill (13). If patients prefer their depression or thought disorder, that remains a matter of their choice as long as they are not dangerous.

The ED staff and psychiatrist are ethically and legally required to protect the patient's confidentiality. The patient's identity, the information he or she discloses, the diagnosis, and the patient's record are all matters for strict confidentiality. Staff must not disclose or release any information about the patient without the patient's permission (14). Only in cases of danger, child abuse, and court orders can the personnel use the patient's communications without permission.

Confidentiality protects patients and permits them the opportunity to talk openly about themselves. Patients' disclosures to a psychiatrist are privileged communications. The psychiatrist is bound by law and ethics not to pass along the patient's information without the patient's permission.

A PATIENT-CARE ORIENTATION

A positive patient-care orientation remains the cornerstone of the entire treatment. It is impossible to list all the legal implications that pertain to emergency psychiatry. But a concerned, patient-oriented approach by EMTs and ED staff toward each patient and family is always necessary and appropriate.

Patient-care orientation involves and combines the approaches discussed in Chapter 3 and the 12 subsequent chapters. Personnel must introduce and identify themselves. They must address the patient by the patient's formal name. They must interview the patient first, alone, and in privacy. They must ask appropriate questions and then, more importantly, must listen to the patient. In short, all emergency personnel must treat the patient and family with dignity and respect. These people want help; staff must strive to be of assistance.

MEDICOLEGAL PRINCIPLES

Emergency personnel must adopt and adhere to medicolegal principles which both provide quality patient care and afford themselves legal protection. They must follow a number of good patient-care principles. These principles cover six aspects: protocols, documentation, evaluation, judgment and reactions, candor and openness, and training.

Protocols serve as guides to patient care and ensure staff protection. These written procedures provide staff with accepted methods of treatment (15). They reflect the recommendations of experts and also the community standards. Many states have developed EMT protocols, and EDs have instituted standardized procedures (16). By following these protocols staff not only pursue established treatment plans but also employ a legally defensible approach to patient care.

Documentation is essential for the comprehensive approach. At each step in the intervention, personnel must record specifically what they have done. The record must reflect the events and the observations; it must be dated, the time must be recorded, and all entries must be signed. In the legal world the EMTs' records and the ED chart loom very large. Often litigation occurs years after the treatment; the chart represents the only "proof" and evidence. The record must be accurate, legible, thorough, and pertinent.

The record must demonstrate many facets of the intervention. It must cover the actual crisis and the treatment rendered. In order to satisfy this requirement, the written report must contain a clear description of what happened, who was present, where it occurred, how the event occurred, and why the intervention was called for. The records must show what medications were given and why. Additionally, the record must indicate who provided the information (eg, mother or probation officer) and how each person provided the data (eg, by telephone or in person).

The record must contain explanations that have been given to the patient, reasons for any delays, consultation notes, and a description of the disposition. The EMTs and ED physician must write down the explanations and instructions they have given to the patient. They must chart the reason for a psychiatric consultation. They must inform the patient of the medication's prominent side effects and record the fact that that explanation has been given. Not infrequently ED staff members restrain a suicidal patient in order to prevent the person from eloping and in order to ensure close observation until the family can be located. The physician must record the reason for the restraint and the delay in finding the family.

The physician must chart consultations obtained, including those secured by telephone. Finally, he or she must document the disposition: the record must show specifically to whom the patient has been referred and the location, date, and time of the appointment.

Staff must appreciate the concept of the psychiatric evaluation. The evaluation consists of two parts: the patient interview and the information from significant others. The family's history, the friends' reports, and the EMTs' observations constitute valuable parts of the evaluation.

Staff must exercise their judgment and be aware of their reactions. Their judgment is a critical part of the treatment. For example, EMTs may assess the patient's suicide risk as very high, based upon the patient's statements, a "goodbye" note, and the family's report. They must follow their judgment, record it, and transport the patient. Similarly, staff reactions and feelings provide valuable information. Personnel must appreciate their own responses to the patient. Staff must monitor, record, and use their reactions.

Emergency personnel must deal openly and honestly with all patients and families throughout the intervention (12). Misstatements and misinformation destroy trust. Patients recall and react to what they perceive as deceit. Staff must explain and inform the patient and family about each step in the treatment.

Training provides a major means for emergency personnel to serve their patients and themselves. Courses, programs, and schools offer pertinent training. These instruction programs enhance staff knowledge and proficiency and provide them with certification. Certification demonstrates that the worker has met national and community standards of training.

REFERENCES

1. Bedford S: *The Faces of Justice: A Traveller's Report.* New York, Simon & Schuster, 1961.

2. Derrett JD: *An Introduction to Legal Systems.* New York, Praeger, 1968.

3. Mills JS: *On Liberty.* New York, Appleton-Century-Crofts, 1947.

4. Ennis B: *Prisoners of Psychiatry.* New York, Harper & Row, 1970.

5. Szasz, TS: *The Manufacture of Madness.* New York, Harper & Row, 1970.

6. Monahan J: Prediction research and emergency commitment of dangerous mentally ill persons: A reconsideration. *Am J Psychiatry* 135:198–201, 1978.

7. Roth LH: A commitment law for patients, doctors, and lawyers. *Am J Psychiatry* 136:1121–1127, 1979.

8. Gurevitz H: *Tarasoff:* Protective privilege versus public peril. *Am J Psychiatry* 134:289–292, 1977.

9. Roth LH, Meisel A: Dangerousness, confidentiality, and the duty to warn. *Am J Psychiatry* 134:508–511, 1977.

10. Curran WF: Failure to diagnose battered-child syndrome. *N Engl J Med* 296:795–796, 1977.

11. An act concerning child abuse and neglect. *Legislative Document No. 775.* One-hundred-ninth Legislature, State of Maine, 1979.

12. Slovenko R: *Psychiatry and Law.* Boston, Little Brown & Co, 1973.

13. Lebensohn ZM: Defensive psychiatry, or how to treat the mentally ill without being a lawyer, in Barton WE, Sanborn CJ (eds): *Law and the Mental Health Professions.* New York, International Universities Press, 1978, pp 19–46.

14. Slaby AE, Lieb J, Tancredi LR: *Handbook of Psychiatric Emergencies.* Flushing NY, Medical Examination Publishing Co, 1975.

15. MacDonald JR, Kinder P: *Department of Emergency Medicine Guideline Manual, Policies and Procedures.* St Louis, CV Mosby Co, 1979.

16. *Treatment, Triage, and Transfer Protocols.* Augusta ME, Medical Care Development Inc, 1978.

18

Overview:
The Further Development of
Emergency Psychiatric Services

This final chapter considers several phenomena that must shape the delivery of emergency psychiatric care. First are the phenomenal increase in numbers of patients requiring crisis intervention and the response of the emergency health care system to this need. Another is the inherent nature of emergency psychiatry. Finally, this chapter looks at the ED's critical role in the community.

THE NEED AND THE RESPONSE TO IT

In ever-growing numbers, patients seek emergency psychiatric assistance. Patient numbers increase both in absolute terms and in their percentage of all ED admissions (1). The emergency health care system has responded to the increased demand for psychiatric services. In the EMT arena, in EDs, and among psychiatrists there have been giant strides to address the needs of patients in emotional crisis. The changes have included recognition of the situation and the development of training programs.

The Emergency Medical Services System has from its inception recognized the significance of behavioral emergencies and designated it as one of the six critical areas of care (2). In recent years the people who mold policy in emergency care have strengthened their interest and concern in crisis intervention. Both educational and service programs prominently feature behavioral issues.

EMTs in their work have realized the importance of the patient in emotional crisis. Their training programs have started to emphasize approaches to emergency psychiatry. EMTs are eager to learn better ways of dealing with psychiatric patients.

281

EDs have become aware of their major role in the treatment of psychiatric patients (3). They have constructed quiet rooms; they have trained their personnel; and they have added psychiatric consultants, social workers, and psychiatric nurses to their staffs. Emergency medical physicians receive psychiatric training during their residencies.

Psychiatry has also recognized the importance of the patient in crisis. The American Psychiatric Association (APA) has offered several courses and included many papers about emergency psychiatry at its annual meetings. The APA has developed a task force on emergency care issues. Psychiatric training programs devote time to teaching residents emergency psychiatry. Emergency psychiatry is emerging as a subspecialty (4).

CHARACTERISTICS OF EMERGENCY PSYCHIATRY

Three features characterize a significant part of emergency medicine and psychiatry. These are a strong orientation to action, a rapid response to and reflection of community changes, and emerging scholarship.

Emergency medicine and psychiatry are *action* medicine and psychiatry. The EMTs and the ED staff are primed and geared for rapid treatment, quick decisions, and prompt responses. Their training and their basic orientation to their work focus on action — doing something. As a result, EMTs and ED personnel sometimes find themselves frustrated by a long, complicated psychiatric case. They must exercise skill and discipline in being able to "just" talk with and, most importantly, "just" listen to patients in crisis.

The emergency system rapidly reflects community changes and trends. Emergency psychiatry serves as a barometer of these societal alterations. The presence of a new "street" drug is first appreciated by the ED staff. The effects of premature psychiatric hospital discharges are promptly noted in an increase in ED psychiatric admissions. The emergency system provides a means for promptly assessing community changes.

The psychiatric emergency system is now beginning to produce its own scholarship. Because of its infancy, the needs to establish itself, and its action orientation, the system has only recently started to examine and present an overview of itself. In the 1980s the system will come of age scholastically. It will continue to document and explore its dimensions, power, and impact.

EMERGENCY CARE WITHIN THE TREATMENT NETWORK

The EMTs, EDs, and psychiatric consultants play a critical role in the community's mental health treatment network by correcting imbalances in it (5). The emergency system has the capacity to handle crises when the other elements of the network for a variety of reasons cannot. A crisis develops in the home and the patient has no physician. The EMTs do respond. On occasion patients find themselves rebuffed by long waiting lists and delays at other care facilities. But the ED remains accessible and open 24 hours a day.

The emergency system has begun to take an active role in anticipating and defining the crises that occur in the community. It goes beyond its function of correcting the imbalance and reacting to events. EMTs communicate with the ED, informing them about the patient, the emergency, and the estimated time of arrival. Physicians refer patients directly to the ED for an emergency psychiatric consultation and call ahead with information.

THE CHALLENGE

The EMTs, EDs, and their psychiatric consultants have twin responsibilities: to provide effective crisis intervention and to function as an integral, coordinated part of the community's treatment network. They possess special skills, capabilities, and powers and have a unique opportunity for therapeutic intervention. They also serve as a focal point and key component of the treatment network. They must appreciate and coordinate their role within the network. The challenge of emergency psychiatry is for the EMTs, ED personnel, and their psychiatric consultants to provide their unique intervention for patients and families during crises and to serve in a coordinated manner as a complement to the rest of the community's treatment network.

REFERENCES

1. Spitz L: The evolution of a psychiatric emergency crisis-intervention service in a medical emergency room setting. *Compr Psychiatry* 17:99–113, 1976.
2. Noble JH Jr, Wechsler H, LaMontagne ME (eds): *Emergency Medical Services: Behavioral and Planning Perspectives.* New York, Behavioral Publications, 1973.
3. Soreff S: Psychiatric consultation in the emergency department. *Psychiatric Annals* 8:189–194, 1978.
4. Fauman BJ: Psychiatry in the emergency room. *JAMA* 242:1401, 1979.
5. Gibson G: The social system of emergency medical care, in Noble JH Jr, Wechsler H, LaMontagne ME (eds): *Emergency Medical Services: Behavioral and Planning Perspectives.* New York, Behavioral Publications, 1973, pp 85–125.

Index

285